Cancer, Radiation Therapy, and the Market

Appraising cancer as a major medical market in the 2010s, Wall Street investors placed their bets on single-technology treatment facilities costing $100–$300 million each. Critics inside medicine called the widely publicized proton-center boom "crazy medicine and unsustainable public policy." There was no valid evidence, they claimed, that proton beams were more effective than less costly alternatives. But developers expected insurance to cover their centers' staggeringly high costs and debts. Was speculation like this new to health care?

Cancer, Radiation Therapy, and the Market shows how the radiation therapy specialty in the United States (later called radiation oncology) coevolved with its device industry throughout the 20th century. Academic engineers and physicians acquired financing to develop increasingly powerful radiation devices, initiated companies to manufacture the devices competitively, and designed hospital and freestanding procedure units to utilize them. In the process, they incorporated market strategies into medical organization and practice. Although palliative benefits and striking tumor reductions fueled hopes of curing cancer, scientific research all too often found serious patient harm and disappointing beneficial impact on cancer survival. This thoroughly documented and provocative inquiry concludes that public health policy needs to re-evaluate market-driven high-tech medicine and build evidence-based health care systems.

Barbara Bridgman Perkins is the author of *The Medical Delivery Business: Health Reform, Childbirth, and the Economic Order* and articles in medical history and public health policy.

Routledge Studies in the History of Science, Technology and Medicine

Edited by John Krige, Georgia Institute of Technology, Atlanta, USA

23. The Historiography of Science, Technology and Medicine
Writing Recent Science
Edited by Ron Doel and Thomas Söderqvist

24. International Science between the World Wars
The Case of Genetics
Nikolai Krementsov

25. The Social Construction of Disease
From Scrapie to Prion
Kiheung Kim

26. Public Understanding of Science
A History of Communicating Scientific Ideas
David Knight

27. Global Science and National Sovereignty
Studies in Historical Sociology of Science
Edited by Grégoire Mallard, Catherine Paradeise and Ashveen Peerbaye

28. Vaccinations and Public Concern in History
Legend, Rumor, and Risk Perception
Andrea Kitta

29. Spatializing the History of Ecology
Sites, journeys, mappings
Edited by Raf de Bont and Jens Lachmund

30. Cancer, Radiation Therapy, and the Market
Barbara Bridgman Perkins

Also published by Routledge in hardback and paperback:

Science and Ideology
A Comparative History
Mark Walker

Cancer, Radiation Therapy, and the Market

Barbara Bridgman Perkins

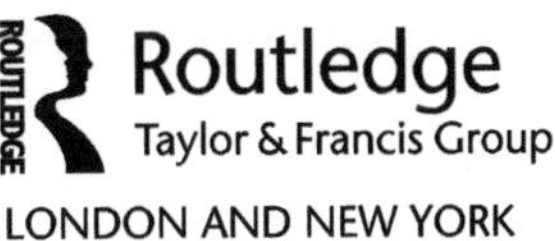

LONDON AND NEW YORK

First published 2017 by Routledge

2 Park Square, Milton Park, Abingdon, Oxfordshire OX14 4RN
52 Vanderbilt Avenue, New York, NY 10017

Routledge is an imprint of the Taylor & Francis Group, an informa business

First issued in paperback 2019

British Library Cataloguing in Publication Data
A catalogue record for this book is available from the British Library

Library of Congress Cataloging in Publication Data
Names: Perkins, Barbara Bridgman, author.
Title: Cancer, radiation therapy, and the market / Barbara Bridgman Perkins.
Other titles: Routledge studies in the history of science, technology, and medicine.
Description: Abingdon, Oxon; New York, NY: Routledge, 2017. |
Series: Routledge studies in the history of science, technology and medicine |
Includes bibliographical references and index.
Identifiers: LCCN 2017001662 | ISBN 9781138285248 (hardback: alk. paper) |
ISBN 9781315269139 (ebook)
Subjects: | MESH: Radiation Oncology–history | Technology, Radiologic–history | Technology, Radiologic–economics | Neoplasms–radiotherapy |
History, 20th Century | History, 21st Century | United States
Classification: LCC RC270.3.R33 | NLM QZ 11 AA1 |
DDC 616.99/40757–dc23
LC record available at https://lccn.loc.gov/2017001662

ISBN: 978-1-138-28524-8 (hbk)
ISBN: 978-0-367-34855-7 (pbk)

Typeset in Times New Roman
by Deanta Global Publishing Services, Chennai, India

Contents

Figures

1 Medical Care as Trade

Management consultants and business school professors advised American doctors, hospital administrators, and health care entrepreneurs in the late 20th century to make medical services more like Jiffy Lube® stations.[1] Patients also noted a resemblance; a breast cancer patient undergoing surgery, radiation, and chemotherapy blogged that she felt "like a car going thru Jiffy Lube."[2] The consultants may have noticed that services specializing in clinical procedures like MRI scanning, kidney dialysis, colonoscopy, keratoplasty, cardiac catheterization, and radiation therapy had already applied market strategies to medical delivery. It would have been hard to miss the massive advertising.

Drive down a city street, open a newspaper, turn on the television, or go on the Internet, and you will be hit with a barrage of advertisements for doctors, drugs, and devices. Radiation therapy ads proclaim that their devices and treatment methods destroy tumors faster and protect surrounding tissues from radiation damage better than those of their competitors.[3] One company exorbitantly claimed that patients receiving its new method of applying radiation became "cancer free in less than 3 hours."[4] Advertising like this misleads people with deceptive claims of treatment effectiveness. A Utah billboard featuring a brand-name device at a nearby hospital claimed "superior results" due to "superior technology."[5] What are the superior results, you might somewhat skeptically ask? But hospital ads are not legally required to base their claims on evidence.[6] Although the ads reinforce popular (and professional) beliefs that there is scientific evidence demonstrating that the latest, most powerful (and most costly) treatments are the safest and most effective, it is not necessarily the case—as this book will show.

The *New York Times Magazine* provides a prominent platform for advertising medical services to the same market as its ads for diamond necklaces and wealth management. Many of its specialty service ads display the *US News and World Report*'s "best hospital" logo like a *Good Housekeeping* seal of approval. The *Report*'s major criterion for determining "best" cancer services—accounting for one-third of the total score—is reputation among its specialists (as conducted in a mail survey with a 37 percent response rate).[7] Availability of the latest technology is another criterion (not unrelated to reputation). Patient survival is taken into account, but only survival for 30 days after hospital admission, which primarily means survival of the hospital experience itself—not an insignificant measure, to be sure. Some hospitals receiving the highest rating in every non-reputation factor still received low rankings. "Best hospital," it seems, circularly identifies prestigious specialty services as best because they are prestigious. Prestige is the product being sold, and it trumps scientific evidence. "Best" hospitals are also profitable.

Markets and the Medical Business System

Business strategies and their market theories have infused their values into every sphere of society, permeating institutions and professions ostensibly dedicated to service. The recent advertisements are just the latest manifestations of a long history of medical marketing, much of which came out of the pharmaceutical industry and patent medicines before that.[8] Earlier radiation therapy promotions included newspaper and magazine stories purporting the mysterious healing powers of radiation[9] and went on to feature movie stars publicizing the latest treatment device (Figure 5.1). The ads reveal the extent to which medical services are commodities for sale in the market.

Medical delivery has long been a market in which buyers with financial means purchase services that sellers choose to offer.[10] The 19th century was noted for its "free trade in doctoring," as historian Nancy Tomes observed.[11] At the turn of the 20th century, leaders sought to disassociate medical care from its commercial image and identify it as a science-driven *profession* dedicated to helping people. Elite American doctors' travel to Europe to learn precepts of experimental science changed medical diagnostics.[12] Treatment in many areas, however, remained based on trial-and-error experience (which the medical profession confusingly calls *empirical*). The professionalization project supplemented more than it substituted for medicine's commercial heritage. Medical leaders persuaded states to establish licensing laws that conferred monopoly status on graduates of schools that taught the new medical sciences. Monopoly strategy was intrinsic to the concept of profession. The claim that medicine rose above commerce, as economist Kenneth Arrow later noted, was itself part of professional marketing.[13]

My identification of 20th-century medicine as market driven contributes to a minority, but growing, view within the history of medical care and policy. In *The Medical Delivery Business*, I showed how evolving business environments shaped the specialties and practices of obstetrics and neonatology. James Schafer's *Business of Private Medical Practice* mapped how market forces shaped the distribution of private specialists' offices.[14] Joseph Gabriel in *Medical Monopoly* called the development of American medicine in the early 1900s "part of the broader story of the rise of corporate capitalism."[15] *Cancer, Radiation Therapy, and the Market* shows how market strategies and interests shaped the development of American radiation therapy. The processes of specialization and professionalization embedded the economy into medical care as well as medical care into the economy.

This view means that the medical profession did not suddenly undergo an economic transformation in the 1970s, as many (pro and con) analysts saw it; it had emulated contemporary economic environments all along.[16] But the profession had succeeded so well in convincing scholars, the public, and itself of its scientific and altruistic nature that rulings in the mid-1970s came as a shock. The US Federal Trade Commission (FTC) and Supreme Court used antitrust law to open up the medical market by once again defining medical care as *trade.*[17] Prohibiting medical association restrictions against overt advertising, patient solicitation, and contract practice, the antitrust rulings (selectively) applied market rules to medical care. The rulings reinforced the development of medical care as business by treating it as such.

Medical discourse, however, did distinctly change in the 1970s. Some medical leaders celebrated the newly respectable precepts of self-interest, pronouncing that "the market has spoken,"[18] even when it led to inequities and overtreatment. Others vigorously denounced greedy doctors. A 2013 *New York Times* opinion piece, signed by 22 medical and policy leaders, accused oncologists of using the latest drugs and radiation devices on their cancer patients—despite recognizing that cheaper alternatives led to equivalent results—because they made more money in the fee-for-service insurance payment system.[19] The *Wall Street Journal* disclosed the following year that cancer specialists in radio- and chemotherapy were among the top beneficiaries of Medicare payments.[20]

My analysis of the development of medicine as business does not necessarily imply that money drives individual physician decision-making. Like all population groups, doctors represent a broad spectrum of humanity. Paul Kalanithi, dying of lung cancer in his mid-thirties, wrote that he had chosen medicine as a link to human suffering and as a means of probing the meaning of life in the face of death.[21] While greed has shaped medicine as much as other fields of work (contrary to professional theory), the individual incentive argument is simplistic and conceals a more profound reality.

It is the *medical business system*, which combines doctors and hospitals with manufacturers and Wall Street financial firms, that is greedy. My use of this term extends a (by now) conventional understanding of *medical industrial complex*[22] to mean not just linkages between industry and medical care but also integrating industrial elements into the structure of medical care. The medical business system designs high-priced products and services for the market. It has made cancer a commercial product line that seeks to maximize productivity, profits, prestige, and market power. A high-tech hospital cancer unit advertisement, which popped up on my computer beside the online version of the *Times*' opinion piece mentioned above, revealed the pervasiveness of the medical business system. (It also vied with the message of the piece.) In exploiting the public's all-too-real fears of cancer, competitive growth of such specialty units multiplies remunerative entities needlessly and inflates medical costs with little gain in terms of people's health. This system has been evolving for a long time and has shaped medical practice for over a century.

The timing question depends largely on definition. In *The Social Transformation of American Medicine*, Paul Starr influentially dated the "making of a vast industry" from the mid-1960s by arguing that corporate forms of medical care started to supplant professional sovereignty around that time.[23] Despite fond memories (which I share) of family doctors making house calls, *Cancer, Radiation Therapy, and the Market* argues for an older business development of medicine by identifying different economic features. Throughout the 20th century, medical specialties divvied up markets and wove features of industry, commerce, and finance into medical care organization and practice.

Just as investigators have struggled with (or avoided) naming the contemporary economic system, no adequate label exists to describe medicine's economic development. Its components encompass *industrial* divisions of labor in hierarchically managed institutions and technology-based production units that maximize productivity.[24] It employs strategies of *business* in valuing everything in monetary terms, producing for the market, seeking economies of scale and scope, and integrating institutions vertically and/ or horizontally.[25] It becomes *capitalist* or *corporate* by privatizing services, building complex delivery systems, prioritizing profits, and importing "forms of organization, governance, finance, compensation, and marketing from the larger corporate sector into medicine."[26] To further obfuscate the issue, the term *market* may be applied to any or all of these economic strategies. Also overlapping with these terms, *neoliberal* theory prioritizes private property, promotes corporate roles, rejects government regulation (selectively), and holds that there is no alternative to a market economy.[27] While recognizing that the theoretical ideal market does not exist, I use the broad definitions of *market* and *business* when describing the incorporation of the economic elements identified above into medical care and particularly into medical specialties.[28]

Medical Specialties and High-Cost Procedure Units

As the fundamental structure of 20th-century medical care, specialties contributed a great deal to its scientific progress. At the same time, they were products of the economies of their times. Specialties carved out the more lucrative portions of the medical market early in the century as they targeted selected technologies, organs, diseases, and populations. Although growth in scientific knowledge calls for (and is a product of) subdivision, the logic of modern specialty organization does not derive principally from medical science; it derives from medicine's economic development. Physician–historian George Rosen held in 1944 that specialization resulted "at least as much" from economic and social factors as from scientific ones.[29] "Science and technology are not independent constructs that 'cause' scientific subdivision," noted specialization scholar Rosemary Stevens, "rather they are embedded in a social process that may be driven by multiple personal, economic, and organizational agendas."[30] In the monopolization process called *professionalization*, specialties actively controlled entry into their fields, standardized knowledge and production, produced distinctive products, enhanced demand, and eliminated competing products.[31]

Specialization commodified medical interventions by turning them into discrete, marketable surgical and technological *procedures*—although that was not necessarily leaders' conscious intent. Many specialists and hospital administrators instead assumed that market strategies would enhance medical care's efficiency and productivity without significantly altering its practices. Intertwined with specialty development, capital investment (including foundation funding) fueled consolidation of medical institutions creating large (academic) medical centers. Specialty services in these centers packaged clinical procedures in revenue-generating units. Becoming profit centers or strategic business units, *specialty procedure units* became the hub of hospital care, as later exemplified by the "best hospital" ads. Fee-for-service payment systems fueled their growth by itemizing charges for each procedure.

Inspired in part by American examples, specialized clinics in British teaching hospitals underwent similar development. Historian Roger Cooter described orthopedic surgeons' fracture clinics between World Wars I and II not so much in terms of technology development and diffusion but in terms of the application of scientific management and efficient production techniques to medical care organization. The new clinic was "essentially a political innovation with significant implications for the distribution of power and authority in medicine."[32] Swiss hospitals around the same time also applied business strategies in organizing "rationalized X-ray institutes that operated according to a hierarchic structured division of labor."[33]

Enterprising physicians, managers, and investors in America later carved out procedure units as freestanding retail outlets like Jiffy Lube stations, as cartooned in Figure 1.1, often locating the units in shopping malls and industrial parks. Freestanding procedure units also resulted from private-practice growth as single-specialty medical groups purchased more and more equipment for their office-based practices. Specialty procedure units eventually grew into high-cost cancer centers and proton treatment facilities across America and Europe.

SECOND OPINION
BY ROB ROGERS
DOC IN A BOX
I'LL TAKE TWO CHOLESTEROL SCREENINGS, ONE COLONOSCOPY AND ONE CHEST X-RAY.
I MISS THE DAYS WHEN QUALITY WAS AS IMPORTANT AS VOLUME.
DRIVE THRU
ROGERS ©2013

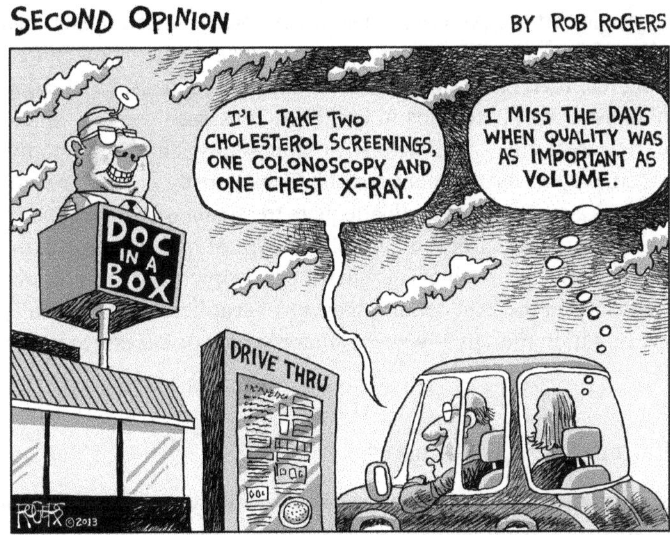

Figure 1.1 Jiffy Lube Medicine.

Source: © 2013 Rob Rogers. Reprinted with permission.

The cost problem in health care is not just the high cost *of* medicine, but the growth of *high-cost medicine* as a strategic entity. Many hospital services were designed to be high cost.[34] High-cost medicine comprises highly capitalized, highly specialized services that escalate clinical intensity and price. It is a major wheel in the medical business system, and the flow of capital is its motor. Requiring capital investment to build and clinical revenues to operate, high-tech specialty units reinforced the role of finance in medical care development. The private insurance industry has provided both by investing surplus income in hospitals and reimbursing their services. As early as the 1910s, insurance companies provided the capital and revenues hospitals required to purchase new technologies like X-ray and to build specialty services.[35] The insurance industry became the primary purchaser of hospital debt via its mortgage and investment departments.[36] Specialty units' growing high-tech expenditures inflated hospitals' fixed capital and overhead costs, requiring them to raise their prices.

Capital investment was a powerful force in shaping 20th-century medical specialties and institutions. Capital infusions tightened bonds between the hospital industry and the finance industry, and the latter took the opportunity to support specialty unit organization. Creditors encouraged selective growth of the more profitable services and technologies. Financial involvement means that the concept of *technological imperative* in medicine in large part expresses a *capital imperative*. Hospitals and specialists had to use their technologies on more and more patients in order to amortize their higher costs. Investors sought to increase *value*, which they variously defined in professional, clinical, and/or monetary terms. Highly trained specialists, their devices, and their medical school and hospital departments embodied the capital invested in medical care.

Multi-billion–dollar medical specialties and specialty service lines came to account for a large portion of the American health care pie.[37] Their unrestrained growth led not only to high costs but also to excessive use of their procedures. There has been a long recorded history of the overuse of procedures such as radiation treatments, diagnostic X-ray, forceps in childbirth, cesarean section, dilatation and curettage, hysterectomy, tonsillectomy, colonoscopy, cholecystectomy, and even open heart surgery. Overtreatment not only does (mostly insured) recipients a disservice, it plays a large role in the inadequate treatment of un- and underinsured people by pricing them out of the market. Growth of high-cost medicine leads to neglect of primary care—which is what most people need most of the time. Critics charged early in the 21st century that the overutilization of specialty services—including radiation therapy—was the major source of excessive health care costs.[38]

Building a Radiation Therapy Industry

Examining the historical development of one medical specialty can reveal fundamental problems of specialty medicine itself and illuminate potential pathways for reform. The history of radiology, which irradiates the human body for both diagnostic and therapeutic purposes, is more complex than conventional accolades of 50 and 100 years of continuous scientific progress have recorded. In visually opening up the body, diagnostic imaging has contributed a great deal to modern medicine by revealing broken bones, tumors, and additional problems otherwise hidden from view. At the same time, it has become vastly overused and has significantly increased health care costs, complications, and unnecessary population exposure to radiation.[39]

This book investigates the use of radiation in medical treatment from the discovery of powerful new forms of energy in the 1890s to the skyrocketing costs of proton centers in the 1990s. Other books fill out other parts of the cancer story. *The Emperor of All Maladies: A Biography of Cancer* compellingly summarizes contemporary ideas about cancer and its treatment. *Cancer Wars: How Politics Shapes What We Know and Don't Know About Cancer* indicts environmental causes of cancer. Many books focus on breast cancer, the most common cancer in the United States (excluding non-life-threatening skin cancers), in order to explore questions of medical treatment and patient experience. *First, You Cry* is a major early book from the patient perspective, and many important books have followed. *Unnatural History: Breast Cancer and American Society* argues that medicine and society have overemphasized the risk of dying from breast cancer as well as the effectiveness of its screening and treatment methods.[40]

Radiation therapy (also called *radiotherapy*), the treatment of disease conditions (usually cancer) with X-rays, radioactive elements, and high-energy particles, grew primarily—but not entirely—out of radiology. Even as its training programs and hospital departments diverged from those of diagnostic radiology, the profession that would rename itself *radiation oncology* remained closely intertwined with radiology.

But the history of medicine is not just the story of what doctors did. Researchers and managers in hospitals, universities, manufacturing companies, and financial firms also drove medical care development. *Cancer, Radiation Therapy, and the Market* tells the stories of how a variety of participants collaborated in a variety of ways to exploit the technical advances, prestige, and money generated by high-voltage and nuclear technologies. Each device story offers new information about the economic development of radiation therapy. Often taking the lead, engineers acquired financing to build new radiation devices, connected with academic radiologists to test them, linked with—or launched—companies to manufacture them, and coordinated with—or operated their own—hospital and freestanding procedure units. Each new device and over-exuberant claims of curing cancer fueled the growth of a radiation therapy industry.

This interconnected development means that the radiation therapy specialty coevolved with the radiation device industry. Each venture brought together university, hospital, and corporate entrepreneurship as well as scientific expertise and engineering ingenuity. Working relationships among the participants involved contractual agreements, shared personnel, social networks, equipment exchange, patent trades, and overlapping directorships. Different mixes of dedication to service as well as institutional and individual ambition, economic motivation, professional hubris, personality conflict, and clinical adventurism individually flavored each initiative. Requiring constant innovation and capital investment infusions, competition fueled an arms race to build higher- and higher-powered cancer guns and procedure units to accommodate them. The ventures integrated business methods as well as devices into medical care organization and practice.

Hospital radiology departments installing high-cost devices employed business modes of operation from the beginning.[41] As physician–historian Joel Howell noted, radiology administrators started charging separately for diagnostic and treatment procedures and employing industrial cost-accounting methods to assess their units in monetary terms early in the 20th century.[42] The spread of radiology's procedure unit model and managerial strategies to other specialties turned medicine into a collection of clinical service stations. Different specialties worked with different industries to devise radiological instruments, pharmaceutical products, surgical supplies, electronic devices, and artificial implants.[43] They also engaged in political activities that promoted the growth of the medical services that used these products.

While reproducing the economic environment may seem a natural, desirable, and even inevitable process, this book demonstrates tensions between the widespread growth of radiation therapy and the specialty's own scientific evidence. Initially acclaimed as a major medical advance, each new device raised medical intensity and price without fulfilling all the hopes invested in it.

Science and Practice

The medical profession and the media often portray 20th-century medicine in terms of cumulative scientific triumph. But, while complex technology confers an aura of science on medicine, the definition of scientific medicine has come to require confirmation that its treatments actually work in particular situations. A scientific approach takes a skeptical view of each new intervention until studies produce good evidence that confirms (or disconfirms) its effectiveness. Expert opinion and premature consensus based on incomplete evidence close further investigation of, and even thought about, medical practices. Progress requires constant questioning.

Evidence-based medicine—a phrase that ought to be redundant—calls for coordinating medical practice with scientific evidence. That is, of course, a great deal easier said than done. Although the medical literature is exhaustive, much of the work on effectiveness is methodologically flawed and inconclusive. The Institute of Medicine's 2009 report, *Value in Health Care*, maintained that 20–30 percent of US health care expenditures represented "over-, under-, or misutilization of medical treatments and technologies, relative to the evidence of their effectiveness."[44] Critics contended in 2011 that the United States was spending $200 billion a year on medical overtreatment.[45]

As policy analysts constantly remind us, US health care spending averages more per person than that of any other country. National health care expenditures hit $1 trillion around 1995, $2 trillion just 10 years later, and $3 trillion in the following decade. But, with the nation consistently ranking last among developed countries in medical quality, equality, and efficiency, we do not buy better health or better health care.[46] It is widely noted—both inside and outside of the profession—that a significant portion of medical treatment is not scientifically justified and that some of it is harmful.[47] Radiation therapy is an important example of a treatment that has not always been used appropriately.

Diagnostic and therapeutic use of radiation could not have arisen, of course, without the discovery in the 1890s of two entirely unexpected forms of energy. Wilhelm Roentgen concluded that some previously unknown force must be emanating from the cathode tubes he was investigating in Germany in 1895 and named it "X-ray." In France the following year, Henri Becquerel discovered that some chemical elements spontaneously emit energy, a phenomenon Marie Curie called *radioactivity*. Both forms of energy severely burned living tissue, as investigators discovered at their own peril.[48] The damaging effects of radiation pointed to a new treatment concept and at the same time forewarned of its dangers. Practitioners sought to corral radiation and use it to damage diseased tissues selectively.

Early radiation therapists, like early radiographers, were not necessarily physicians. Chicago cathode-tube manufacturer and homeopathic medical student Emil Grubbé purportedly used X-rays to treat a cancer patient just 23 days after Roentgen's announcement. He did so at the behest of one of his professors, who, observing Grubbé's hands blistered from working with X-rays, applied a principle of his profession. The immediate result of the treatment seemed to confirm the homeopathic principle that an agent causing disease can also cure it. "Any physical agent capable of doing so much damage to normal or healthy cells and tissues," the professor reasoned, must have clinical potential in treating cancer.[49] The breast cancer of the patient that Grubbé treated shrank, giving rise to hope that a cure for cancer had at last been found, but the patient died of metastases shortly thereafter. This pattern of striking initial response with little longer-term benefit would recur over and over in radiation therapy and would mislead radiotherapists again and again. Whether or not Grubbé was the first to apply X-rays against cancer—and it is disputed—it is clear that early radiation treatments were not, and could not have been, based on scientific methods of the time.

Radiologists have recognized that their use of radiation frequently exceeded contemporary scientific evidence of effectiveness and all too often inflicted serious patient harm. Canadian radiation oncologist Charles Hayter called North American radiation therapy the "ultimate rebuke to proponents of scientific medicine, for it was a treatment that was grounded completely in experience."[50] Medical historian Caroline Murphy made a similar case regarding British radiotherapy.[51] Historian John Pickstone held that cancer treatments throughout the 20th century in the United Kingdom and the United States were essentially experimental.[52] As a newly trained radiologist in 1946, Henry Kaplan asserted that radiation treatment up to then had "evolved by trial and error" rather than by scientific study.[53] Kaplan aspired to change that situation, but he would not always succeed—even in his own practices (Chapter 7).

Practitioners initially applied radiation (by trial and considerable error) to patients with asthma, anemia, migraine, epilepsy, and a wide range of skin, infectious, inflammatory, and menstrual conditions.[54] Doctors irradiated the scalps of children with ringworm as late as the 1950s. Disproportionate numbers of children so treated subsequently suffered leukemias as well as thyroid, skin, and brain cancers.[55] After nearly half a century of broad radiation use, physicians conceded that they were often inflicting more harm than good and increasingly focused their radiation beams on cancer.

The latest developments in radiation therapy have periodically fueled extravagant promises of curing cancer. Mass-market magazines such as *Life*, *Time*, *Fortune*, and *Newsweek* pronounced each new cancer gun to be the ultimate in scientific progress—although they also conceded its limitations. Innovative devices and therapeutic strategies brought so many hopes and hypes that, if true, they would collectively have cured cancer many times over. The popular articles may have led (and misled) patients and the public into thinking that radiation treatments were scientifically demonstrated to be effective. "The initial responses of skin cancers and other superficial neoplasms treated by irradiation were so dramatic," Kaplan later wrote, "that they generated the unrealistic expectations that a miraculous cure for all cancers had finally been discovered."[56] He noted, however, that most tumors tended to recur and/or metastasize after their remarkable initial regression.

Even as they invoked magic and miracle, radiotherapists tended to view each new device as the epitome of modern scientific medicine. But machines alone do not make medicine scientific. Published studies revealed (often inadvertently) how radiation treatments were not based on scientific evidence—nor could they have been, as adequate evidence was not available. This means that in many cases we simply have not known—and in fact still do not know—how effective and how damaging radiation treatments are.

Some radiation oncologists, physicists, and engineers may take issue with my skeptical analysis of the literature, interpreting the same reports—as did many of their authors—as supporting the use of radiation. I ask them to take a closer look at the reports. But I also recognize that highly trained physicians may disagree with each other. Two prominent oncologists recently wrote about men who died of prostate cancer after suffering complications from a series of treatments. Otis Webb Brawley, former chief medical officer of the American Cancer Society, suggested that the quality of life of his friend's final decade would have been better without the chemotherapy and surgery he had received. "Millions of patients [are] exposed to harm," Brawley held, when treated with profitable but insufficiently tested pharmaceuticals.[57] In contrast, former National Cancer Institute director Vincent DeVita—who played a major role in developing chemotherapy—suggested that if only his friend could have received the very latest drug, he might have lived a little longer.[58] Valuing different outcomes, both of them may have been right from their points of view.

Despite considerable progress in understanding cancer, the progress has not always extended to its treatment. There are many unknowns, and many treatments are based on hope, desperation, and a placebo effect. I appreciate the oft-quoted aphorism that the practice of medicine is an art as well as a science. Doctors have to measure the harms that their treatments may inflict on patients against the risk of those patients suffering and dying from their disease in the near future. Yet as a patient, a purchaser, a public health professional, and a history scholar, I want to know—and I believe the public deserves to know—what the available evidence does and does not say concerning the medical interventions on offer.

In studying radiation therapy, I do not mean to imply that other cancer treatments are more scientifically justified. There is, in fact, shockingly little scientific support for routine radical surgery, radiation rays, and chemotherapy cocktails (or what some critics call slash, burn, and poison). But, because this book does not examine other treatment modalities, it can only observe that many radiation treatments have been insufficiently tested and have harmed patients, and that their long-term effects are in large part unknown.

Although the damage that X-rays and radioactive elements inflict is the basis of their therapeutic use, both forms of radiation turned out to be more damaging than their users had imagined. Radiation's disruption of cell division destroys cancer cells, but it also destroys normally regenerating cells. Severe consequences can include anemia, compromised immune systems, gastro-intestinal injuries, internal scarring, and new cancers. Concurrent with devising (later rejected) theories that radiation damaged cancerous tissues selectively, clinicians in the early years accepted that healthy tissues were always afflicted and that some patients would die from their treatments rather than their cancers. While medical mistakes and machine malfunctions have led to well-publicized patient harms from radiotherapy, the harms described in this book come from its standard use.

Ensuring safe and effective treatment is a public health as well as a medical responsibility. While practicing physicians are (necessarily) concerned with the patients in front of them, the field of public health is concerned with the health of communities and effective health care delivery systems. Although many of their efforts have met with resistance from organized medicine and business, public health programs in the United States have striven to improve the outcomes of cancer.

Cancer and Radiation Therapy in the United States

On June 29, 2016, Congressman Mark DeSaulnier, himself diagnosed with cancer the previous year, hosted one of the 270 meetings held across the United States to launch President Obama's and Vice-President Biden's Cancer Moonshot. Although it echoed President Nixon's much-hyped 1970 War on Cancer, the Moonshot's goals were ostensibly more modest: achieve a decade's worth of progress in cancer research in half that time. The nearly 300 medical providers, scientific researchers, company executives, cancer activists, and patients who attended the sometimes emotional meeting in Concord, California expressed a wide range of concerns, but all wanted to participate in cancer policy making. Some used the occasion to call for universal health care. Some companies used the Moonshot to sell their products and appreciated the call for more connections between industry and academia.[59] Most attendees had high hopes that investing more resources in cancer research would improve its treatment.

Because cancer can be frightening and life-threatening, it is tempting to hurl the entire therapeutic armamentarium at it. Many physicians and their patients feel that the threat of cancer overrides treatment risks.[60] Chances are high that a newly diagnosed cancer patient in the United States will receive radiation treatments, although no one actually knows how high. One data set covering 70 percent of cancer patients reported that 31 percent of them diagnosed between 2000 and 2011 received radiation in the first round of treatment (compared to 62 percent undergoing surgery, 26 percent chemotherapy, and 17 percent hormone therapy).[61] Adding the patients receiving radiation later in the course of their disease—often after initial treatment failure—it is thought that somewhere around one million Americans receive radiation treatments each year. (Other data sets report other figures, as discussed in Chapter 10.) Treatment combinations have increased in recent decades, and, in most cases, radiation supplements other therapies. Only 7 percent of patients received radiation as the sole treatment in the first round.

The latest cancer intervention rates do not signify a final reckoning of scientific progress, nor do they offer benchmarks for judging past—or future—interventions. They merely describe practices as of the first decade of the 21st century, and they will continue to change. Would more treatment lead to better outcomes? If so, which treatments? (The answer often depends on the specialty of the respondent.) Would less treatment be better for patients? No one really knows the answers to these questions. What is clear, however, is that uncertainty regarding these questions has spurred cancer entrepreneurialism.

Radiation therapy has become a successful industry. The field's clinical inadequacies have contributed to ongoing growth as it searched for a gun that would finally shoot a magic bullet. Growing capital investment fueled a race to build higher and higher-powered guns, and, in so doing, augmented the power and wealth of participating universities, hospitals, specialties, manufacturers, and financial firms.

Treating cancer has itself become a major medical business in the United States, second only to cardiac care and with faster-rising expenditures.[62] The country is expected to spend $174 billion in the year 2020 on 1.6 million newly diagnosed patients and 18 million total cancer patients (over half a million of whom will die of cancer that year).[63] These figures mean that cancer is a huge medical market, and it is especially so in countries with large numbers of older people. The disease is fundamentally a loss of control over the body's normal and necessary regenerative processes, and this loss expands with age; of people who die from cancer in the United States, 70 percent are 65 or over. Since, biologically, death is necessary for the existence of life, should we not be more realistic about the limitations of cancer treatment and include quality of life in medical treatment decisions?

It is distinctly not comfortable—nor is it comforting—to talk about inadequacies of cancer care when millions of people, including some close to me, are fervently hoping for more encouragement. A physician once explained that when his publisher questioned his proposal for a book on the "stupidities" of medicine on the grounds that it would be a "downer," he instead wrote one on medicine's technological progress.[64] Such an approach to medical discourse (and publishing) is part of the problem. Promoting technology as an antidote to medical limitations and failures adds to individual suffering as well as to social costs. The real "upper" entails reforming health care in ways that actually improve people's health—and that requires acknowledging some hard realities. One reality is the limited value of what we are getting for our $174 billion a year in cancer-care expenditures, which, contrary to popular and professional belief, have played only a small role in the recent improvements in cancer outcomes.

Although the measured overall cancer mortality rate in the United States rose continuously throughout most of the 20th century's growth in medical care, it started to decline in the early 1990s. The decline was largely due to a receding of the tobacco-induced lung-cancer epidemic. But it was also, in part, a result of earlier diagnosis and treatment of several other major cancers, particularly those of the uterine cervix, breast, and colon. Chapters 4, 8, and 10 discuss cancer data and outcomes in more detail and show that improvements in cancer outcomes were not generally due to increasingly sophisticated medical treatments. The data do, however, suggest hope for the prevention of certain cancers, earlier diagnosis, and a limited selection of treatments. At issue is what societies choose to do with the information they have available.

Markets and Policy

Market assumptions, values, and ideologies have dominated health policy one way or another over the past century. Leaders have alternately assumed *laissez-faire*, actively promoted market strategies, or sponsored reforms designed to reverse market failures. All three policy approaches have asked the same (limited) question: How much should third parties—private and/or public—intervene in the relationships between consumers and sellers in the health care market?

Labor and other progressive leaders called for national health insurance in the 1910s; in the following decade, medical and business leaders called for growth in private health insurance. Private insurance, which spends a portion of its intake on services rendered and invests the remainder in the financial markets, prevailed. The resulting conflict of interest between service and profit may explain why so many Americans feel that their health insurance plans—if they have them—are not designed to meet their health care needs. They're not. They are designed to meet the needs of the medical and insurance industries. When insurance plans build in higher deductions and co-payments, insured as well as uninsured people find that bills for costly services can have a serious impact on their access to health care.

Civil-rights activists in the 1960s insisted that all people in a democratic society had a right to equal access to health care. Not choosing any of the national health insurance or national health service proposals on the table, Congress passed the Medicare program, which entitled social-security beneficiaries to reimbursement for medical services; and the Medicaid program, which expanded medical welfare programs for low-income people.[65] As many citizens eagerly joined the Medicare and Medicaid rolls, there were strong political reactions against the programs. Critics lambasted the principle of equal rights in the name of the market. A 1971 opinion piece in the *New England Journal of Medicine*, for example, refuted health care rights and held that medical care was no different from any other commodity in the marketplace.[66]

Idealizations of *the market* continued to denigrate government involvement in health care. "Just as the market revived our flagging manufacturing sector," business school professor (and advocate of the Jiffy Lube model of medical care) Regina Herzlinger advised in the 1990s, "the market and only the market can provide the health care that the American people want at a price they are willing to pay."[67] The market implosion and ensuing recession a decade later revealed the poverty of these ideas—not to mention that of people otherwise "willing" to pay.

In repudiating government regulation, free-market advocates neglected the crucial role governments have played in maintaining the stability of market systems.[68] Licensing, antitrust laws, bankruptcy protection, product safety reviews, and the many supply and demand subsidies have defined the medical market and funded its growth. Free-market advocates have obscured the active role that interested parties play in shaping the medical market in the first place. *Cancer, Radiation Therapy, and the Market* shows how market interests and strategies drove the development of 20th-century medical care. It illustrates how leading providers, manufacturers, insurers, and financiers comprised the market "forces" that built a medical specialty.

The turn of the 21st century brought a staggering leap in medical costs and profits based on proton-beam therapy. This book explores the following questions: How did America come to spend so much of its resources on medical interventions of marginal benefit? What are the human consequences? What are the international implications? And what might we do about it?

Outline of the Book

Cancer, Radiation Therapy, and the Market investigates effects of evolving economic and political environments on the development of a medical specialty, its technology, and its practices. Although the book offers some international comparisons, its North American perspective—which includes leading Canadian contributions—skimps on concurrent and prior developments in the rest of the world. France, for instance, initiated a radium industry and radium treatments, Germany pioneered X-rays, German and Swiss companies manufactured betatrons, the United Kingdom developed linear accelerators, the USSR built synchrotrons, and Belgium and Japan pioneered particle accelerators. US technologies were not necessarily better than those of its international rivals—but the country's large industrial infrastructure, research universities, investor wealth, and affluent market sustained a domestic radiation-therapy industry that influenced world radiotherapy development. In the 1980s, the United States accounted for 60 percent of the global production and consumption of medical devices.[69]

Crossing disciplinary boundaries of medical and business history, clinical research, and public health policy, the work draws upon archival resources, medical literature, professional and governmental reports, financial statements, media stories, and advertising. Its three parts cover successive time periods between 1895 and the 2010s. Each part opens with a section on the economic and political environment of the time, and every chapter relates radiotherapy development and/or policy to this environment. The first period largely implemented entrepreneurship, the second competition, and the third finance—although, of course, all three factors played roles in each period. Most chapters examine how academic, medical, hospital, industrial, and financial interests combined in different ways to build new devices and clinical procedure units for the devices. Clinical practices in each time period raised interventional intensity and patient exposure to radiation, but the practices were not always consistent with contemporary research findings on effectiveness.

Part I, "Radiation Enterprise, 1895 to World War II," covers the period from the discovery of X-rays in 1895 and radioactivity in 1896 to World War II. A time of enormous economic change, this period saw the rise of mass production, big business, and the corporation. Foundations and other large accumulations of wealth redesigned educational and medical institutions along the lines of the industrial economy.

Chapter 2, "The Medical Radium Industry," shows how the radium industry played a major role in radium therapy development. Industrialists in France and the United States organized clinics and published journals dedicated to using the radioactive element medically. The US Standard Chemical Company founded the American Radium Society to promote the company's product and to establish its own scientific and medical credentials. The limited supply of radium was an international geopolitical issue, and a competing US company, the National Radium Institute, actively molded national mining policy in its own interests. Mining executive James Douglas, benefactor of Memorial Hospital of New York, and Johns Hopkins University gynecologist Howard Kelly sought government assistance to build the institute solely for the purpose of accruing radium for Memorial Hospital and the private practice Howard A. Kelly Hospital. The chapter briefly summarizes contemporary research findings that questioned the intensive medical uses of radium and demonstrated its many dangers. Most of the ensuing chapters of the book investigate developments in external beam irradiation or *teletherapy*.

Chapter 3, "The General Electric Company Dominates X-ray," investigates the US General Electric Company's dynamic role in developing radiation equipment and shaping institutions purchasing the equipment. After inventing a kilovoltage X-ray tube specifically for medical treatment, the company bought the Victor X-ray Company to secure its position in the radiology market. GE then escalated the voltage of its X-ray devices as it competed in the "million-volts or bust" race. The company advertised a broad product line of devices and placed articles in mass-distribution magazines to promote their popular acceptance. GE built close ties with New York's Memorial Hospital, and academic medical center competition accelerated the growth of the medical X-ray. GE instructed hospital and radiology administrators in principles of business management and designed hospital radiology units along industrial lines to maximize productivity and equipment placement. In extending its planning strategies to the national economy, the company shaped future planning efforts.

Chapter 4, "Competing Research Universities," examines the development of high-powered radiation therapy devices in industry-aligned laboratories in three research universities. Physicists at the California Institute of Technology built a high-voltage X-ray tube and invited American College of Radiology founder Albert Soiland to send his cancer patients to their laboratory for treatment. At the University of California, physicist Ernest Lawrence and colleagues built a supervoltage X-ray machine for the university's medical school in San Francisco. Appreciating that cancer treatment significantly enhanced fundraising, Lawrence's team also treated patients with neutrons emanating from laboratory cyclotrons. Having treated patients with both California technologies, radiologist Robert Stone came to advise against continuing neutron therapy due to severe patient damage. Massachusetts Institute of Technology (MIT) engineer John Trump developed MIT's Van de Graaff X-ray generator for medical purposes and worked with radiologists to use it clinically. Although photographs in the medical literature documented stunning tumor reductions with radiation therapy, the field's own scientific research did not, for the most part, demonstrate notably better patient outcomes using radium, neutrons, or supervoltage X-rays compared with kilovoltage X-rays, and it often found significant patient harm. It did note slightly better patient outcomes with radiation compared to the radical hysterectomy of the time for cancer of the uterine cervix, which accounted for a large portion of radiotherapy patients at the time.

Part II, "Competitive Megavoltage: World War II to the 1970s," starts with the booming economy of World War II and ends with the declining economy of the 1970s. Government funding added to economic growth supported huge expansion in private health insurance, complex medical centers, and specialty departments. The 1950 International Congress of Radiology in London revealed international competition in high-voltage radiotherapy. Megavoltage attained iconic status when the May 5, 1958 cover of *Life* magazine featured a 2 million volt (2MeV) device.

Chapter 5, "Megavoltage Competition in Academia and Industry," follows the postwar activities of the General Electric Company, the Massachusetts Institute of Technology, and the University of California in applying their megavoltage triumphs to medical care. GE advertised radiation therapy to the public, continued to instruct hospital and radiology administrators in business management, and held options on virtually every megavoltage technology. Its own resonance transformer, however, did not sell well—despite movie-star endorsement.

Partnering with manufacturing, medicine, and finance in the form of the fledgling venture capital company American Research & Development Corporation, MIT's John Trump commercialized the Van de Graaff accelerator by establishing the High Voltage Engineering Corporation to manufacture the device and developing his High Voltage Research Laboratory to specialize in radiotherapy research, treatment planning, and clinical consultation. Trump built a treatment facility at MIT to use the Van de Graaff accelerator in conjunction with the Lahey

Clinic. Accusing the Trump team of false advertising, California's Robert Stone inveighed against flamboyant publicity that exaggerated clinical benefits of the Van de Graaff device. Stone installed GE's ultra-high-powered synchrotron in his own department, only to find that it added more to the cost of radiation treatment than to its effectiveness. For a variety of reasons, none of the devices appearing in this chapter enjoyed major success in the medical marketplace. It was another device entirely that led to a radiotherapy sales boom.

Chapter 6, "Medicine's Nuclear Arms Race," studies the competition to use cobalt-60 teletherapy devices to treat cancer. Two Canadian teams and one ambitious US medical center raced to build and use devices employing the artificially radioactive isotope created in reactors made for the atomic bomb. Eldorado Mining and Refining sales manager Roy Errington acquired exclusive rights to market Canada's cobalt-60 production and invited Ontario physician Ivan Smith to work with him in constructing and using a new medical device. The Ontario team beat a competing Saskatchewan team by days and widely broadcast the first use of a "cobalt bomb." Errington partnered with the Canadian government to form Atomic Energy of Canada, Ltd. (AECL), which became the world's largest seller of cobalt-60 devices.

In the United States, radiologist Gilbert Fletcher at Texas Medical Center's M. D. Anderson Hospital allied with General Electric—with money from the federal government—to build the third cobalt bomb. The large and increasingly affluent North American market and the device's relatively low price for its energy level supported the first teletherapy boom since kilovoltage, although it was AECL, not GE, that benefitted most. Expanding international sales of the new technology were not due to strong evidence that it significantly improved cancer survival over other megavoltage-level devices. It was economic and professional factors that drove the cobalt boom—just as they would drive a linear accelerator boom.

Chapter 7, "An Economic Success Story at Stanford," investigates how Stanford's medical linear accelerator (colloquially called *linac*) developed in the context of building a successful research university, an industrial park, and a new research- and practice-funded medical school. Rising to positions that enabled him to foster his maxim that "higher education is a highly competitive business," Frederick Terman sponsored engineer Edward Ginzton's work on the linear accelerator, and Ginzton collaborated with radiology department executive Henry Kaplan to adapt the instrument for medical use. Kaplan's program to use his new linac to treat Hodgkin's Lymphoma furthered the device's acceptance. Although Kaplan's aggressive treatment program (which included chemo- as well as radiotherapy) severely damaged many patients, it also came to lower the disease's mortality rates. Ginzton became president of Varian Associates, the company manufacturing the Stanford linac, and Varian's close connection with Stanford and its location in Stanford's industrial park favored the company on Wall Street and facilitated worldwide acceptance of its accelerator.

Chapter 8, "Radiation Therapy Politics," briefly reviews mid-century epidemiological data and professional discourse regarding the relative effectiveness of higher-powered devices. Radiation therapists—now calling themselves radiation oncologists—used temporal correlations between voltage increases and cancer survival gains, particularly those of cervical cancer, to claim a (spurious) causal connection between the two. But the linear accelerator was never demonstrated to be significantly more effective in treating cancer than cobalt-60 or other competing megavoltage devices.

The specialty actively engaged in political activities and promoted programs that funded its latest devices and supported its leading centers. Regional Medical Programs (RMP) added to the coffers of specialties treating cancer (as well as heart disease and stroke). Varian Associates exploited the Conquest of Cancer's dubious claim that wider radiotherapy use could reduce the total cancer death rate by 15–25 percent over the subsequent five years. Radiotherapy leaders participated in health planning and Certificate of Need activities in order to protect their services from concerns of excessive costs and supply. Applications to purchase costly radiotherapy devices submitted to New York City's Cobalt Committee and Washington State's Certificate of Need program illustrated the competitive pressures on hospitals and radiation oncologists to constantly upgrade their technologies.

Part III, "Financializing Medicine, 1970s to the 2010s," covers the era that saw the decline of the nation's economy and the rise of the financial industry and its market theories. A growing cadre of management consulting companies cropped up to teach medicine how to make its services more like business, specifically Jiffy Lube.

Chapter 9, "Speculating on Proton Therapy," investigates an organizational innovation that skyrocketed radiation therapy to new energy and new cost heights. Although physics laboratories had long treated cancer patients with proton beams, the race was on after California's Loma Linda Medical Center announced its new hospital-based proton treatment center. Growing numbers of manufacturers, management companies, property developers, and financial firms partnered with enterprising radiation oncology groups and hospital administrators to build proton centers of their own. In requiring capital investments up to $300 million (each) and new forms of business organization, proton centers integrated the financial industry into medical delivery more than ever before and further opened the door to corporate medicine. It did not take long for competing manufacturers to put smaller, cheaper devices on the market.

Although many proton centers' business plans counted on treating large numbers of men with prostate cancer, insurance companies began to restrict payments on grounds of inadequate scientific evidence of the greater effectiveness of the more costly device. Instead of evidence, proton-therapy growth was predicated on an *a priori* assumption that a better-measured dose distribution was bound to lead to better patient outcomes. Health policy in the market era has been unwilling or unable to restrict medical care growth on grounds of effectiveness. Manufacturers have marketed their devices worldwide and have partnered with development companies to build increasing numbers of particle centers in Europe and Asia. Spread of American proton center innovation meant that the most market-driven health care system in the developed world was imposing its private, high-debt mode of operation upon the rest of it. As an ongoing process, proton-center development is a moving target, and any description of it as of the mid-2010s is necessarily provisional.

Chapter 10, "Rationalizing Radiation Therapy, Reforming Health Care," briefly reviews US cancer incidence, mortality, and survival data as of the early 21st century and summarizes key health care reform efforts. The American College of Radiology's Patterns of Care project aimed at strengthening the radiation oncology profession and its services. Contrary to widespread claims, however, the national declines in cancer mortality starting in the 1990s were not primarily due to advances in cancer treatment. They were due in large part to the reduced incidence of tobacco-related cancers and early diagnosis of a few other cancers. Cancer screening has added to the early diagnosis, but it may lead to excessive intervention in some cancers. Cochrane Collaboration reviews of international literature have revealed a patchwork of randomized controlled trials that have collectively found small survival gains with the use of radiation under certain conditions for certain categories of patients with Hodgkin's, cervical, breast, and prostate cancers; some significant harms; and many uncertainties.

The chapter then summarizes US reforms aimed at paying for medical care, measuring its effectiveness, prioritizing capital investment, protecting patient safety, directing specialty growth, and mitigating professional conflicts of interest. Although each policy approach improved medical delivery to a certain extent, none has fully addressed the problems identified. They have maintained a discriminatory insurance system, shied away from clinical effectiveness, adopted professional policies that conferred competitive advantages, applied loopholes in device regulation, and built market principles into health planning and Certificate of Need. A political inability in the 1990s to come to a consensus on the ethics of extremely damaging radiation treatments raised questions about practice standards and standard radiation-therapy practices.

Chapter 11, "Choosing Health Over Wealth," summarizes the key market strategies driving medical care discussed in this book. Some of the strategies are characteristics of specialization itself. Some apply managerial and financial principles to medical delivery in the name of competition. Some lead to excessive investment in high-cost technologies relative to their assessed effectiveness. Cumulatively, the market strategies have built a medical business system that determines access by price and that measures value by technological and capital intensity.

The market revolution in health care is a capital coup. Market strategies mean that Wall Street has become a major planner and a major beneficiary of health care. Even when inspired by ideals of equity in terms of justice, many health care reforms have augmented investor equity. Significant reform requires challenging the market strategies embedded in medical care and taking control of capital investment. It can start by asking fundamental questions about the current medical delivery system, such as who benefits from the market strategies and what the evidence is that competition improves health care. Democratic processes to frame alternative ways of delivering health care are pivotal in creating a more effective, equitable, and efficient health care system.

Notes

1 Regina E. Herzlinger, *Market-Driven Health Care: Who Wins, Who Loses in the Transformation of America's Largest Service Industry* (Reading, MA: Addison-Wesley, 1997), 163, 166.
2 Meredith K. Biegel, "Breast Cancer: My Story," November 1, 2001. http://www.oncolink.org/coping/article.cfm?c=398&id=107 accessed November 29, 2015.
3 Amol K. Narang, Edwin Lam, Martin A. Makary, *et al.*, "Accuracy of Marketing Claims by Providers of Stereotactic Radiation Therapy," *Journal of Oncology Practice* 9 (2013): 57–62.
4 Marc David, "Cancer Free in Less than 3 Hours," *WA Health Magazine* May 2006: 26–27.
5 Gamma West Cancer Services. http://www.robertsstudio.net/advertising/files/page4–1004-full.html accessed November 22, 2013.
6 Natasha Singer, "Cancer Center Ads Use Emotion More Than Fact," *New York Times* December 18, 2009.
7 "U.S. News & World Report Releases 2013–14 Best Hospitals Rankings," *U.S. News and World Report* July 16. 2013.
8 Jeremy A. Greene and David Herzberg, "Hidden in Plain Sight: Marketing Prescription Drugs to Consumers in the Twentieth Century," *American Journal of Public Health* 100 (2010): 793–806.
9 Matthew Lavine, "The Early Clinical X-Ray in the United States: Patient Experiences and Public Perceptions," *Journal of the History of Medicine and Allied Sciences* 67 (2012): 587–625.
10 Donald A. Barr, *Introduction to U.S. Health Policy: The Organization, Financing, and Delivery of Health Care in America* (Baltimore: Johns Hopkins University Press, 2011), 32.
11 Nancy Tomes, *Remaking the American Patient: How Madison Avenue and Modern Medicine Turned Patients into Consumers* (Chapel Hill: University of North Carolina Press, 2016), 19.
12 John Harley Warner, *The Therapeutic Perspective: Medical Practice, Knowledge, and Identity in America, 1820–1885* (Cambridge, MA: Harvard University Press, 1986), 1, 12, 244, 261; George Weisz, *Divide and Conquer: A Comparative History of Medical Specialization* (New York: Oxford University Press, 2006), 71–72.
13 Kenneth J. Arrow, "Uncertainty and the Welfare Economics of Medical Care," *The American Economic Review* 53 (1963): 941–973.
14 James A. Schafer, *The Business of Private Medical Practice: Doctors, Specialization, and Urban Change in Philadelphia, 1900–1940* (New Brunswick, NJ: Rutgers University Press, 2014), 12.
15 Joseph M. Gabriel, *Medical Monopoly: Intellectual Property Rights and the Origins of the Modern Pharmaceutical Industry* (Chicago: University of Chicago Press, 2014), 3.
16 Rosemary Stevens, *American Medicine and the Public Interest* (Berkeley, CA: University of California Press, updated ed. 1998); Morris J. Vogel, *The Invention of the Modern Hospital: Boston, 1870–1930* (Chicago: University of Chicago Press, 1980); David Rosner, *A Once Charitable Enterprise: Hospitals and Health Care in Brooklyn and New York 1885–1915* (Cambridge: Cambridge University Press, 1982).
17 US Supreme Court, *Goldfarb v. Virginia State Bar* (421 U.S. 773 [1975]); Clark C. Havighurst, *Deregulating the Health Care Industry: Planning for Competition* (Cambridge, MA: Ballinger, 1982), 98–106, 131–137; Carl E. Ameringer, *The Health Care Revolution: From Medical Monopoly to Market Competition* (Berkeley, CA: University of California Press, 2008), 100–103, 197–198.
18 Malik M. Hasan, "Sounding Board: Let's End the Nonprofit Charade," *New England Journal of Medicine* 334 (1996): 1055–1057.

19 Ezekiel J. Emanuel and 21 other signatories, "A Plan to Fix Cancer Care," *New York Times* March 24, 2013, SR14.
20 Christopher Weaver, Tom McGinty, and Louise Radnofsky, "Small Slice of Doctors Account for Big Chunk of Medicare Costs," *The Wall Street Journal* April 9, 2014, A1, A5.
21 Paul Kalanithi, *When Breath Becomes Air* (New York: Random House, 2016), 42.
22 Robb Burlage, "Editorial: The Medical Industrial Complex," *Health PAC Bulletin* November 1969, 1–2; Arnold S. Relman, "The New Medical-Industrial Complex," *New England Journal of Medicine* 303 (1980): 963–970.
23 Paul Starr, *The Social Transformation of American Medicine: The Rise of a Sovereign Profession and the Making of a Vast Industry* (New York: Basic Books, 1982), 420.
24 Eliot Freidson, *Profession of Medicine: A Study of the Sociology of Applied Knowledge* (New York: Harper and Row, 1970), 116; Theodore Levitt, *The Marketing Imagination* (New York: Free Press, 1986), 50, 61.
25 Thomas C. Cochran, *The American Business System: A Historical Perspective, 1900–1955* (New York: Harper and Row, 1957), vi–vii; Alfred D. Chandler, *The Visible Hand: The Managerial Revolution in American Business* (Cambridge: Harvard University Press, 1977), 1–12; Glenn Porter, *The Rise of Big Business 1860–1920* (Arlington Heights, IL: Harlan Davidson, 1992).
26 Thomas K. McCraw, ed., *Creating Modern Capitalism: How Entrepreneurs, Companies, and Countries Triumphed in Three Industrial Revolutions* (Cambridge, MA: Harvard University Press, 1997), 1–16; James C. Robinson, *The Corporate Practice of Medicine: Competition and Innovation in Health Care* (Berkeley, CA: University of California Press, 1999), 13–15, 233.
27 Colin Crouch, *The Strange Non-Death of Neoliberalism* (Cambridge: Polity, 2011), 16, 167, 176; David M. Kotz, *The Rise and Fall of Neoliberal Capitalism* (Cambridge, MA: Harvard University Press, 2015).
28 Barbara Bridgman Perkins, *The Medical Delivery Business: Health Reform, Childbirth, and the Economic Order* (New Brunswick, NJ: Rutgers University Press, 2004), 3–8.
29 George Rosen, *The Specialization of Medicine with Particular Reference to Ophthalmology* (New York: Froben, 1944), 31.
30 Rosemary Stevens, *American Medicine and the Public Interest* (Berkeley, CA: University of California Press, updated ed. 1998), xv–xvi.
31 Jeffrey Lionel Berlant, *Profession and Monopoly: A Study of Medicine in the United States and Great Britain* (Berkeley, CA: University of California Press, 1975).
32 Roger Cooter, "The Politics of a Spatial Innovation: Fracture Clinics in Inter-War Britain," In John V. Pickstone, ed., *Medical Innovations in Historical Perspective* (New York: St. Martin's Press, 1992), 146–164.
33 Monika Dommann, "From Danger to Risk: The Perception and Regulation of X-Rays in Switzerland, 1896–1970," In Thomas Schlich and Ulrich Tröhler, eds., *The Risks of Medical Innovation: Risk Perception and Assessment in Historical Context* (London: Routledge, 2006), 93–115.
34 Rosemary Stevens, *In Sickness and In Wealth: American Hospitals in the Twentieth Century* (New York: Basic Books, 1989), 37.
35 Beth Mintz and Michael Schwartz, "Capital Formation and the United States Health Care System: The Relationship between the Private and the Public Sector," *Research in the Sociology of Health Care* 18 (2000): 229–248.
36 Gordon MacLeod and Mark Perlman, *Health Care Capital: Competition and Control* (Cambridge, MA: Ballinger, 1978), 296.
37 Robert A. Berenson, Thomas Bodenheimer, and Hoangmai H. Pham, "Specialty-Service Lines: Salvos in the New Medical Arms Race," Health Affairs 25 (2006): w337–w343; Lewis G. Sandy. Thomas Bodenheimer, L. Gregory Pawlson, and Barbara Starfield, "The Political Economy of U.S. Primary Care," Health Affairs 28 (2009): 1136–1145.

38 Ezekiel J. Emanuel and Victor R. Fuchs, "The Perfect Storm of Overutilization," *JAMA* 299 (2008): 2789–2791.

39 John K. Iglehart, "Health Insurers and Medical-imaging Policy—A Work in Progress, *New England Journal of Medicine* 360 (2009):1030–1037; Vijay M. Rao and David C. Levin, "The Overuse of Diagnostic Imaging and the Choosing Wisely Initiative," *Annals of Internal Medicine* 157 (2012): 574–576.

40 Robert Aronowitz, *Unnatural History: Breast Cancer and American Society* (Cambridge: Cambridge University Press, 2007), 3–8, 257.

41 Bettyann Holtzmann Kevles, *Naked to the Bone: Medical Imaging in the Twentieth Century* (Reading, MA: Addison-Wesley, 1997), 54–55; Pierre-Yves Donzé, "Making Medicine a Business in Japan: Shimadzu Co. and the Diffusion of Radiology (1900–1960)," *Gesnerus* 67 (2010): 241–262.

42 Joel D. Howell, *Technology in the Hospital: Transforming Patient Care in the Early Twentieth Century* (Baltimore: Johns Hopkins University Press, 1995), 125.

43 Stuart S. Blume, *Insight and Industry: On the Dynamics of Technological Change in Medicine* (Cambridge, MA: MIT Press, 1992), 260; Jeffrey Kirk, *Machines in Our Hearts: The Cardiac Pacemaker, the Implantable Defibrillator, and American Health Care* (Baltimore: Johns Hopkins University Press, 2001); Thomas Schlich, *Surgery, Science and Industry: A Revolution in Fracture Care, 1950s–1970s* (Basingstoke: Palgrave Macmillan, 2002), 62; Julie Anderson, Francis Neary, and John V. Pickstone in collaboration with James Raferty, *Surgeons, Manufacturers and Patients* (Basingstoke, Hampshire: Palgrave Macmillan, 2007), 75–76; Dominique A. Tobbell, *Pills, Power, and Policy: The Struggle for Drug Reform in Cold War America and its Consequences* (Berkeley, CA: University of California Press, 2012).

44 Institute of Medicine (US), *Value in Health Care: Accounting for Cost, Quality, Safety, Outcomes, and Innovation* (Washington: National Academies, 2009), 2.

45 Donald M. Berwick and Andrew D. Hackbarth, "Eliminating Waste in U.S. Health Care," *JAMA* 307 (2012): 1512–1516.

46 Karen Davis, Kristof Stremikis, David Squires, and Cathy Schoen, *Mirror, Mirror, on the Wall: How the U.S. Health Care System Compares Internationally* (New York: Commonwealth Fund, 2014).

47 Virginia A. Sharpe and Alan I. Faden, *Medical Harm: Historical, Conceptual, and Ethical Dimensions of Iatrogenic Illness* (Cambridge: Cambridge University Press, 1998); Atul Gawande, *Complications: A Surgeon's Notes on an Imperfect Science* (New York: Picador, 2002); Shannon Brownlee, *Overtreated: Why Too Much Medicine is Making Us Sicker and Poorer* (New York: Bloomsbury, 2007); H. Gilbert Welch, Lisa M. Schwartz, and Steven Woloshin, *Overdiagnosed: Making People Sick in the Pursuit of Health* (Boston: Beacon, 2011); Henry Marsh, *Do No Harm: Stories of Life, Death, and Brain Surgery* (New York: St. Martin's, 2014).

48 Daniel S. Goldberg, "Suffering and Death among Early American Roentgenologists: The Power of Remotely Anatomizing the Living Body in Fin de Siècle America," *Bulletin of the History of Medicine* 85 (2011): 1–28.

49 Emil Grubbé, *X-Ray Treatment: Its Origin, Birth, and Early History* (St. Paul, MN: Bruce, 1949), x, 45; James T. Case, "History of Radiation Therapy," In Franz Buschke, ed., *Progress in Radiation Therapy* (New York: Grune & Stratton, 1958), 13–41; Juan A. del Regato, "Albert Soiland and the Early Development of Therapeutic Radiology in the United States," *International Journal of Radiation Oncology Biology Physics* 9 (1983): 243–254. This is the US version of an early and perhaps first use of X-ray in medical treatment, but there are challenges to it and competing versions. In *The Fight Against Cancer: France 1890–1940*, Patrice Pinell attributed the first to Dr Despignes of Lyons. (London: Routledge, 2002), 23. The Grubbé story has been questioned on the grounds that he was not a physician, was not a reliable reporter, may not have manufactured cathode tubes, and made his bid for X-ray fame 37 years after the putative treatment. Konrad Leszczynski and Susan Boyko, "On the Controversies

Surrounding the Origins of Radiation Therapy," *Radiotherapy and Oncology* 42 (1997): 213–217.
50 Charles Hayter, *An Element of Hope: Radium and the Response to Cancer in Canada, 1900–1940* (Montreal: McGill-Queen's University Press, 2005), 28.
51 Caroline Claire Scanlon Murphy, "A History of Radiotherapy to 1950: Cancer and Radiotherapy in Britain 1830–1950," PhD thesis, University of Manchester, 1986, Chapter 2.
52 John V. Pickstone, "Contested Cumulations: Configurations of Cancer Treatments through the Twentieth Century," *Bulletin of the History of Medicine* 81 (2007): 164–96.
53 Henry S. Kaplan and Hugh M. Wilson, "The Present Status of Radiation Therapy of Cancer," *Connecticut State Medical Journal* 10 (1946): 183–186.
54 Ira I. Kaplan, *Practical Radiation Therapy* (Philadelphia: W.B. Saunders, 1931), 125; Richard F. Mould, *A Century of X-rays and Radioactivity in Medicine* (Philadelphia: Institute of Physics Publishing, 1993), 31.
55 Catherine Caulfield, *Multiple Exposures: Chronicles of the Radiation Age* (Chicago: University of Chicago Press, 1989), 141.
56 Henry S. Kaplan, "Historic Milestones in Radiobiology and Radiation Therapy," *Seminars in Oncology* 6 (1979): 479–489.
57 Otis Webb Brawley with Paul Goldberg, *How We Do Harm: A Doctor Breaks Ranks about Being Sick in America* (New York: St. Martin's Griffin, 2011), 91, 231–239.
58 Vincent T. DeVita and Elizabeth DeVita-Raeburn, *The Death of Cancer* (New York: Farrar, Straus and Giroux, 2015), 13–31.
59 Mevion Medical Systems, "On Heels of Biden's Cancer Moonshot, Revolutionary Cancer Treatment Comes to Nation's Capital," press release, February 16, 2016. http://www.mevion.com/newsroom/press-releaseson-heels-of-bidens-cancer-moonshot-revolutionary-cancer-treatment-comes-to-nations-capital accessed June 9, 2016.
60 Jean-Paul Gaudillière, "Hormones at Risk: Cancer and the Medical Uses of Industrially-produced Sex Steroids in Germany, 1930–1960," In Thomas Schlich and Ulrich Tröhler, eds., *The Risks of Medical Innovation: Risk Perception and Assessment in Historical Context* (London: Routledge, 2006), 148–169.
61 American College of Surgeons, National Cancer Data Base (NCDB) Public Benchmark Reports, 2000–2011. https://www.facs.org accessed December 3, 2013.
62 Thomas J. Smith and Bruce E. Hillner, "Bending the Cost Curve in Cancer Care," *New England Journal of Medicine* 364 (2011): 2060–2065.
63 National Institutes of Health, "Cancer Costs Projected to Reach at Least $158 Billion in 2020," news release, January 12, 2011. http://www.nih.gov/news/health/jan2011/nci-12.htm accessed September 27, 2014.
64 William Hanson, *The Edge of Medicine: The Technology that Will Change Our Lives* (New York: Palgrave Macmillan, 2008), vii.
65 Robert B. Stevens and Rosemary Stevens, *Welfare Medicine in America: A Case Study of Medicaid* (New Brunswick, NJ: Transaction, 2003); Beatrix Hoffman, *The Wages of Sickness: The Politics of Health Insurance in Progressive America* (Chapel Hill: University of North Carolina Press, 2001), 182–184.
66 Robert M. Sade, "Medical Care as a Right: A Refutation," *New England Journal of Medicine* 285 (1971): 1288–1292.
67 Regina E. Herzlinger, *Market-Driven Health Care* (Reading, MA: Addison-Wesley, 1997), ix.
68 Karl Polanyi, *The Great Transformation* (Boston, Beacon, 1944); Rosemary Stevens, *The Public–Private Health Care State: Essays on the History of American Health Care Policy* (New Brunswick, NJ: Transaction, 2007), 178; Leo Panitch and Sam Gindlin, *The Making of Global Capitalism: The Political Economy of American Empire* (London: Verso, 2012), 1.
69 Michael Moran, *Governing the Health Care State* (Manchester: Manchester University Press, 1999), 138.

Part I

Radiation Enterprise, 1895 to World War II

"Wealth and Science Joining Hands for the Conquest of Cancer"
—*New York Times*

Part I investigates the active development of radiation therapy following the discoveries of X-rays and radioactivity. The specialty and its practices did not emerge just from the scientific discoveries and internal forces within medicine; they were also products of the economic and political environment. Competing research universities and companies industrialized radium production, manufactured X-ray tubes designed for medical treatment, and raced to achieve a million volts.

Political and Economic Environment

Worldwide economic development underwent momentous change in the late 19th and early 20th centuries. Cities lit up, factories thrummed with electricity, and radio messages crossed the Atlantic. Financial and manufacturing interests consolidated companies, built bigger production plants, and created mass markets for mass production.[1] Establishing big business and the big corporation, they also had a profound impact on nations' institutions.

As Andrew Carnegie celebrated in his *Gospel of Wealth*, the vast accumulations of wealth brought with them the power to mold society. Business magnates and foundations funded by Gilded Age fortunes rebuilt social institutions and integrated them into the new economy. They transformed education and health care by creating what they saw as "higher" levels in the forms of research universities and complex medical centers. Companies and foundations endowed university laboratories and technical institutes like the Massachusetts and the California Institutes of Technology with the mission of linking technological invention to industrial production.[2] The best way to achieve that goal, they advised scientists and engineers, was for the institutions themselves to apply industrial production and business management techniques.[3]

Business interests also shaped medical care development. Not long after the industrial merger mania of the late 1800s, wealthy patrons, local businesses, and foundations set about consolidating small hospitals, clinics, and research institutes and combining them with medical schools. In the process, they constructed the academic medical center. After the 1910 Carnegie-funded Flexner report envisioned a national network of such centers, the Rockefeller and other foundations funded expansions in size, specialization, and technological complexity of medical schools and their affiliated hospitals.[4] The increasingly complex hospitals found it necessary to adopt business techniques to manage their growing capital investments.[5]

Local business and medical leaders added to the national project by devising facility surveys and equipment inventories to bind medical care to hospitals and direct its technological growth and economic performance.[6] The market-oriented strategies converted hospitals from places that cared for sick people into collections of specialty treatment centers. The 1920 Cleveland Hospital and Health Survey, for example, advised that highly capitalized departments like radiology had the capacity and the responsibility to help raise hospital revenues.[7]

Donors and investors also endowed their beneficiaries with faith in the market as the means of progress and economic growth its goal. One physicist called the contemporary buzz of techno-entrepreneurial activity a "fever of commercialized science" aimed at increasing national economic growth.[8] In forging strong ties between research universities and the electrical, chemical, and mechanical industries, "the needs, values, and priorities of big business came to influence the entire realm of institutions of higher learning."[9]

Specialty areas such as radiology and cancer care were shaped by, and at the same time reinforced, the business transformation of medical care. A *New York Times* illustration allegorizing "Wealth and Science Joining Hands for the Conquest of Cancer" (Figure I.1) announced the 1909 bequest of George Crocker, heir to the Crocker railroad fortune, establishing an Institute for Cancer Research at Columbia University. The announcement came not long after Cornell University, Columbia's major medical competitor, had established the C. P. Huntington Fund for Cancer Research—which owed its existence to another railroad fortune.[10]

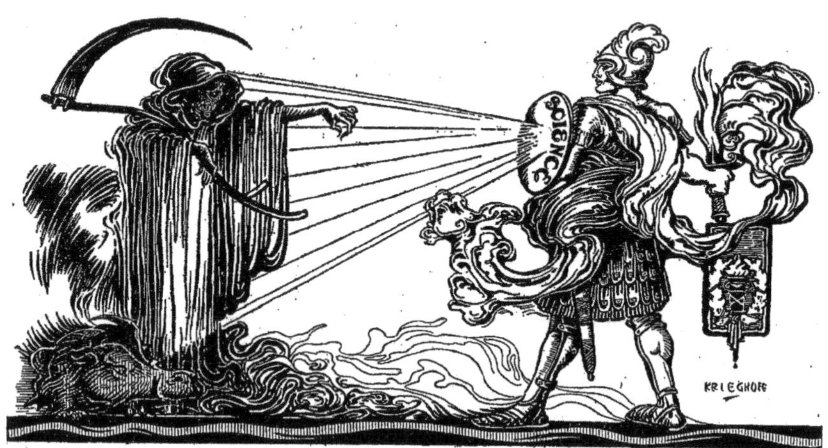

Figure I.1 "Wealth and Science Joining Hands for the Conquest of Cancer."
Source: *New York Times*, December 19, 1909.

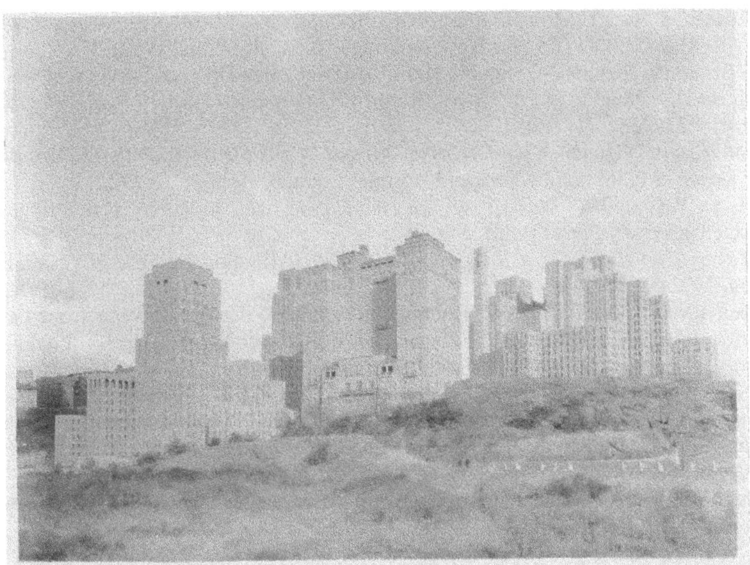

Figure I.2 A New View of Medical Delivery: Columbia-Presbyterian Medical Center, circa 1930.

Photo: Underwood and Underwood. Courtesy Archives & Special Collections, Columbia University Health Sciences Library.

The Crocker Institute added another component to Columbia-Presbyterian Hospital's growing academic medical center. An X-ray company advertising in *Hospital Progress* used the soon-to-be iconic view of Columbia-Presbyterian (Figure I.2) to publicize hospital purchase of its equipment.[11] In so doing, it demonstrated not only how hospital complexes changed medical delivery but also how they changed the market for medical equipment.

In short, the early 20th century industrial economy transformed not only the production of goods, it profoundly transformed the production of educational and medical services. As the *Hospital Progress* ad suggested, hospitals centralized X-ray equipment in radiology procedure units dedicated to using the technology for diagnostic and therapeutic purposes. At the same time, surgeons and gynecologists competed with radiologists in using radium as a new treatment modality.

Notes

1 Glenn Porter, *The Rise of Big Business 1860–1920* (Arlington Heights, IL: Harlan Davidson, 1992), 79–92.
2 David F. Noble, *America by Design: Science, Technology, and the Rise of Corporate Capitalism* (Oxford: Oxford University Press, 1977), 128–147.
3 Roger L. Geiger, *To Advance Knowledge: The Growth of American Research Universities, 1900–1940* (New York: Oxford University Press, 1986), 174–177.
4 Steven C. Wheatley, *The Politics of Philanthropy: Abraham Flexner and Medical Education* (Madison, WI: University of Wisconsin Press, 1988).

5 David Rosner, *A Once Charitable Enterprise: Hospitals and Health Care in Brooklyn and New York 1885–1915* (Cambridge: Cambridge University Press, 1982), 37.

6 Barbara Bridgman Perkins, "Designing High-Cost Medicine: Hospital Surveys, Health Planning, and the Paradox of Progressive Reform," *American Journal of Public Health* 100 (2010): 223–333.

7 Cleveland Hospital Council, *Cleveland Hospital and Health Survey, Part Ten, Hospitals and Dispensaries* (Cleveland: Cleveland Hospital Council, 1920), 819–992.

8 Leonard S. Reich, *The Making of American Industrial Research* (Cambridge: Cambridge University Press, 1985), 249, 252.

9 Glenn Porter, *The Rise of Big Business 1860–1920* (Arlington Heights, IL: Harlan Davidson, 1992), 111–2.

10 In making the gift, Mrs. Collis P. Huntington stipulated that the income from the fund support cancer research under James Ewing's direction at Cornell's Loomis Laboratory. A grateful Memorial Hospital announced the gift in the *New York Times*. "Mrs. C.P. Huntington's Gift," *New York Times* May 24, 1902. Established in 1886, the Loomis Laboratory was named for Cornell professor Henry P. Loomis and not, as some recent histories have held, for banker Alfred L. Loomis, who, while he did gain his wealth at a precociously early age and set up an eponymous laboratory, was born in 1887.

11 "Seventeen Wappler X-ray Machines in the World's Largest Hospital Group," advertisement in *Hospital Progress* January, 1929, 50A.

2 The Medical Radium Industry

Radium is a rare, naturally radioactive element that is damaging to the body and expensive to extract. Paradoxically, perhaps, both of these qualities contributed to its medical allure as well as to its problems. Radium was the first very high-cost medical technology, and its exorbitant price bestowed an elite status on its possessors and shut competing physicians and institutions out of the market. It also severely burned living tissues, but doctors hoped they could control it to burn diseased cells selectively. As a trial-and-error process, the initiation of clinical radium involved neither the relation of treatment to specific disease processes nor the carrying out of laboratory testing prior to widespread diffusion.[1]

Producing radium for medical use mandated its industrial development. The tiny amounts occurring in nature required business organization and management to locate higher quality ores, acquire mining rights, extract the ores, develop refining processes, access capital to build factories, develop markets, and build clinics to use it. Industry was heavily involved in coordinating these activities—first in France.

Radium Pioneering

Chemists Marie and Pierre Curie discovered radium in 1898 and laboriously extracted it from the tons of ore shipped to their Paris laboratory. After a vial of radium in his pocket burned his adjacent skin, physicist Henri Becquerel suggested using it to treat cancer.[2] The Curies encouraged both commercial development and clinical use of the element. They taught industrialists how to purify it and donated small quantities of it to favored physicians. Their refusal to patent their extraction processes eschewed personal financial gain and served as a gift to the industrialists. The Curies' exchange of expertise and personnel with industrialist Émile Armet de Lisle enabled him to build a refinery that provided the Curies with more radium. It also enabled the nonphysician industrialist to pioneer a radium clinic, publish a radium treatment journal, and write the first textbook on radium therapy.[3] Academic medicine in France followed, not led, the industrial pursuit.[4]

Radium prompted a form of medical tourism. North Americans who could afford the trip flocked to Paris to learn about radium and to get some. Industrialists James Douglas and Joseph Flannery, as well as physicians William Aikins of

Toronto, Robert Abbé and James Ewing of New York, Howard Kelly of Baltimore, Albert Soiland of Los Angeles, and John Harvey Kellogg of Battle Creek—most of whom reappear in this book—all made the pilgrimage. Some returned bearing small vials of radium along with concerns that their continent lagged behind Europe in its clinical use.

Many of the radium-seeking doctors specialized in surgery, the field that took the lead in the radioactive element's clinical use. With surgical removal as its primary treatment, cancer was already within surgery's professional domain. The development of anesthesia and antisepsis in the 19th century had driven a rise in surgery, much of which was dedicated to removing tumors. Although it was apparently engineer Alexander Graham Bell who first proposed the idea,[5] Robert Abbé, Henry Janeway, and other surgeons started implanting radium or tubes containing its radon-gas decay product directly into (or onto) tumors. They would call this technique brachytherapy.[6]

The radium therapy leaders initiated political efforts to professionalize their field and to control radium use. In the same year that wealth and science joined hands at Columbia (1909), medical leaders joined hands at the New York Yacht Club to form the Radium Institute of America. They dedicated their new institute to furthering medical use of radium and establishing standards that excluded patent-medicine salesmen.[7] In so doing, the profession was trying to distinguish "quackery" and "commercial" use of radium from what it deemed legitimate (and noncommercial) medical usage. The distinctions remained murky. Medical journals advertised radium treatments along with the physicians offering them, and radium became a fad used by a wide range of therapists. Radium's use was severely restricted, however, by the element's tiny quantities and soaring prices.

The supply of radium was an international political issue, and a series of monopolies maintained its astronomically high prices. The element's natural rarity meant that possessors of the richest ore and the means to extract it, ship it, and refine it controlled world trade in radium and its medical use. The Austro-Hungarian Empire had controlled the richest known ore at the time, the Bohemian pitchblende that the Curies used. When the empire imposed an exportation embargo, its Vienna refinery drove up prices and achieved worldwide domination of the radium supply. Companies in other European countries turned to lower-grade ores in the western United States and shipped vast quantities of the carnotite they extracted to refineries in Europe.[8] Consequently, Americans had to pay extremely high prices to Europe for radium originating on American land. This situation contributed to two major domestic radium companies and one major political uproar.

The Standard Chemical Company

The two competing US companies both combined the powers of industry, medicine, government, and academia but in different proportions. Pittsburgh's Standard Chemical Company and its subsidiary, the Radium Chemical Company, followed the more conventional industrial model. When Standard founder Joseph

Flannery couldn't buy radium in the quantity deemed necessary to treat his sister, who would die of cancer, he decided to get into the business of extracting radium from Colorado carnotite himself. Figure 2.1 depicts the rather glorified version of his story that appeared in a series of ads in the *Southern Medical Journal*, luring doctors to "The Romance of Radium."

Wealthy already from mining vanadium for steel, Flannery set out to extract radium from the same ores. He started shipping the ores to his refinery in 1911, hired chemists from American universities and European companies to develop purification processes, and put his radium on the market in 1913.[9] He built a grand office building in close proximity to the University of Pittsburgh and the Carnegie Institute of Technology to house the family companies. The Oakland Bank, founded to meet the financial needs of the companies and directed by Flannery's brother, occupied the ground floor. As befitting a high-value currency, the Standard Chemical Company's radium was stored in the vault of the Oakland Bank. Medical radium was a highly polluting industry. Seventy years later, nearby residents blamed their cancers on the higher than normal radioactivity levels persisting at the former factory site.[10] A *Scientific American* article noted that cleanup had become the major radium industry.[11]

The Standard Chemical Company had "actively shaped the way radium was marketed, prescribed, and consumed," according to historian Maria Rentetzi.[12] As soon as it had a product to sell, its subsidiary, the Radium Chemical Company, set out to broaden the market for it. Following the Parisian precedent, Radium Chemical built a research laboratory and a radium clinic to study and simultaneously promote medical use of the radioactive element. The company hired physician William Cameron to direct the clinic, edit its journal *Radium*, and in general stimulate radium sales. The dual purpose of the journal, sent to doctors free of charge, was to legitimize the company as a participant in the field of radiation therapy as well as to market its products. The company played a leading role in developing medical radium and in advising doctors how to use its product (as illustrated in the small print in Figure 2.1). Cameron informed clinicians and researchers at a 1914 meeting at New York City's Waldorf-Astoria hotel that radium had "seemingly cured" patients at the company clinic in Pittsburgh. The *New York Times*'s enthusiastic announcement did not inform the public of Cameron's or the clinic's potential conflict-of-interest links with the company.[13]

The Standard Chemical Company founded the American Radium Society as another means of promoting its product and establishing its scientific and medical credentials.[14] Leaders in radiology and surgery readily participated in the Radium Society and proudly delivered its prestigious Janeway lectures. The society's internal histories have in large part expunged its commercial origins and glorified its scientific ones.[15] At its 1966 Golden Anniversary, it neglected to mention the society's origin in the Standard Chemical Company and unabashedly (if a bit incoherently) celebrated the "Valhalla of its pioneer members, who in their unswerving devotion to science with indomitable idealism blazed the trail of a high endeavor."[16] The society attributed its origins instead to professional demand for such an organization.

Vol. XV No. 11 SOUTHERN MEDICAL JOURNAL 11

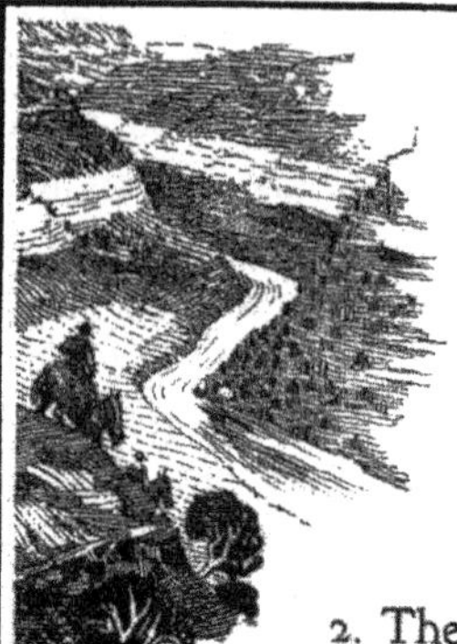

The Romance of Radium

2. The First Production in America

IN 1911, Joseph M. Flannery of Pittsburgh, Pa., after much study and investigation, decided that the world needed more Radium and set about in his characteristically energetic way to produce it on a big scale in this country, and founded the Standard Chemical Co.

Our Service

An immediately available supply of standard radium tubes, needles and plaques, under seal of the United States Bureau of Standards; quality guaranteed by the Standard Chemical Company, the pioneer American and world's largest producer of radium.

Necessary instruments and screens for the safe handling and application of radium.

A comprehensive and scientific course of instruction in the physics and therapeutic use of radium.

A loose-leaf Compendium of Abstracts of professional papers showing the technic and results of radium treatment, with supplements as issued.

"RADIUM"—a quarterly journal, the oldest publication devoted exclusively to the therapeutics of radium.

Complete installations of the latest apparatus for the collection, purification, tubing and measurement of radium emanation.

Medical and technical experts always available for conference or for advice by letter.

Skilled assistance in seeking lost radium.

Deposits of Radium bearing ore (Carnotite) were discovered in southwestern Colorado and southeastern Utah, regions very wild and difficult of access. But Mr. Flannery found a way of getting out the ore and of refining it. And after two years of almost super-human effort, the first Radium to be produced on a commercial scale was refined in the Pittsburgh laboratory of Mr. Flannery's company, which has since produced about three-fourths of all the Radium now in use.

Radium Chemical Co.
Pittsburgh

BOSTON, LITTLE BUILDING — NEW YORK, 501 FIFTH AVENUE — CHICAGO, MARSHALL FIELD ANNEX BLDG. — SAN FRANCISCO, FLOOD BUILDING

Figure 2.1 The Radium Chemical Company Idealizes Its Product.

Source: *Southern Medical Journal* 15 (1922): 11.

In establishing laboratories, clinics, journals, and professional societies, the radium industry actively shaped the development of radiation therapy. The medical profession adopted many of the instruments and practices developed in Standard's laboratories—while at the same time accusing the company of indiscriminately using radium.

Standard Chemical designed methods to expose the human body to radium by every means and via every orifice possible, including inhalation, ingestion, and injection. Company physician C. Everett Field was a fervent proselytizer of intravenous radium. These means of administering radium vastly expanded the number of customers for the product, many of whom would suffer severe radium toxicity. Only after a well-publicized horrific death from radium's use as a tonic in 1932 did the US Food and Drug Administration begin to control radium, and then primarily in patent medicines.[17] Looking at Field's and others' popular practices through the retrospectoscope of history, it is easy to conclude that many of them inflicted more harm than good. But that was also the case with the mainstream medical use of radium, which some of its leaders acknowledged (as discussed later in this chapter). Meanwhile, a different business model for producing medical radium was emerging.

A Public–Private Joint Venture

The limited availability of radium, along with Standard's high price, set in motion a competing radium business that would heavily involve the federal government and shape national mining policy. The same year that Standard Chemical put its radium on the market (1913), a mining magnate and a leading academic physician formed a joint venture that sought government assistance to produce radium solely for the benefit of two hospitals. James Douglas, president of the mining company Phelps Dodge and also a (nonpracticing) physician, had already directed a company chemist to work on commercial processes for refining radium.[18]

Douglas had become involved with the Memorial Hospital of New York after his daughter died of cancer. He connected with Memorial pathologist James Ewing and sponsored their trip to Europe together to investigate radium. Motivated by a substantial donation from Douglas, Memorial's board redefined its mission back to its original focus on cancer, appointed Ewing president of its medical board, and strengthened its ties with Cornell medical school.[19] Cornell's connection with Memorial—and radium—would help build the competing academic medical center on the opposite side of Manhattan from Columbia.

Douglas also joined forces with Johns Hopkins University gynecologist Howard Kelly, who (contrary to Hopkins's new policy) continued to operate his own private hospital in Baltimore and sought to acquire radium for it. Although Ewing and Kelly had each accumulated a significant radium supply, neither had enough of the element to support its latest treatment technique. German reports of applying large amounts of radium to uterine tumors in "packs" positioned a few centimeters from the body (also called teleradium) had led to a leap in medical demand for the element.[20] Standard Chemical's William Cameron used company radium to upstage the Kelly and Memorial Hospitals in using pack radium. The hospitals' ambition to use this technique, together with an all-time high price for radium of $180,000 per gram,[21] provided strong incentives for the two hospitals to build their own company to produce radium more cheaply. They turned to government expertise.

Phelps Dodge president James Douglas was the joint venture's link to the new (1910) US Bureau of Mines, which connected radium therapy and federal oversight of the nation's mineral resources.[22] Shortly after its inception, the bureau made the price of radium a national political issue, calling it "humiliating" that the United States had to pay enormous prices to European suppliers for radium originating in carnotite-bearing lands in Colorado. Oddly ignoring the Standard Chemical Company, the Bureau of Mines announced that it would support a domestic radium industry, by which it meant the Douglas–Kelly company.[23]

Douglas and Kelly leased mining claims and incorporated their own company, which they misleadingly named the National Radium Institute. It was not a national institute in the sense of being established by or for the nation; it was designed to supply only Memorial Hospital and the Howard A. Kelly Hospital. Douglas and Kelly put up the necessary capital (less than the market price of one gram of radium) and served as company directors. The institute formally proposed a plan for extracting and producing radium from Colorado ores, and the Bureau of Mines approved it within weeks. The institute expected to benefit from governmental scientific and technological expertise, and the Bureau of Mines agreed to build and staff a laboratory in Denver to develop the necessary concentration processes.[24] It seems likely that the Denver lab would have shared its knowledge with the Phelps Dodge chemist who visited it.

The National Radium Institute presented itself to the government and to the public as philanthropy on the grounds that it would not commercially market radium. The *New York Times* picked up the refrain, headlining "great philanthropic move" and "radium cure free to all"—neither of which was intended.[25] Far from being philanthropic, the Radium Institute conferred competitive advantages on two hospitals. The Phelps Dodge/ Johns Hopkins/ Bureau of Mines collaboration then tried to take its control of radium supplies a step further.

Geopolitics and Medical Radium

Nationalizing ores on public lands was an idea that served the interests of both the National Radium Institute and President Woodrow Wilson's new administration. On the eve of the US entry into World War I, Douglas, Kelly, and the Bureau of Mines identified radium as an issue of national security. They deemed it an "imperative duty of the Federal Government to take possession at once of all the radium-bearing ore in the country for the public good."[26] It was "almost a patriotic duty," they claimed, to develop a radium industry in the United States in order to reduce the nation's dependence on foreign radium supplies.[27]

The Wilson administration backed a Congressional bill to nationalize radium, calling the plan "supplementary to" the Douglas–Kelly institute.[28] The purpose of the bill, the Bureau of Mines noted in its cooperative agreement with the National Radium Institute, was to demonstrate that radium could be produced at approximately one-third the market (Standard Chemical's) price.[29] The bill proposed withdrawing public areas containing radium ores from the mining laws governing public lands and restricting their availability.[30] A number of prominent radium-using physicians testified to Congress in support of the bill.[31] Not surprisingly, the Standard Chemical Company did not agree with a proposal that gave a substantial advantage to its competition, and the Congressional hearings heated up. Each side (accurately) hurled accusations of monopoly against the other.[32]

Both sides of the battle also exploited the serious cancer illness of Congressman Robert Bremner, who was at the time receiving radium treatments in Kelly's hospital. The *New York Times* initially predicted that Bremner's very public treatment would increase national support for the land withdrawal proposal.[33] Lobbying a Congressional group in support of the proposal, Kelly advised that although he had already inserted tubes containing radon-gas emanations from his entire radium supply into Bremner's tumor, more radium might produce better results.[34] He also not so subtly reminded the group that Bremner was a personal friend of President Wilson. The nation watched as Bremner deteriorated, and the interested parties further exploited his death.[35] The Wilson administration used the death to call for more radium and more federal action,[36] while Memorial's James Ewing publically contended that a radium overdose had killed Bremner.[37] Ewing's criticism may seem to contradict his own radium efforts and those of his hospital, but, as a pathologist studying autopsy material, he reported that he was finding serious healthy tissue destruction alongside of tumor damage.[38] Although the debate did not clarify whether more radium would have cured Bremner or killed him faster, it did illustrate how medical use of radium had become a political issue.

Howard Kelly's propensity for getting into the newspapers led to professional disgruntlement. The Committee on Honor of the Maryland state medical society demanded that he appear at a hearing to respond to charges of violating medical ethics in publicizing his treatments and in overtly behaving in a competitive manner.[39] Suddenly, in the midst of the Congressional hearings, medical society charges, and his famous dying patient's treatment, Kelly sailed to Europe—radioing the *New York Times* that his trip had "nothing to do with radium."[40] A slightly abashed Kelly returned five weeks later, reporting (to the *Times*) that he would henceforth restrain his public statements in the interests of purging medicine of quackery—except to say that it was a shame that the price of radium was still so artificially high.[41]

Although the land withdrawal bills failed, the Phelps Dodge/Johns Hopkins/Bureau of Mines joint venture had served its purpose. It produced a large quantity of radium for the two hospital beneficiaries at a cost considerably lower than Standard's price—even, apparently, when taking into account the monetary value of the government expertise involved.[42] Kelly and Douglas multiplied their initial capital investment by a factor of 8.5. The agreement had been that Kelly and Memorial would split the first 7 grams of radium their company produced and that the Bureau of Mines would get any excess. When production totaled 8.5 grams, however, Kelly and Memorial wanted all of it.

The dispute rose to the desk of the US Attorney General, who ruled that contractual exchange of radium in return for technical assistance was illegal and that the Bureau's share had to be a voluntary gift. Douglas and Kelly declined to gift any more than half a gram, requiring the bureau to renege on its earlier offer to provide radium to federal hospitals.[43] Despite the public-utility implications of its name, the National Radium Institute appeared to be no less economically motivated than the national radium industry. Memorial Hospital and Howard Kelly would owe much of their medical leadership to their politico-entrepreneurial activities.

Howard Kelly became the world's most radium-rich physician, enabling him to expand his clinical use of pack radium.[44] Shifting his therapeutics away from surgical intervention, he applied radium to a wide range of gynecological problems, including uterine fibroids and excessive menstrual bleeding. The radium treatments did stop the bleeding, but a third of one group of young women he irradiated never menstruated again, and many of the remainder suffered sequential miscarriages.[45] Kelly's use of radium contributed to his personal wealth, and he enjoyed the lifestyle it accorded him—to the extent of resigning his Johns Hopkins professorship in 1919 in order to maintain it. Yet it would be simplistic to attribute his motives in acquiring, using, and promoting radium solely to lining his own pockets, as industry representatives did in the Congressional hearings. Kelly was consciously building a profession and its institutions as well as his position in them.

Memorial Hospital secured a leading reputation in radiation therapy as it became the world's most radium-rich hospital, and it built a teletherapy "radium bomb" in 1917.[46] James Ewing would equate the reputation of Memorial Hospital and the field of radiation therapy as the hospital assumed a leadership position in radium therapy.[47] Cornell University Medical College distributed copies of *Radium Therapy in Cancer at the Memorial Hospital* to medical schools across the country. Hedging against treatment failure, the report cautioned that determination of optimal dosage was critical and that even small deviations could make large differences in therapeutic success and in the avoidance of serious complications.[48] Continuing concentration on dosage would blame many treatment failures on individual therapists and distract attention from the overrated effectiveness and damaging consequences of the treatment itself.

The two radium companies exemplified the ways in which medicine, business, and politics intersected in building a medical technology. The National Radium Institute and Standard Chemical Company each sought political and economic control of a natural resource and its clinical use. Although the institute did so in the name of philanthropy, it was a business venture that used the public sector to meet private interests. James Douglas may have hoped to use the institute's experience to take Phelps Dodge into the radium business, but he died in 1918 of a blood condition that may have arisen from his personal use of radium as a tonic. The stories of the two companies demonstrate how medical radium served institutional and political goals.

With the dismantling of the National Radium Institute as well as the Austro-Hungarian Empire, the Standard Chemical Company came to account for over half of the world's supply of radium. But its monopoly was short lived. High-grade ores discovered in Belgium's colony in the African Congo caused the price of radium to fall and enabled more and more physicians and hospitals to use it medically. Then Canada discovered high-grade ores. Although it had failed in the venture for which it was named, the Canadian company Eldorado Gold Mines, Ltd. found gold of another kind and began extracting radium. The Toronto Stock Market responded jubilantly.[49] Canada formed a cartel with Belgium to divvy up the world market and prevent the price of radium from falling below $25,000 per gram.[50] At such a (relative) bargain-basement price, hospitals across Europe and North America aspired to get some.

Sponsoring an International Conference on Cancer in London in 1928, the British Empire Cancer Campaign feared that it lagged internationally in the use of radium.[51] The Medical Research Council subsequently found that the use of radium (and X-ray) to treat cancer occurred largely in the more entrepreneurial special hospitals.[52] Approximately one-third of cancer patients in Britain were being treated with radiation alone or in combination with surgery by 1939.[53] Radium therapy, historians have held, played a significant role in shifting the environmental approach to cancer previously taken by British public health authorities to a managerial and technological one.[54]

Governments played a significant role in spreading radium therapy. In addition to Britain in 1929, radium distribution programs were instigated by New York State in 1920, Québec in 1922, and the United States in 1938. New York initially purchased radium for the State Institute for the Study of Malignant Disease at Buffalo, which, the state announced, would provide free radium treatments for any resident who traveled to Buffalo to receive them.[55] Québec initiated its program to demonstrate the province's growing technological prowess as well as its commitment to health care.[56] The US National Cancer Institute (NCI) applied half its first-year budget to purchase radium to loan to hospitals. Although NCI subsequently shifted its funding from treatment to research, the initial investment covered radium loans to 75 US hospitals over the next three decades.[57] While tumor reductions were encouraging, researchers were coming to think that radium therapy might all too often lead to more harm than good.

Questions of Radium Use and Its Clinical Effectiveness

The publicity surrounding the National Radium Institute had supported radium therapy with well-timed newspaper articles portraying it in a positive light. The *New York Times* featured a spread announcing "Marvelous Cures of Cancer Attributed to Radium" just as the institute was starting up.[58] Days before the introduction of the Congressional land withdrawal bill, the paper reported that both Abbé and Kelly believed that sufficient quantities of radium would cure cancer, almost regardless of the type or stage of the cancer being treated.[59] Solely on the grounds of so many professional reputations at stake, the paper suggested that the answer to the question, "Is cancer at last conquered?" must be "yes."[60]

To give it its due, the *Times* also registered doubts about radium treatment, if not with such exuberant coverage. The paper reported that the Harvard Cancer Commission had concluded from research at Boston's Collis P. Huntington Hospital that radium seemed curative only in certain limited cases. It also reported that the New England Society for the Control of Cancer had contended that there was "too much faith" in radium.[61] Stronger opinions called the medical use of radium a fraud. Strangely ignoring French leadership in the field, a Parisian physician charged that most doctors who used radium were charlatans and, reacting to the *Times*'s accolades of Abbé and Kelly, that "Americans are accustomed to do innumerable stupid things for the sake of a new thing."[62]

Radium initially dominated X-ray in the treatment of cancer (at least in countries that took measurements).[63] European as well as American users applied much of their radium on cancers of the uterine cervix—which were plentiful and easily accessible to treatment. Many women did not survive the extensive pelvic surgeries practiced at the time, and radium seemed to offer a more benign solution. With the uterus already in their domain, gynecologists like Howard Kelly took charge of radium treatments to it. At the University of Pennsylvania, gynecologists had started irradiating cervical cancers when radium appeared on the market in 1913, and they ceased operating on that cancer a few years later in favor of radium. In their first decade of radium use, they reported a 40 percent relative 5-year survival rate for stage 1 disease and a 20 percent "salvage" rate for all stages—figures that were roughly comparable to other contemporary reports.[64] Many hospitals in the United States and Europe discontinued radical hysterectomy in favor of radium. The surgery-oriented Mayo Clinic was one facility that did not, having concluded that radium combined with surgery improved outcomes where radium alone was insufficient.[65] Many contemporary reports also neglected to mention complications arising from radium treatment.

Doctors had known from the beginning that radium could inflict serious bodily harm. Ewing had noted reports of severe nausea and vomiting, extreme muscular weakness, diminished urine, impaired wound healing, feeble pulse, and anemia. But he blamed much of this toxicity on inexperienced physicians and their use of excessive dosages rather than on the treatments themselves.[66] Gynecologists seconded Ewing's accusations and further blamed radium company sales forces for inciting untrained doctors to use their product.[67] Gynecologist George Gray Ward advised that mortality from radium treatment itself should not exceed 2 percent, and he accepted 21 percent morbidity as a reasonable benchmark for radium treatment of cervical cancer. Of women treated in his hospital, 10 percent suffered some degree of hemorrhage, 5 percent had bowel and bladder irritability, 4 percent developed uterine infections, and 4 percent developed fistula.[68] "The great irony of these early years of radiotherapy," later noted radiation oncologist Charles Hayter, "was that although the use of radium in medicine originated from observations of its accidental damaging effects, little attention was paid to the damage sustained through its deliberate therapeutic use." [69]

For the most part, however, it was not low effectiveness or high complication rates that reduced radium use; it was the new thing on the market. Radium use was "waning," noted Columbia University's Francis Carter Wood in 1923, due not only to its limited value but also to a new X-ray tube on the market.[70] While some practitioners argued into the 1930s that adding more radium to radium packs would finally give them what they needed, others turned to new high-powered X-rays.[71] Cheaper than radium, high-voltage X-rays presented the newest invention in cancer therapy, and the General Electric Company led the charge.

Notes

1 Charles Hayter, *An Element of Hope: Radium and the Response to Cancer in Canada, 1900–1940* (Montreal: McGill-Queen's University Press, 2005), 25–28.

2 Patrice Pinell, *The Fight Against Cancer: France 1890–1940* (London: Routledge, 2002), 25.

3 Edward R. Landa, "A Brief History of the American Radium Industry and its Ties to the Scientific Community of its Early Twentieth Century," *Environment International* 19 (1993): 503–508; Xavier Roqué, "Marie Curie and the Radium Industry: A Preliminary Sketch," *History and Technology* 13 (1997): 267–291.

4 Patrice Pinell, *The Fight Against Cancer: France 1890–1940* (London: Routledge, 2002), 37–38, 55.

5 Richard F. Mould, *A Century of X-rays and Radioactivity in Medicine* (Philadelphia: Institute of Physics Publishing, 1993), 127.

6 R. B. Stark, "Robert Abbé and his Contributions to Plastic Surgery," *Plastic and Reconstructive Surgery* 12 (1953): 41–58.

7 "Medical News: Radium Institute of America," *Journal of the American Medical Association* 53 (1909): 1923.

8 Edward R. Landa, "The First Nuclear Industry," *Scientific American* 247 (November 1982): 180–193.

9 Edward R. Landa, "Buried Treasure to Buried Waste: The Rise and Fall of the Radium Industry," *Colorado School of Mines Quarterly* 82 (1987): i–viii, 1–76. In addition to medical use, the Radium Chemical Company also painted watch dials with radium, tragically leading to large numbers of women painters ingesting lethal quantities of radium.

10 "Town Lives with Uranium Wastes and Fears," *New York Times* September 12, 1982. The site had been used for other radioactive projects in the meantime.

11 Edward R. Landa, "The First Nuclear Industry," *Scientific American* 247: (November 1982): 180–193.

12 Maria Rentetzi, "The U.S. Radium Industry: Industrial In-House Research and the Commercialization of Science," *Minerva* 46 (2008): 437–462.

13 "Finds Radium Kills the Cells of Cancer," *New York Times* February 5, 1914.

14 Roger Robison, "Historical Vignette: American Radium Engenders Telecurie Therapy during World War I," *Medical Physics* 27 (2000): 1212–1216; Maria Rentetzi, "The U.S. Radium Industry: Industrial In-House Research and the Commercialization of Science," *Minerva* 46 (2008): 437–462.

15 J. Frank Wilson, "An Historical Perspective: American Radium Society, 1916–1995: Years of Distinction," *American Journal of Clinical Oncology* 20 (1997): 530–535.

16 T. Leucutia, "The American Radium Society and the Journal: Fifty Years of Scientific Advancement," *American Journal of Roentgenology, Radium Therapy and Nuclear Medicine* 96 (1966): 804–806. It also neglected to mention the destruction of Richard Wagner's Valhalla palace built for gods and heroes with stolen gold in a blaze fueled by abuse of power.

17 Stephen S. Hall, *A Commotion in the Blood: Life, Death, and the Immune System* (New York: Henry Holt and Company, 1997), 77.
18 Edward R. Landa, "Buried Treasure to Buried Waste: The Rise and Fall of the Radium Industry," *Colorado School of Mines Quarterly* 82 (1987): i–viii, 1–76.
19 Roger F. Robison, *Mining and Selling Radium and Uranium* (Cham, Switzerland: Springer, 2015), 164–165. Memorial Hospital would become Memorial Sloan-Kettering Cancer Center on merging with the General Motors executives' eponymous research institute.
20 James T. Case, "The Early History of Radium Therapy and the American Radium Society," *American Journal of Roentgenology, Radiation Therapy and Nuclear Medicine* 82 (1959): 574–585.
21 Joel O. Lubenau and Richard F. Mould, "The Roller Coaster Price of Radium," *Journal of Oncology* 59 (2009): 148e–154e.
22 Arty R. Zantinga and Max J. Coppes, "James Ewing (1866–1943): 'The Chief,'" *Medical and Pediatric Oncology* 21 (1993): 505–510.
23 "America Ignores Her Radium Mines," *New York Times* May 5, 1913.
24 Maria Rentetzi, "The U.S. Radium Industry: Industrial In-House Research and the Commercialization of Science," *Minerva* 46 (2008): 437–462.
25 "Radium Cure Free to All," *New York Times* October 24, 1913; "May Give Radium to Many Hospitals," *New York Times* October 25, 1913.
26 *New York Times* December 19, 1913, no title.
27 "Scientists' Eyes on Radium Test," *New York Times* December 28, 1913.
28 "Lane Wants Radium Deposits Protected," *New York Times* December 30, 1913.
29 Charles L. Parsons, *et al.*, *Extraction and Recovery of Uranium, Radium, and Vanadium from Carnotite* (Washington: US Bureau of Mines, 1915).
30 Edward R. Landa, "Buried Treasure to Buried Waste: The Rise and Fall of the Radium Industry," *Colorado School of Mines Quarterly* 82 (1987): i–viii, 1–76.
31 "Control of Radium Urged on Congress," *New York Times* January 20, 1914.
32 "Against Radium Monopoly," *New York Times* January 12, 1914.
33 "Scientists' Eyes on Radium Test," *New York Times* December 28, 1913.
34 Jesse N. Aronowitz and Roger F. Robison, "Howard Kelly Establishes Gynecologic Brachytherapy in the United States," *Brachytherapy* 9 (2010): 178–184.
35 "Bremner Sends Message to Public," *New York Times* January 12, 1914.
36 "Plea for Radium Cure," *New York Times* February 7, 1914.
37 "Experts Disagree on Treating Cancer," *New York Times* March 24, 1914.
38 James Ewing, "Radium Therapy in Cancer," *Journal of the American Medical Association* 68 (1917): 1238–1247.
39 "Vexed with Dr. H. A. Kelly," *New York Times* January 11, 1914.
40 "Wireless Message from Howard A. Kelly, on Board the Steamship Minnewaska," *New York Times* January 25, 1914.
41 "Dr. Kelly Reticent: Radium Expert Admits Restraint by Professional Ethics," *New York Times* March 1, 1914.
42 Charles L. Parsons, *et al.*, *Extraction and Recovery of Uranium, Radium, and Vanadium from Carnotite* (Washington: US Bureau of Mines, 1915).
43 Edward R. Landa, "Buried Treasure to Buried Waste: The Rise and Fall of the Radium Industry," *Colorado School of Mines Quarterly* 82 (1987): i–viii, 1–76.
44 Roger F. Robison, "Howard Atwood Kelly (1858–1943): Founding Professor of Gynecology at Johns Hopkins Hospital and Pioneer American Radium Therapist," *Journal of Oncology* 60 (2010): 21e–35e.
45 Howard A. Kelly, "Radium in the Treatment of Menstrual Disorders," *Journal of the American Medical Association* 97 (1931): 760–763.
46 Richard F. Mould, *A Century of X-rays and Radioactivity in Medicine* (Philadelphia: Institute of Physics Publishing, 1993), 120.
47 Stephen S. Hall, *A Commotion in the Blood: Life, Death, and the Immune System* (New York: Henry Holt and Company, 1997), 88.

48 Henry H. Janeway, *Radium Therapy in Cancer at the Memorial Hospital in New York* (New York: Paul B. Hoeber, 1917), 57.
49 Paul Litt, *Isotopes and Innovation: MDS Nordion's First Fifty Years, 1946–1996* (Montreal: Published for MDS Nordion by McGill-Queen's University Press, 2000), 9.
50 Edward R. Landa, "The First Nuclear Industry," *Scientific American* 247 (1982): 180–193; Joel O. Lubenau and Richard F. Mould, "The Roller Coaster Price of Radium," *Journal of Oncology* 59 (2009): 148e–154e.
51 Caroline Claire Scanlon Murphy, "A History of Radiotherapy to 1950: Cancer and Radiotherapy in Britain 1830–1950," PhD thesis, University of Manchester, 1986, 1.33, 5.30.
52 Medical Research Council, *Medical Uses of Radium: Summary of Reports from Research Centres for 1938* Special Report Series no. 236, (London: Medical Research Council, HMSO, 1939).
53 Sholto Mackenzie, *Cancer: An Inquiry into the Extent to which Patients Receive Treatment* Reports on Public Health and Medical Subjects No. 89, (London: Ministry of Health, HMSO, 1939).
54 Rosa M. Medina Domenech and Claudia Castañeda, "Redefining Cancer During the Interwar Period: British Medical Officers of Health, State Policy, Managerialism, and Public Health," *American Journal of Public Health* 97 (2007): 1563–1571.
55 "Free Radium for Cancer Ready Oct. 15," *New York Times* August 2, 1920.
56 Charles Hayter, "Tarnished Adornment: The Troubled History of Québec's Institute du Radium," *Canadian Bulletin of Medical History* 20 (2003): 343–365.
57 David Cantor, "Radium and the Origins of the National Cancer Institute," In Caroline Hannaway, ed., *Biomedicine in the Twentieth Century: Practices, Policies, and Politics* (Amsterdam: IOS, 2008), 95–146.
58 "Marvelous Cures of Cancer Attributed to Radium," *New York Times* September 28, 1913.
59 "Is Cancer at Last Conquered?" *New York Times* December 17, 1913.
60 "Dr. Jacobi Cured of Cancer by Radium," *New York Times* December 29, 1913; "Dr. Mayo Hopeful of Radium Results," January 10, 1914.
61 "Too Much Faith in Radium," *New York Times* February 4, 1914; "Radium's Use in Cancer. Harvard Report Says it Cures in Superficial Cases Only," *New York Times* May 3, 1915.
62 "Radium a 'Fraud' Asserts Dr. [Eugene] Doyen," *New York Times* April 19, 1914.
63 Medical Research Council, *Medical Uses of Radium: Summary of Reports from Research Centres for 1930* Special Report Series No. 160. (London: HMSO, 1931), 5.
64 Floyd E. Keene and Robert A. Kimbrough, "End-results of Radium Therapy in Carcinoma of the Cervix," *American Journal of Obstetrics and Gynecology* 23 (1932): 838–841.
65 James W. Ross, "A Clinical Study of Cancer of the Uterine Cervix: Summary of the Results Obtained by Various Methods of Treatment," *Canadian Medical Association Journal* 7 (1922): 772–780.
66 James Ewing, "Radium Therapy in Cancer," *Journal of the American Medical Association* 68 (1917): 1238–1247.
67 Palmer Findley, "Complications and Disappointments in Radium Therapy for Cancer of the Uterus," *Canadian Medical Association Journal* 32 (1935): 154–161.
68 George Gray Ward, "The Complications of Radium Therapy in Gynecology." *American Journal of Obstetrics and Gynecology* 25 (1933): 1–10.
69 Charles Hayter, *An Element of Hope: Radium and the Response to Cancer in Canada, 1900–1940* (Montreal: McGill-Queen's University Press, 2005), 32.
70 Francis Carter Wood, "Recent Cancer Therapy," *Canadian Medical Association Journal* 13 (1923): 152–159.
71 Burton T. Simpson and Melvin C. Reinhard, "Advantages and Disadvantages of Radium Packs," *American Journal of Roentgenology and Radium Therapy* 35 (1936): 513–521.

3 The General Electric Company Dominates X-ray

The General Electric X-ray Company played a dynamic role in developing X-ray therapy. General Electric (GE) and the Victor Electric Company each entered the medical X-ray business within a year or two of Roentgen's 1895 discovery.[1] Victor started small, making the first electric dental drill in a founder's basement. GE, in contrast, was born big in the finance-funded industrial merger mania of the 1890s. The 1892 merger of Edison Electric and Thomson-Houston Electric was bonded by their combined patents and J. P. Morgan capital.[2] It was banker Morgan, not inventor Thomas Edison, who took control of the new company. Defining its business model in terms of competitive advantage rather than competition, GE employed patent controls, mutual licensing agreements, and the purchase of competitors to monopolize the markets it chose to engage in.[3] The mergers stifled competition from existing companies, and the patent controls protected the company from new competitors.[4] Finding that competing companies were still producing a cheaper tube, GE (temporarily) dropped X-ray in favor of other inventions.

General Electric established its Research Laboratories in 1900 in order to develop in-house engineering expertise. GE engineer Charles Steinmetz and lawyer Albert Davis expected that the laboratories would reduce dependence on other companies' patents. Where GE could not claim basic inventions, the labs patented improvements on other companies' products. Adding a twist to science and wealth joining hands, *Time* magazine would portray the GE labs as "Science Working for Wealth."[5]

Shortly after coming to the GE labs from the Massachusetts Institute of Technology (MIT), engineer William Coolidge developed a tungsten alloy that made light-bulb filaments more durable. The engineering advance plus its marketing led to GE's overpowering domination of the incandescent lamp market, exceeding 90 percent in the 1920s.[6] The company may have tried to reach the same level of dominance in the X-ray market. Coolidge applied ductile tungsten (along with ideas very like those that German physicist Julius Lilienfeld was in the process of patenting[7]) to X-ray tubes. The tungsten significantly increased X-ray tubes' stability and durability. Cornell radiologist Lewis Gregory Cole tested the new tube for GE and hosted a 1913 dinner where Coolidge demonstrated the tube to other New York radiologists.[8] The technologic advance reputedly marked the decline of X-ray devices that were "loud, sparking, smelly," and all too likely to seriously burn or shock the patient or the operator.[9] GE sold the Coolidge tube through companies like Victor Electric. Subsequent lawsuits overturned GE X-ray patents on grounds of false claims of originality, but they had served their purpose. The company had its foot in the door and maintained dominance with vigorous marketing and by continuously developing upgraded models with new features.

A New Therapy Tube Brings GE Back into the X-Ray Business

While physicians were using their lower-powered X-ray tubes for both diagnosis and treatment, Coolidge went on to construct a more powerful 200,000 volt (200 kilovolt, or kv) X-ray tube. Designed specifically for therapy, the new tube emitted X-rays that reached deeper into the body and delivered higher radiation doses with less skin burn than the previous devices. Kilovoltage would drive a sales boom and "revolutionize the whole X-ray business," company managers enthused in 1920.[10] With such a promising technology in its domain, the company decided to get back into the X-ray business.

After surveying the competition, GE honed in on Victor Electric, which had a sales and service network already in place. GE could compete directly with Victor, its managers deliberated, but it would take a great deal of time and money.[11] So GE bought the company instead. Victor contributed all of its assets to the new entity, which was for a few years named Victor X-ray Company. GE purchased a majority on its board of directors with its capital, patents, and "good will." A few years later, it reorganized the company as a wholly-owned subsidiary named General Electric X-ray Company.[12]

Even as the merger was in process, GE's then vice president, Owen Young, hired an advertising firm to instruct him in medical marketing. The firm suggested putting advertisements aimed at doctors in medical journals and strategically placing articles designed to teach patients to accept diagnostic and therapeutic X-ray procedures (as well as separate charges for them) in popular magazines.[13] The periodical pieces should emphasize humanitarian aspects of treating cancer, the advertising firm advised—as well as seek to dispel allegations that the merger of GE and Victor had violated antitrust laws.

It was not company advertising, however, that led to the 200 kv treatment tube's first clinical use; it was personal contacts. Michigan's Battle Creek Sanitarium, known for its wide range of popular physico-, hydro-, electro-, and radiotherapies, seems to have been the first to use the new Coolidge tube. The sanitarium was already using radium and a set of X-ray tubes that Coolidge had personally delivered in 1913. As Battle Creek radiologist James Case told the 1921 story, a gentleman brought his wife in to receive the very latest in X-ray treatment. Case explained that although Coolidge had a 200 kv tube, it wasn't yet released to the market. The husband, who happened to manage the regional GE branch, called Coolidge, and a 200 kv tube arrived two days later. When the new tube burned out Case's transformer, GE sent a more powerful one. Case treated the patient within days, not taking time to calibrate or test the new device. Much later, he acknowledged that each voltage increment in X-ray treatment initially caused severe health problems and even patient prostration due to excessive doses.[14]

When GE entered the market with its new tube, it took Madison Avenue's advice and placed full-page advertisements in journals such as *Hospital Management*. One such ad illustrated the company's international marketing prowess, showing photos of hospitals that had adopted Victor X-ray equipment in Japan, the Philippines, Australia, China, Cuba, and Brazil.[15] GE sales representatives demonstrated company wares at medical conventions, where they made personal contacts with physicians in, or hoping to get into, radiation therapy. Such direct connections with physicians were instrumental not only in selling equipment but also in obtaining suggestions for upgrades, and GE patented a broad line of accessories for its machines.[16] GE lab physicists reported on their devices at medical and physics meetings and to business groups like the Radiological Society of the National Association of Manufacturers. Coolidge himself publicized his tubes at professional meetings; in return, the professions medaled him and invited him to deliver prestigious endowed lectures.

Accepting a gold medal from the Franklin Institute of Philadelphia, Coolidge took the opportunity to describe his proposed method of using cathode tubes to generate electron beams for clinical treatment instead of smashing the electrons against a metal target to produce X-rays. He informed the 1926 gathering that doctors at Cornell and the Albany Medical School were already experimenting with the new method. Unfortunately for GE, *Time* magazine reported that the Cornell researchers considered the electron beam to be "practically useless" therapeutically.[17] Electron therapy did not rise at this time, although it would experience several reincarnations and occupy a small niche at the end of the century.

Voltage in the 200–220 kv range rapidly became the "work horse" of X-ray therapy. The higher energy rays penetrated into the body and (unlike the predecessors) permitted X-ray treatment of deeper tumors without frying the skin. Many radiotherapists came to use kilovoltage as a supplement to radium. Standard procedure for treating patients with cancers of the uterine corpus at Memorial Hospital around 1930, for example, first used radium, then high-voltage X-ray, then hysterectomy, and finally postoperative radiation.[18] Meanwhile, GE industriously marketed new products based on increasing X-ray voltages.

GE Escalates Voltage and Builds a Product Line

Not satisfied with relying on existing—and sometimes negative—media reports, GE started publishing its own 8–12-page newsletter in 1929. Sent free to hospitals and interested doctors, the newsletter, called *Victor News* long after the company's name change, served to advertise GE products within the medical community. It featured each increase in power and compactness as the latest in scientific achievement and justified the company's relatively high prices by equating the GE trademark with progress.[19]

Each higher-powered, higher-cost machine upped the capital investment necessary for manufacturers and medical providers to stay in the X-ray treatment business. For manufacturers, escalating voltages and competitive upgrades were planned obsolescence strategies that sold more machines. For providers, higher voltage attracted doctors and patients and raised the ante for competitors to remain in the game. Photo spreads in *Victor News* ramped up competition by graphically illustrating to radiologists and hospital administrators how other radiotherapy units were getting ahead of them. GE marketing, added to the technological superiority of Coolidge tubes, allowed the company to claim 50 percent of the US X-ray market by 1935.[20]

The *Wall Street Journal* joined *Victor News* in publicizing that Coolidge had announced at the 1930 American Roentgen Ray Society meeting that he had sent a 500,000-volt X-ray device to Cornell for testing.[21] Cornell's Floyd Richtmyer, one of many physicists who moved fluidly between industry and academia, tested the new tube in his laboratory built with General Electric aid.[22] Coolidge further revealed that the company was about to send a device nearly (but not quite) twice as powerful as the 500 kv one to Memorial Hospital for purposes of investigational treatments. The Works Project Administration of the Depression's economic recovery program (ironically) supported the installation of the new machine at the well-endowed institution.[23] *Victor News* reported that the device was an important step in the company's quest for a million volts.[24]

GE was running in the "million volts or bust" race that had, mostly for PR purposes, set that milestone as its goal. Although contestants knew there was nothing clinically significant about crossing the million-volt line—and that radium emitted more than an equivalent energy—each X-ray power increment escalated the prestige, price, and competitive advantage of its manufacturers and purchasers. Contestants garnered firsts (with considerable fudging) in announcing million-volt devices, patenting them, building them, installing them, using them clinically, using them on particular types of cancer, and then actually using them at or above a million volts. St. Bartholomew's Hospital in London, for example, announced the installation of its Metropolitan-Vickers "Million" in 1937, although the machine did not operate at a million volts until 1939.[25] By that time, there were prior claims of million-volt treatment from General Electric and, as discussed in Chapter 4, from universities in California and Massachusetts (and at least one of those claims appeared to be true.)

With the headline "Chicago Hospital to Have Million Volt X-ray Unit," GE had proclaimed in 1932 that it had achieved the million-volt goal.[26] Mercy Hospital's latest acquisition, *Victor News* announced, enhanced Chicago's reputation as a "real medical center" and enabled the city to surpass even New York. The company demonstrated its machine at Chicago's 1933 World's Fair.[27] Expressing what was undoubtedly GE's ambition, a Mercy Hospital radiation therapist maintained at a meeting of the American Radium Society that a national supply of such supervoltage machines would be much more cost-efficient than widespread diffusion of radium.[28] (The term *supervoltage* was generally used to describe all voltages higher than 400 kv, while *megavoltage* meant voltages at a million volts and higher.) Seattle's Swedish Hospital purchased a GE device similar to Mercy Hospital's and operated it at 800 kv. The Washington State governor attended the gala opening of the department featuring the new device, and a city newspaper stirred up interurban competition by claiming that the new machine made Seattle the "medical center of the West."[29] Political ambitions in Chicago, Seattle, and other cities clearly had spurred the diffusion of high-powered radiotherapy devices.

GE's 1932 announcement had been premature, however, and 7 years later, the company again publicized a million-volt breakthrough. *Victor News* announced in 1939 that James Ewing at New York's Memorial Hospital was installing an "entirely new type" of GE transformer that, combined with a multisectional Coolidge tube, achieved one million volts.[30] After having considered the cyclotron and the Van de Graaff device, Ewing wrote University of California physicist E. O. Lawrence that he regarded GE's new resonance transformer as the best route to supervoltage treatment.[31] The new machine arrived at Memorial 2 years after Columbia-Presbyterian Hospital had installed a University of California device of purportedly equivalent voltage (described in Chapter 4). GE engineers spread the news of its new million-volt machine at the 1939 annual meeting of the Radiological Society of North America.[32] The device brought the hospital that had based so much of its reputation on radium into the megavoltage era.

New York's Memorial Hospital was a logical alliance for GE—and vice versa. The hospital provided the clinical capacity that the company lacked, and GE labs served (partly) as a physics department for Cornell's medical school, which was isolated from the university's main campus in Ithaca. The hospital had close ties with GE from its beginning.[33] Radiation physicists at Memorial tested GE's radiotherapy devices clinically and attested to their reliability. The company's hospital linkage provided it with academic status and research capacity. The hospital's ties with Cornell strengthened when J. D. Rockefeller, Jr. donated funds for a new building as well as land located across the street from Cornell's growing medical center and the Rockefeller Institute for Medical Research. The combined institutions formed a formidable academic medical complex in competition with Columbia-Presbyterian's burgeoning center on the other side of Manhattan. Memorial purchased five more GE X-ray devices for its new facility, bringing its total to 14. *Victor News* used Memorial's brand loyalty to advertise GE's product line and the competition between Columbia and Cornell to stimulate X-ray department growth.[34]

While hospitals like Memorial could afford the company's most powerful products, lower kilovoltage machines—by then called "ortho" or "conventional" voltage devices—remained GE X-ray's bread and butter. Emulating General Motors' price and power levels ranging from Chevrolet to Cadillac, General Electric built a line of radiotherapy devices rising in voltage and cost. Entering also into financial services, GE financed purchases—particularly during the Depression.[35] GE's product line shaped the market and the practice of X-ray therapy.

In the mid-1930s, *Victor News* advertised a new 200 kv machine in its Maximar® line, reformulated specifically for doctors' offices and smaller hospitals. They were so inexpensive, the company advised, that "scores upon scores of hospitals and clinics" could now get into radiation therapy.[36] GE developed its 220 kv Maximar as an intermediate step and introduced the top of its mid-level line, the 400 kv Maximar. These machines were followed by a 250 kv Maximar, sold as the deluxe device of the lower kilovolt range. Each new device added to the overhead costs of radiation therapy units and had to be offset by increasing utilization rates and charges. Augmenting professional descriptions of properly organized radiology departments, GE (like its rival Westinghouse) established consultation services that designed radiology procedure units that maximized equipment placement and patient throughput.

Many clinicians purchasing a range of devices felt that voltage increases above 220 kv did not significantly improve patient outcomes.[37] The equipment proliferation particularly exasperated public health physician Roswell Pettit. Radiologists should try adjusting their existing machines, Pettit admonished attendees at a meeting of the Illinois state medical society, "before succumbing to the pressure exerted by super-high voltage representatives of X-ray manufacturers."[38]

General Electric maintained market presence—and pressure—by expanding the network of sales and service stations it had inherited from Victor Electric. Local representatives frequently visited doctors and hospital administrators to advise them on purchasing new machines, maintaining them, and replacing them. Pettit evidently felt that they applied high-powered pressure to buy more high-powered equipment. Like general practice medicine and pediatrics around that time, the company instigated routine checkups to ensure that customers would return. Checkups, *Victor News* advised, helped hospitals operate their units at top efficiency and attain their "full share of the electro-medical equipment business."[39]

GE continued to expand the X-ray market. Filling in the lower end of the company's product line, ads began to appear for a 60–140 kv apparatus—essentially the voltage range of the original X-ray devices—but now specifically labeled for "superficial and intermediate" therapy. GE also introduced a mobile version of this machine, designed to treat localized infections at patients' bedsides.[40] Every hospital performing surgery needed to purchase such a machine, the company suggested, on the grounds that it controlled postsurgical infection. GE's infection-control rationale was not supported in the scientific literature, which had already concluded that X-rays did not have a bactericidal effect; its rationale was based instead on the advice of one (unnamed) "eminent authority."[41] The potential market for postsurgical use was huge, however, and *Victor News* raved that the mobile unit could open up a "vast field of therapy which is practically unexplored."[42]

Salesmanship permeated the highest corporate levels. Owen Young got involved in selling GE X-ray equipment even as chairman of the board. On hearing that Westinghouse and Kelley-Koett had outbid a "less aggressive" GE salesman in Florida, Young contacted an administrator friend at the hospital involved, stating he was willing to write a personal check to make up the difference between GE's higher bid and those of the competing companies. The hospital quickly took him up on his offer, and Young had to quash its grateful trustees' offer of a commemorative plaque, insisting that his (competition-busting) contribution remain anonymous.[43] Favoring market domination over competition, the company taught its business strategies to medicine—and to the nation.

The Company Promotes Business Strategies in Medicine (and Beyond)

GE reinforced medical specialization's functional division of labor. Like the work organization that made factory work more efficient, academic medical centers had developed a hierarchy of staff and trainees to perform a hierarchy of patient care tasks.[44] *Victor News* suggested that the machines' easy adjustability was particularly suitable for operation by nurses, and its photographs showed nurses aiming machines at patients and operating control panels.

The radiology profession codified functional division of labor in *Practical Radiation Therapy*. "Properly organized" departments, the textbook instructed, assigned a managerial role to physicians and the actual treatment of patients to interns and technicians.[45] This organization required a full range of medical staff, from the senior resident who managed the treatment process down through the ranks to the junior intern, who should perform routine preparations and take patients' histories. Fully trained radiologists should read films and plan treatments in the privacy of their offices. Such a division of labor, in which radiologists never have to lay eyes—let alone hands—on patients, eventually led to outsourcing radio-diagnosis to computer monitors across the globe.

New York's Memorial Hospital took the factory division of labor too far, MIT engineer John Trump would later charge, by "excessively routiniz[ing] its radiation procedure to handle mass numbers of patients." "The diagnostician marks the suggested treatment on a chart and usually does not see the patient again," Trump claimed, and "the treatment is administered by technicians on the basis of the chart."[46] Although such an organization may enhance institutional productivity, it misses opportunities for doctors to learn how the machines actually functioned and malfunctioned—not to mention patient response to treatment. A radiation oncologist noted in 2011 that many of his colleagues continued to practice without examining their patients receiving radiation therapy.[47]

General Electric actively encouraged a managerial approach to medical care, holding that medical care had much to learn from industry. *Victor News* called on the burgeoning field of business management to teach doctors and hospital administrators how to think and act like businessmen. One editorial advised that high-cost assets boosted financial gains.[48] Higher-powered machines, the company instructed potential customers in the late 1930s, could treat more patients per day at lower unit costs and thus generate higher revenues per patient.[49] Of course, this required treating higher total numbers of (paying) patients.

The returns on investment could be professional as well as monetary.[50] "He who serves best profits best," GE was fond of intoning. It was advisable (and possible) to apply "good business principles to the practice of medicine," the company advised in a mantra that the medical profession would make more overt 50 years later, "without detracting in the least from established standards."[51] Neither the company nor the physicians who worked with it seemed to consider the reciprocal: that business principles might shape medical standards themselves.

Hospital administrators learned quickly, and they came to cite higher productivity and cost-efficiency as a major justification when submitting equipment requests to their trustees. In actively instructing its customers in capital accounting rules and business principles, GE ventured to remake medical delivery in its own image. If that was not ambitious enough, company leaders also aspired to remake the national economy in the GE image. Their methods would shape many public planning efforts in the decades to come, including those of health planning.

Top GE executives during the Depression and the New Deal era envisioned a broad planning program to stimulate the national economy. Believing the corporation to be the fundamental institution of society, GE engineer Charles Steinmetz proposed extending "methods of economic efficiency from the individual industrial corporation to the national organism as a whole."[52] GE president Gerard Swope and chairman Owen Young (also at times director of General Motors, director of the Federal Reserve Bank, and trustee of several universities) promoted a form of national planning in which major industries would use their own trade associations to regulate their markets.[53] Relieved from antitrust laws under lenient Federal Trade Commission oversight, the idea went, trade associations and related corporations would use governmental enforcement powers to build industrial oligopolies.[54] A writer for the progressively-oriented *Survey* magazine admired Swope's proposal for transforming private enterprises into what he defined as quasi-public utilities.[55] Although this form of progressivism promoted economic planning over *laissez-faire*, it was caught in the dilemma of defining progress in terms of corporate organization and its continued growth. That dilemma would warp medical institutional development as well as ongoing health reform.

Academia, particularly the research university, which was itself growing more and more like industry, was a key player in medical-industry growth. Research universities actively competed with General Electric in the million-volt race. Educational institutions combined with industry to convert their research into products and with physicians willing to use them experimentally on patients. Would any of their new devices become the goose that laid the golden egg or the gun that shot the magic bullet?

Notes

1 Albert G. Davis to E. W. Rice, February 3, 1920. Owen D. Young Papers, Box 6. Schenectady Museum Archives, Schenectady, NY.

2 Sameer Kumar and Jeffrey L. Ricker, "General Electric, a Model of Corporate Citizenship and Business Evolution," *International Journal of Energy Technology and Policy* 2 (2004): 354–368.

3 Leonard S. Reich, *The Making of American Industrial Research* (Cambridge: Cambridge University Press, 1985), 52, 74, 86; Rebecca Edwards, *New Spirits: Americans in the Gilded Age 1865–1905* (New York: Oxford University Press, 2006), 239, 159.

4 George Wise, *Willis R. Whitney, General Electric, and the Origins of U.S. Industrial Research* (New York: Columbia University Press, 1985), 2, 72, 73, 117.

5 "Science: Chemical Engineers," *Time* June 27, 1932.

6 Leonard S. Reich, *The Making of American Industrial Research* (Cambridge: Cambridge University Press, 1985), 86; George Wise, *Willis R. Whitney, General Electric, and the Origins of U.S. Industrial Research* (New York: Columbia University Press, 1985), 215.

7 Robert G. Arns, "The High-Vacuum X-Ray Tube: Technological Change in Social Context," *Technology and Culture* 38 (1997): 852–890.
8 E. Dale Trout, "History of Radiation Sources for Cancer Therapy," In Franz Buschke, ed., *Progress in Radiation Therapy* (New York: Grune & Stratton, 1958), 42–61.
9 Matthew Lavine, "The Early Clinical X-Ray in the United States: Patient Experiences and Public Perceptions," *Journal of the History of Medicine and Allied Sciences* 67 (2012): 587–625.
10 Albert G. Davis to E. W. Rice, May 19, 1920. Owen D. Young Papers, Box 6. Schenectady Museum Archives, Schenectady, New York.
11 Albert G. Davis to E. W. Rice, February 3, 1920. Owen D. Young Papers, Box 6. Schenectady Museum Archives, Schenectady, New York.
12 "GE to Control X-ray Corporation," *Bridgeport Telegram* October 9, 1920. Owen D. Young Papers, Box 6. Schenectady Museum Archives, Schenectady, New York.
13 Thomas F. Logan to C. F. Samms, November 19, 1920. Owen D. Young Papers, Box 6. Schenectady Museum Archives, Schenectady, New York.
14 James T. Case, "Some Early Experiences in Therapeutic Radiology: Formation of the American Radium Society," *American Journal of Roentgenology and Radium Therapy* 70 (1953): 487–491.
15 "Why Do Many Leading Physicians and Hospitals in Foreign Countries Buy Victor X-Ray Equipment?" advertisement in *Hospital Management* February 1928, 77.
16 S. Reid Warren and Roderick L. Tondreau, "The Retrospectoscope: The Good Old Days with William J. Hogan," *RadioGraphics* 6 (1985): 515–520.
17 "Science: Cathode Rays," *Time* November 1, 1926.
18 William P. Healy, "Evaluation of Radiation Therapy in Malignant Disease of the Female Generative Tract," *American Journal of Obstetrics and Gynecology* 26 (1933): 789–803.
19 "Editorial: Coolidge Tubes," *Victor News* September 2, 1929.
20 Kendall Birr, *Pioneering in Industrial Research; The Story of the General Electric Research Laboratory* (Washington: Public Affairs Press, 1957), 153. As this author noted, GE kept its data closely guarded, and few figures have been available concerning the X-ray industry and its sales.
21 "GE New X-ray Tube," *Wall Street Journal* September 25, 1930, 4; W. D. Coolidge, "The Development of Modern Roentgen-ray Generating Apparatus," *American Journal of Roentgenology and Radium Therapy* 24 (1930): 605–620.
22 F. K. Richtmyer, H. A. Barton, and M. T. Jones, "A 600 kv X-ray Plant," *British Journal of Radiology* 5 (1932): 214.
23 Milford D. Schulz, "The Supervoltage Story," *American Journal of Roentgenology, Radium Therapy & Nuclear Medicine* 124 (1975): 541–559.
24 "A 900,000 Volt X-ray Tube," *Victor News* May–June, 1931.
25 Arthur Jones, "The Development of Megavoltage X-ray Therapy at St. Bartholomew's Hospital," In P. N. Plowman and A. N. Harnett, eds., "Megavoltage Radiotherapy 1937-1987, Proceedings of a Conference," *British Journal of Radiology* Supplement no. 22, 1988, 3–10; G. S. Innes, "The One Million Volt X-ray Therapy Equipment at St. Bartholomew's Hospital, 1936–1960," In P. N. Plowman and A. N. Harnett, eds., "Megavoltage Radiotherapy 1937–1987, Proceedings of a Conference," *British Journal of Radiology* Supplement no. 22, 1988, 11–16.
26 "Chicago Hospital to Have Million Volt X-ray Unit," *Victor News* March, 1932.
27 "Medicine's Century of Progress Shown at Chicago Exposition," *Victor News* June, 1933.
28 Burton T. Simpson and Melvin C. Reinhard, "Advantages and Disadvantages of Radium Packs," *American Journal of Roentgenology and Radium Therapy* 35 (1936): 513–521. Henry Schmitz in discussion.
29 "800.000 Volt X-ray Unit Installed at Seattle's Swedish Hospital," *Victor News* April, 1934.

30 "Memorial Hospital's New Million-Volt Apparatus," *Victor News* January, 1939.
31 James Ewing to E. O. Lawrence, October 11, 1938. Ernest O. Lawrence papers, BANC FILM 2248. The Bancroft Library, University of California, Berkeley, CA.
32 E. E. Charlton, W. F. Westendorp, L. E. Dempster, and George Hotaling, "A Million Volt X-ray Unit," *Radiology* 35 (1940): 585–597.
33 Otha W. Linton, *Radiology at Memorial Sloan-Kettering Cancer Center* (New York: Department of Radiology, Memorial Sloan-Kettering Cancer Center, 2006), 41, 60.
34 "New High Voltage Therapy Units," *Victor News* July, 1939.
35 "'New Coolidge Tubes for Old' is General Electric Policy," *Victor News* January, 1933; "Editorial: Credit," *Victor News* March, 1933.
36 No title, *Victor News* October, 1937.
37 Robert S. Stone, "Skin Reactions Caused by 1,000 Kilovolt and 200 Kilovolt Radiations," *Radiology* 30 (1938), 88–93.
38 Ruth Brecher and Edward Brecher, *The Rays: A History of Radiology in the United States and Canada* (Baltimore: Williams and Wilkins, 1969), 355.
39 No title, *Victor News* September–October, 1932.
40 "Mobile X-ray Therapy Unit Facilitates Bedside Treatment," *Victor News* January, 1939.
41 Manuel Lederman, "The Early History of Radiotherapy: 1895–1939," *International Journal of Radiation Oncology Biology Physics* 7 (1981): 639–648; "A Boon to Surgeons in the Treatment of Infections," *Victor News* June, 1940.
42 No title, *Victor News* October, 1939.
43 Owen Young to J. R. Clough, April 1, 1937; John D. Thompson to Owen D. Young, April 16, 1937; Owen Young to John D. Thompson, May 4, 1937; Owen Young to John D. Thompson, May 18, 1937. Owen D. Young Papers, Folder 2-150-C. Schenectady Museum Archives, Schenectady, New York.
44 Barbara Bridgman Perkins, "Shaping Institution-based Specialism: Early Twentieth-century Economic Organization of Medicine," *Social History of Medicine* 10 (1997): 419–435.
45 Ira I. Kaplan, *Practical Radiation Therapy* (Philadelphia: W.B. Saunders, 1931), 331.
46 John Trump to Karl Compton, February 16, 1948. John G. Trump papers, MC 223, Box 7. Massachusetts Institute of Technology. Institute Archives and Special Collections, MIT Libraries, Cambridge, MA.
47 James Cox, "ASTRO Interview," June 17, 2011. https://www.astro.org/About-ASTRO/History/James-Cox/ accessed May 18, 2016.
48 "Editorial: Coolidge Tubes," *Victor News* September 2, 1929.
49 No title, *Victor News* February, 1938.
50 "Editorial: Investments," *Victor News* December 2, 1929.
51 "Editorial: Reputation," *Victor News* December, 1931.
52 Patrick J. McGrath, *Scientists, Business, and the State, 1890–1960* (Chapel Hill: University of North Carolina Press, 2002), 22; James Gilbert, *Designing the Industrial State: The Intellectual Pursuit of Collectivism in America, 1880–1940* (Chicago: Quadrangle Books. 1972), 181.
53 Kim McQuaid, "Competition, Cartelization and the Corporate Ethic: General Electric's Leadership during the New Deal Era, 1933–1940," *American Journal of Economics and Sociology* 36 (1977): 417–428; Patrick D. Reagan, *Designing a New America: The Origins of New Deal Planning, 1890–1943* (Amherst: University of Massachusetts Press, 1999).
54 Kim McQuaid, "Corporate Liberalism in the American Business Community, 1920–1940," *Business History Review* 52 (1978): 342–368.
55 Robert W. Bruère, "The Swope Plan and After," *Survey* 67 (1932): 583–585, 647–648, 653.

4 Competing Research Universities

An extravagantly titled article, "Science Will Liberate All Mankind in Next Century," in the *New York Times* in 1934 announced that leading industrialists, scientists, and doctors predicted that high voltage would advance cancer treatment enormously.[1] Achieving the advances, the article advised, required strengthening research universities that commercially exploited their technology innovations.

A scientific industrial complex preceded the medical industrial complex. The California Institute of Technology (Caltech), the University of California, and the Massachusetts Institute of Technology (MIT) in particular led the way in building high-voltage technologies and the industry-aligned research university. All three attracted donors by emphasizing medical as well as industrial use of their new machines, and they connected with physicians willing to send patients for treatment in their laboratories. It was easier for California, which had a medical school—albeit across the San Francisco Bay from its physics department. Caltech's clinical radiation service was short-lived and MIT's would not flourish until after World War II, but they all played key roles in developing supervoltage devices for medical treatment.

Supervoltage Treatment at Caltech

Caltech was the first of the three institutions to build a supervoltage device and an associated clinical service. The Carnegie and Rockefeller Foundations had joined the Edison Company in furnishing such a well-equipped high-voltage laboratory that the well-known physicist Robert Millikan declared he "owed it to physics" to become president of the new institute.[2] Interested in commercial applications from the beginning, Millikan used the laboratory to design and patent income-generating instruments. Lab physicist Charles Lauritsen built an X-ray tube that reached 600,000 volts in 1928.

Millikan attained funding to develop Lauritsen's X-ray tube for therapeutic purposes, and, along with Lauritsen, he proposed to physician Albert Soiland that he send patients for treatment with their supervoltage device.[3] Although Soiland had earlier predicted that maximum therapeutic effects would level out around 300,000 volts,[4] he started sending patients to Caltech in 1930 for treatments that were twice as powerful.

Albert Soiland had taken a common route to medical specialization; he carved out special markets and announced that he was limiting his practice to them. Defining himself first as a surgeon, he honed in on radiology and then narrowed his practice to radiotherapy. He took the radium tour to Paris and after that used radium clinically. After taking on partners, he built the private, freestanding Los Angeles Tumor Institute. He advised physicians to send all their cancer patients to special clinics like his for a "proper course of radiation treatment" prior to surgical removal of their tumors.[5] With a reputation for providing the latest technologies, the Hollywood-based Tumor Institute became famous for treating movie stars such as William Powell (who survived his cancer) and Humphrey Bogart (who did not).

In 1934, Tumor Institute physicians claimed that they had treated patients at full megavoltage.[6] Strangely (since it was considered such a big deal), their report did not offer dates or details to back their claim. Two years later, at a meeting of the International Congress of Scientific and Social Campaign against Cancer, they challenged that "the race is on for higher achievements" in high-voltage therapy. It was "practically an accepted procedure" to treat some cancers by radiation alone, they affirmed, due to "striking immediate results."[7] Accepted procedures and striking immediate results would continue to lead technology development and mislead radiotherapists.

The Tumor Institute advertised its treatments and technologies in brochures and professional journals. Its 1939 brochure described an armamentarium that included two 100 kv X-ray devices, two 200 kv devices, its Lauritsen 600 kv supervoltage apparatus, and a (4-gram) teleradium "bomb." The particular advantage of teleradium over radium implants, the freestanding clinic advised, was that it could be used on an outpatient basis. Despite the availability of more powerful equipment, kilovoltage remained the standard treatment at the Tumor Institute. Of its radiation patients in 1939, 58 percent received 200 kv X-rays, 35 percent received supervoltage X-rays, and 7 percent received radium teletherapy treatments.[8] Many of the 200 kv treatments were for benign uterine fibroids or inflammatory conditions rather than cancer. Around half of the cancer patients had gynecological (usually cervical) cancers, and nearly one-third had skin cancers.

Albert Soiland also played a major role in professionalizing radiology and gaining its monopoly in clinical X-ray. He had instigated the American College of Radiology in 1922 as a means of challenging the competitive threat of nonmedical entrepreneurs' purchasing X-ray machines and hanging out their shingles. Under the college's aegis, he successfully lobbied California's governor not to sign a bill that would have certified non-MD radiographers.[9] The college went on to organize the 1937 Inter-Society Committee for Radiology to "protect the interests of radiology from insurance and the New Deal" and, under Medicare, to win a long battle to escape from the status of hospital employee by billing separately for their hospital-based services.[10] Radiologists would come to appreciate the American College of Radiology for explicitly representing their economic interests.[11]

Although a Los Angeles Tumor Institute physician noted in 1942 that early supervoltage hopes had "not been very well realized,"[12] the Soiland–Caltech collaboration contributed to spreading the "supervoltage gospel," as it was sometimes called, as did one similar and one very different radiation machine in Berkeley.

Academia and Industry at the University of California

University of California (UC) physicist Ernest O. Lawrence demonstrated his diminutive magnetic resonance accelerator at the 1930 meeting of the National Academy of Sciences. Calling the 4-inch device a "proton merry-go-round," he would name its mammoth successors *cyclotron*, short for circular instrument. Lawrence's drive to build ever bigger and more powerful machines required an alliance with industry. It also, biographers have alleged, caused him to miss being first to split the atom and to recognize artificial radioactivity. He still got a Nobel Prize—for the technology itself and its potential medical application.

Accomplished in raising money to develop technology, Lawrence pioneered big science supported by a broad collection of private and public funds. Industry initially supported half of Lawrence's laboratory research with money and materials.[13] Federal Telegraph donated an enormous magnet for the first large cyclotron, the American Smelting and Refining Company gave lead shielding, and General Electric provided other equipment.[14] The university's accolade to *Free Enterprise and University Research* would also name the Rockefeller, John and Mary Markle, Josiah Macy, Jr., and Columbia Foundations as further donors to Lawrence's lab. Cancer research and treatment accounted for a significant portion of foundation funding.

Robert Sproul became university president in the same year (1930) that Lawrence demonstrated his 4-inch cyclotron, and he significantly fostered its growth. Trained as an engineer who believed in a "symbiosis of capitalistic and academic industry," Sproul encouraged applied research that could lead to revenue-generating patents.[15] Like many academicians of the time who felt that their research should be dedicated to public welfare and not to personal, institutional, or corporate wealth, Lawrence initially disdained patenting his cyclotron. He changed his stance, however, upon hearing that the Raytheon company was on the verge of patenting a similar invention. Lawrence turned to the Research Corporation, established to procure patents for academic inventions, manage their licensing, and encourage their manufacturing—while distancing their academic inventors from commerce.[16]

In investing in the Lawrence lab, the Research Corporation purposely challenged the General Electric Company (GE). The Research Corporation also supported the legal challenges that broke GE's patent monopoly on high-voltage X-ray. *Time* magazine accused GE in 1930 of using patent monopolies to charge excessively high prices, hold back the development of potentially useful inventions, and in general retard the profession of radiology.[17] Lawrence went on to develop a device that competed with GE and did not seem to perceive a potential conflict of interest in so doing.

Lawrence's career-long relationship with GE was both competitive and cooperative. He was a good customer for their products, and they for his; GE gave Lawrence price discounts and paid for fellowships in his lab.[18] Lawrence had spent the summer of 1929 in GE's research labs in Schenectady, New York, trading knowledge and equipment with William Coolidge and other GE scientists. Lawrence's radiation laboratory (which would become known as the rad lab, and later, Lawrence Berkeley National Laboratory) intentionally emulated the cross-disciplinary as well as academia–business interactions he'd witnessed at GE.[19] Lawrence also enticed the creative technician David Sloan to become one of his graduate students.

The Sloan Supervoltage Device

Working under a GE-funded fellowship at UC, David Sloan designed a 800 kilovolt X-ray device that competed with GE. Appreciating cancer treatment as a means of funding larger and more complex machines, Lawrence asked the Research Corporation to expedite commercializing the new device, not only for the purpose of producing supervoltage X-rays for medical treatment but also to try to break into the lucrative 200–300 kv X-ray treatment market. General Electric wanted the Sloan accelerator, Lawrence informed the Research Corporation, "but, of course, I hope this can be avoided."[20] Less than a year later, Lawrence wrote Coolidge at GE that "Sloan and I would be only too glad to have you and your organization associated with the commercial development of our X-ray tube."[21] It seems that Lawrence sought commercial development of the Sloan device with or without GE. When the university publicly demonstrated its new X-ray generator in 1932, it attracted a predictable flock of industry representatives from GE, Kelley-Koett, and Westinghouse.

Sloan's supervoltage generator also attracted radiologist Robert Stone from the university's medical school in San Francisco. As *Lawrence and His Laboratory* rather curiously put it, Stone "saw Sloan's rays burn through steel, and desired to use them on his patients."[22] Lawrence sold Stone on the new supervoltage machine on the grounds that it was smaller and cheaper than the Caltech and GE devices.[23] Lawrence's laboratory built a Sloan accelerator for the university's San Francisco hospital, which initiated its clinical use in 1934. Two years later, a journal article describing the hospital's experience indicated that although the machine was generally used at 800 kv, it "has been operated" at a million volts.[24] Such a claim seemed to imply that it had been used clinically at that level. A 1941 paper more clearly specified that the machine had operated clinically at 1000 kv (or one million volts), but so had MIT's new device by then.

Most of the first 300 patients treated on the Sloan machine were already dead, the 1941 paper acknowledged—"but these were desperate cases to begin with." Every patient experienced complications, some of considerable severity. So many breast-cancer patients developed lung fibrosis that the hospital gave up high-voltage treatments on that group of patients. The paper concluded that the Sloan device produced "no striking improvement" in radiation therapy results.[25] In contrast, the long survival of Gunda Lawrence (mother of Ernest and his physician brother John) following treatment on the Sloan device may have reinforced the brothers' beliefs in radiation therapy and in their own devices.[26]

The Sloan Device Goes to Columbia

The Crocker Research Laboratory at Columbia-Presbyterian Hospital installed the only other clinical Sloan instrument in 1937. The installation came despite Columbia radiotherapy leader Francis Carter Wood's criticism of supervoltage two years before at the American Roentgen Ray Society meeting, where he had reminded his colleagues of the "disappointment which followed exaggerated claims" for 200 kv machines.[27] The research literature, Carter Wood had pointed out, suggested that only a few cancer types responded more effectively to the higher voltages. He had advocated a moratorium on new installations of costly supervoltage machines until the field had definitive evidence of effectiveness.

Flying in the face of his earlier critique and proposed moratorium, Carter Wood collaborated with E. O. Lawrence in building a Sloan device for Columbia. He did, however, object to Lawrence's ambition to push the machine to a million volts. Lawrence himself conceded that there was "not much point in X-rays above half a million volts for therapy purposes,"[28] but they were both striving for leadership in their fields. Carter Wood publically demonstrated his new machine in the basement of Columbia-Presbyterian Hospital.[29] *Life* magazine published a large photo of the device, captioned, "Biggest Gun in the War Against Cancer is Crocker Laboratory's 1,250,000-Volt X-ray Machine."[30] According the most powerful machines the most publicity, the media tended to round voltage up—sometimes way up. As reported by *Life*, Columbia's voltage level would have one-upped Memorial Hospital's GE supervoltage machine, also in Manhattan. There was little evidence, however, that the Columbia machine actually operated at the reported level.

Carter Wood called the new device "very promising" after only a few weeks of use.[31] Two years later, when Memorial Hospital went megavoltage with a GE resonant transformer, Carter Wood pronounced that his California device operating at 700 kilovolts was just as effective.[32] California did not develop the Sloan X-ray generator commercially, however, due to patent problems with GE. Even more discouraging (for California), the Research Corporation determined that another of its X-ray investments, the Van de Graaff accelerator, might be more competitive.[33] Meanwhile, California had another technology it employed medically.

Neutron Beam Treatments at California

At the same time he was developing the Sloan device, Lawrence was considering medical applications of his cyclotron. It was physicist Ernest rather than physician John who promoted the clinical use of neutron beams and engaged radiologist Robert Stone in the endeavor. Soon after the 1932 discovery of the neutron, and the cyclotron was found to be spewing large quantities of them, E. O. suggested to John that they use the neutrons for cancer treatment.[34] "I must confess," he wrote Danish physicist Niels Bohr a year later in 1935, "that one reason we have undertaken this biological work is that we thereby have been able to get financial support for all of the work in the laboratory. As you know, it is much easier to get funds for medical research."[35]

E. O. Lawrence publicly declared his intention to treat cancer patients with neutrons at the 1936 meeting of the Radiological Society of North America, and *Time* magazine announced two years later that neutron treatments at Lawrence's lab had begun.[36] While cautioning that the treatment was still in an experimental phase, the US Public Health Service issued a dramatic press release describing how the "amazing penetrating neutron rays may pierce straight to the malignant mass" and kill the "most fiercely active cancer cells."[37]

Now Robert Stone sent his patients the other way across the San Francisco Bay for treatment. Figure 4.1 shows Stone and John Lawrence positioning patient Robert Penny for neutron treatment. Not a few of the patients were well-to-do; one arrived in a limousine bearing chilled champagne for laboratory staff.[38] The National Cancer Institute (NCI) supported Lawrence's medical cyclotron with one of two grants awarded in its first year of operation (in addition to its radium loans). Lawrence wrote physicist friend Arthur Compton, chair of NCI's National Advisory Cancer Council, that it was of "compelling importance" to explore all the treatment possibilities opened up by gamma rays, neutrons, and artificially radioactive substances. In light of what X-rays and radium had already accomplished, he advised, and keeping in mind that neutrons carried energies up to 12 million volts, it was "almost unthinkable that the manifold new radiation and radioactive substances should not greatly extend the successful range of application of radiation therapy."[39] Carrying this message to the council, Compton reported that Lawrence saw more promise in "building sources of neutron rays than for extending X-rays to yet greater voltage ... since it has not yet been possible to demonstrate the superiority of 1,000-kv X-rays over 200-kv rays."[40] Lawrence submitted to the

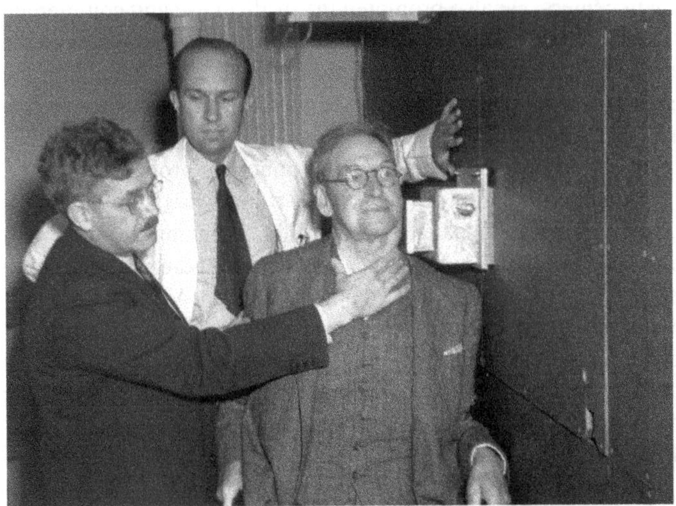

Figure 4.1 Robert Stone and John Lawrence Position Patient Robert Penny for Neutron Treatment.

Photo Courtesy of Lawrence Berkeley National Laboratory, Berkeley, CA.

advisory council's pressure to treat a friend of an influential politician, although he cautioned the council that his neutron treatments were "pure experiment."[41]

Later scholars accused the Lawrence laboratory of unethically using patients to build a medical profession, although it was hardly unique in that regard.[42] The lab scheduled only one day a week for cancer treatment, rendering it impossible to follow the accepted fractionation procedures of the time. Graduate students donned gleaming white lab coats on clinic day and put up temporary walls to make it look more like a medical facility—not to mention to protect patients from the oil-spewing machinery. "Cyclotroneers who complained that the medical research tail had begun to wag the physics dog were not-so-gently reminded by Ernest which end it was that brought in the necessary grants."[43] Physics research needs determined the operation and the energy level of the new machine.

Lawrence then engaged president Sproul in efforts to raise funds for an even bigger "medical" cyclotron. He needed an endowed clinical facility like Caltech's Kellogg Laboratory, he told Sproul, so he could experiment with neutrons and radioactive isotopes produced in the cyclotron. Lawrence, Sproul, and Langley Porter, the dean of the medical school, subsequently dined at the Bohemian Club—whose membership brought together much of San Francisco's wealth and power—to plan the new clinic.[44] Sproul turned to William Crocker—banker, UC regent, and another Crocker railroad heir—to buy them a clinical laboratory.

Continuing to look for other ways his cyclotron could accelerate proceeds as well as protons, Lawrence told the National Advisory Cancer Council that Stone had suggested the lab charge patients for neutron treatments just as the university hospital charged for high-voltage X-ray treatments.[45] Lawrence even envisioned a market for medical cyclotrons someday, a day that would arrive 50 years later with proton treatment centers. He also promoted the medical use and commercial production of elements made radioactive in the cyclotron. He sent samples to the president of American Cynamid and invited him to visit his lab. After his visit, the Cynamid president wrote Lawrence that he envisioned the new radioactive isotopes opening an "entire new field for medical conquest" and sent him (another) generous check.[46] Lawrence also accepted annual retainers of around $5,000—a huge increment to teaching salaries of the time—from American Cynamid, General Electric, and Eastman Kodak in exchange for assigning any resulting patents to the companies. When Philip Reed, GE's chairman of the board, came to town, he got the works: a tour of the cyclotron, dinner at Trader Vic's, a visit with Diego Rivera at work, and a walk through Chinatown, nightcapped, of course, at the famous Top of the Mark restaurant.[47]

Conceding that Robert Stone and his brother John had both warned him against overstating the case for neutrons, Ernest nonetheless predicted in 1942 that "neutron therapy will eventually take an important place along with surgery, X-ray and radium in the treatment of cancer."[48] But his neutron treatments terminated abruptly when the men and machines were commissioned to build an atomic bomb. After the war, Stone reported in a prestigious lecture in 1948 that only 17 of his second group of 226 patients receiving neutron treatments were still alive and that some of them suffered severe radiation damage. "Neutron therapy as administered by us," he advised in a medical association talk, "has resulted in such bad late sequelae in proportion to the few good results that it should not be continued."[49] Stone further advised that the damage the neutron patients suffered "should serve as a warning to those proposing to use protons, multimillion volt beta rays and multimillion volt roentgen rays [another name for X-rays] in the treatment of cancer." He would have been fully aware that some of those proponents were seated in the audience.

Stone had earlier challenged the "common belief, held by both the medical profession and the laity … that higher and higher voltages are synonymous with better and better treatments, and more and more cures of cancer." This belief, he criticized, was "stampeding radiologists into procuring apparatus capable of producing higher and higher voltages."[50] Yet, as discussed in Chapter 5, he would join the stampede and commission the most powerful machine of them all. But first, MIT's Van de Graaff accelerator made an impact.

MIT Enters the Megavoltage Race

The Massachusetts Institute of Technology (MIT) was an industry-oriented research university from the beginning. MIT administrators expected their scientists and engineers to acquire industrial contracts that would cover the expenses of their highly equipped laboratories and turn their scientific work into industrial products.[51] MIT led academia in patent policies and personal connections with industry in pursuit of these goals.[52]

General Electric president Gerard Swope chaired the 1930 search committee that chose Princeton physicist Karl Compton as MIT's new president. Compton had close connections with GE, having learned industrial research in GE's laboratories and served the company on annual retainers.[53] He was, in addition, linked to many other corporations and foundations; at one time or another he served on the boards of the Sloan-Kettering Institute, the Rockefeller Foundation, the Alfred P. Sloan Foundation, and the Ford Foundation. Compton's dual mandate at MIT was to improve its science and to "adjust engineering education to the perceived needs of industry."[54] MIT's translational research role required selecting projects possessing commercial potential.

High voltage was a hot area in physics and engineering at the time, and Compton persuaded his Princeton protégé Robert Van de Graaff to join him at MIT and to bring his new electrostatic generator with him. The Van de Graaff machine became MIT's entry in the high-voltage race. Engineering graduate student John Trump (who would become uncle to Donald J. Trump) joined in, and, with funding from the Research Corporation, Van de Graaff and Trump built a mammoth generator in an aircraft hangar. *Time* magazine announced its spectacular 1933 public presentation (as seen in Figure 4.2).[55] Pronouncing the generator to be the most important development ever in the high-voltage field, Compton sought to develop it commercially. He helped patent it as well as build the company that manufactured it after the war. Trump built a special laboratory at MIT dedicated to refining the machine and developing its applications, particularly in treating cancer.[56]

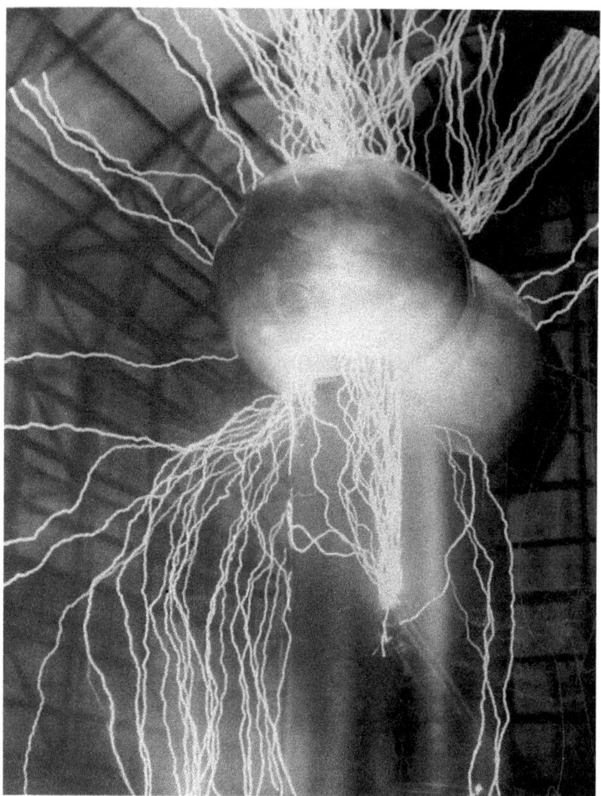

Figure 4.2 The Van de Graaff High-Voltage Generator on Display (Time Exposure).

Courtesy of MIT Libraries, Institute Archives and Special Collections, Cambridge, Massachusetts. Massachusetts Institute of Technology, Office of the President, records of Karl Taylor Compton and James Rhyne Killian.

According to Van de Graaff, it was Trump who instigated medical use of the electrostatic X-ray generator.[57] According to medical histories, radiologists initiated the connection with MIT. It was a combination. In 1932, A Massachusetts General Hospital (Mass General) radiologist spoke at MIT on clinical uses of X-rays. Two years later, Trump and Van de Graaff suggested to Mass General radiologists that they use the high-energy X-rays generated by Van de Graaff's machine for cancer treatment.[58] After another year, Harvard radiologist Richard Dresser took them up on their offer. Trump agreed that his team would build a device for Dresser—but only if his lab could get funding to design it for a million volts.[59]

Disbursing wealth from the mining and railroad industries, representatives from the Boston-based Godfrey M. Hyams Trust were impressed by the spectacle in the hangar. The trust paid for a clinical machine and a new hospital building to house it.[60] In the forefront of the use of radium and kilovoltage, Harvard's Collis

P. Huntington Memorial Hospital for Cancer Research appreciated in 1935 that the new megavoltage device would enable the hospital to maintain its pioneering position in treating cancer.[61] GE's Gerard Swope was less happy with MIT's hospital device and rebuked Compton for "improper commercial competition with GE and its medical instrumentation business."[62] This would not be the last time GE would accuse MIT of improper competition in medical megavoltage.

Trump and Dresser announced their upcoming million-volt machine at the 1936 meeting of the American Roentgen Ray Society. Trump wrote in his notes that Dresser started using the device clinically in March 1937, thereby recording the probable first use of megavoltage X-ray in cancer treatment.[63] In order to assure the milestone in the face of measurement problems, it seems, Dresser had set the machine at 1.2 MeV.[64] A Harvard radiologist referred to the machine's output as "a fairly honest one megavolt."[65] Dresser wrote in the Huntington Hospital's 1937 annual report that patients experienced "surprisingly little" radiation sickness, which, he said, indicated that many could be treated on an outpatient basis. Dresser reported impressive regression or complete disappearance of many tumors, although he suspected—correctly, as it turned out—that many of them would recur.[66]

More positive about the new technology than some of the physicians using it and only 6 months after the first Van de Graaff treatment, Trump wrote (in a grant proposal, a genre known for hyperbole) that "definite evidence is rapidly accumulating indicating that the penetrating radiations produced by this apparatus are more effective for certain types of cancer than those of the 200 and 400 kv installations now commercially available."[67] The Hyams Trust paid for the development of a cheaper and more compact 1.25 MeV Van de Graaff generator to serve as a prototype for a commercial machine.[68] In 1940, Trump's laboratory delivered the new device to the Massachusetts General Hospital, which operated it for the next 15 years. Prior to turning it over to the hospital, the lab had used the machine to study dosimetry, develop clinical techniques, and train radiology residents.[69] A study combining the first eight years of Van de Graaff use at the Huntington and Mass General hospitals concluded that, at best, its treatments may have given patients a few more months of life, with less skin damage than with kilovoltage.[70]

As he finished building his 1.25 MeV X-ray machine, Trump was already writing a grant proposal for a 3 MeV device. The new proposal outlined a "medical radiation program" to be located at MIT using the 3 MeV machine. He expected his new program to bring about a "new order of effectiveness in a field of radiation therapy" as well as establish MIT as a "center of medical radiations and of radiation therapy research."[71] His High Voltage Research Laboratory's clinical radiation program would flourish for many years after the war, as Chapter 5 continues.

Caltech, the University of California, and MIT all depended on foundation and industrial capital to develop their megavoltage technologies. Maintaining mutually advantageous relationships with industry, the radiation engineers did not start their own companies at this time, as some of them would do after the war. By the time of US entry into World War II, MIT, GE, and others outside of the United States had achieved the million-volt goal and had found no substantial therapeutic improvement.

Research on the Use and Therapeutic Effectiveness of Radium and X-ray

A multitude of photographs in the medical literature documented stunning reductions of skin and other superficial tumors treated with radiation. Taken from a radiotherapy textbook, Figure 4.3 illustrates just one of many examples of striking radiation results that may have convinced radiotherapists of the benefits of their technology.

In accounting for a large portion of radiotherapy patients, cancer of the uterine cervix put gynecologists in competition with radiologists. To many women receiving radiation for advanced cervical cancer, radium and X-rays were gifts that could ameliorate distressing and even incapacitating consequences of their cancers.[72] Many women accepted radiation as safer than hysterectomy, which in the early 1920s carried a mortality rate estimated at 18 percent.[73]

A 1927 review of the by-then voluminous international literature was moderately positive regarding the use of radiation on cervical cancer. Radiation alone, the review concluded, sometimes eradicated the cancer, and the 5-year survival rate of women treated with radiation was 22 percent compared to 18 percent of those treated by hysterectomy.[74] The report noted that surgical mortality may have accounted for the difference. The difference could have also been due to differences in disease stage, fast becoming seen as the most important prognostic indicator for cancer.

In 1935, a Memorial Hospital gynecologist reported 5-year "salvage" rates of 55 percent of women whose cervical cancers were diagnosed early, 35 percent of those diagnosed at mid-stage, and 15 percent of those whose cancers were

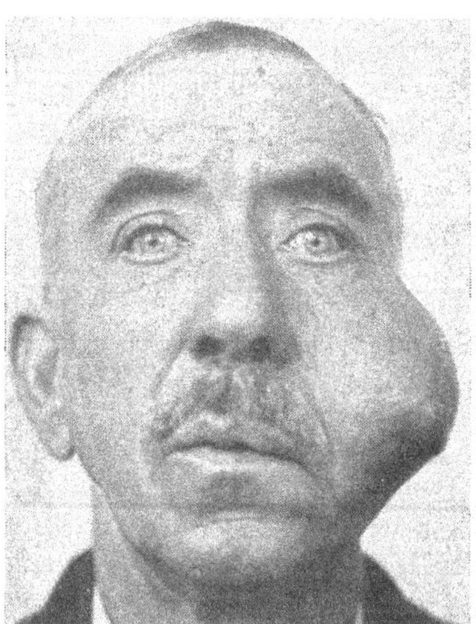

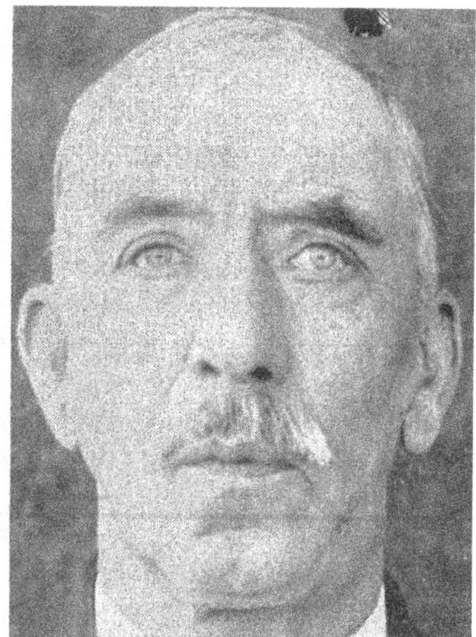

Figure 4.3 Before and After Radiation Treatment of Lymphosarcoma of Cheek.

Source: Walter M. Levitt, *A Handbook of Radiotherapy* (New York: Paul B. Hoeber, 1952), 118. Reprinted with permission, Wolters Kluwer.

advanced when diagnosed.[75] Research studies would continue to find stage at the time of diagnosis to be the most important survival factor, as further discussed in Chapter 8. Observing that breast-cancer outcomes were not as good after radiation, most clinicians did not relinquish surgery as they added radiation to its treatment. Protocols at Memorial and other hospitals sometimes even combined radical mastectomy with radium implants plus radium packs or kilovoltage.[76]

Enthusiastic reports staking claims and stressing achievements appeared in the medical literature shortly after (or even before) the installation of each new device—far too early to evaluate clinical effectiveness. The 1930 chairman of the American Medical Association Section on Radiology criticized the widespread use of radiation therapy prior to scientific study, noting that he received twice as many papers on treatment as he did on diagnosis and that science would be better served the other way around.[77] Summarizing world literature and opinion, the *1932 Year Book of Radiology* observed that pack radium seemed to have increased radium effectiveness, although there was dissent about that in England. The *Year Book* also reported that supervoltage had "no definitive biological results," but that its advocates were "enthusiastic" and German radiologists had reported good results.[78] As leaders suggested that therapeutic practices were not consistent with scientific study, radiotherapists in New York City all reported that their own cure rates were significantly above average.[79]

Radiologists were also aware of severe treatment complications and attempted to counteract them. Combining X-ray and radium (sometimes pack and brachytherapy together) in treating advanced cervical cancer, a Memorial Hospital gynecologist experimented with treatment order in an attempt to reduce radiation-induced patient prostration, tissue sloughing, severe hemorrhage, fistula, and death.[80] Like California, Memorial found pulmonary fibrosis to be a serious consequence of irradiating breast cancers.[81]

Radiotherapists were sometimes devastatingly critical of their earlier work as they learned more about damages their treatments inflicted. "At one period," James Ewing contended in 1934,

> the prescription of dosage was so uncertain and the results apparently so capricious that all one could really do was to place the patient under the machine and hope for the best. Patients were often burned from unexpected leaks and on one or more occasions, it is said, they were actually electrocuted on the treatment table.[82]

Many patients—and therapists—suffered severe bodily harm and early death from radiation. But it was less threatening to see flaws in past practices than it was to criticize contemporary practices. Many leaders, including Ewing, kept the faith.

In the context of the grand opening of the 1939 Memorial Hospital building, Ewing announced that radiation treatment was the "outstanding contribution of medicine to humanity in the present century and outweighs all previous progress in this field."[83] All he needed to cure cancer, he had advised the previous year, was a million dollars (per cancer) to organize research along the lines of the "great industrial research laboratories."[84] Like Millikan, Lawrence, and Trump, Ewing appreciated cancer's role in attracting funding.

The prestige of physics bestowed a mantle of science as well as funding on radiotherapy. Radiologists and radiation physicists built careers, and their services built reputations, on the use of radium, X-rays, and neutrons. But their own research demonstrated that growth of the field owed more to professional, institutional, and industrial aspirations than it did to improved cancer control. Their effectiveness studies did not find markedly better patient outcomes using ever higher-powered and higher-cost devices. In measuring costs of radiation treatment using a 200 kilovoltage machine at $45 or less, $100 for 400 kv treatment, $400 for 700 kv, $175 using a radium pack used at a distance of 10 cm, and $4,000 using a radium pack at 50 cm, a Charlotte, North Carolina radiologist suggested that Americans were paying too much for radiation therapy.[85] Magnifying the cost of medical care and building high-cost medicine, however, conferred high value on radiation therapy and elite status on its providers. The power escalation would continue after the war, with MIT continuing to lead.

Notes

1 "Science Will Liberate all Mankind in Next Century, Leaders Predict," *New York Times* May 26, 1934. It also predicted slumless cities, and, in its sole accurate forecast, ground-directed airplanes.
2 Roger L. Geiger, *To Advance Knowledge: The Growth of American Research Universities, 1900–1940* (New York: Oxford University Press, 1986), 185.
3 Albert Soiland, "Experimental Clinical Research Work with X-ray Voltages Above 500,000, A Preliminary Statement," *Radiology* 20 (1933): 99–102.
4 Albert Soiland, "The Evolution of Roentgen Therapy in Higher Voltages," *California and Western Medicine* 22 (1924): 148–150.
5 Albert Soiland, "Radiology," *California and Western Medicine* 26 (1927): 372–373.
6 Seeley G. Mudd, Clyde K. Emery, Orville M. Meland, and William E. Costolow, "Data Concerning Three Years' Experience with 600 kv (peak) Roentgen Therapy," *American Journal of Roentgenology, Radium Therapy, and Nuclear Medicine* 31 (1934): 520–531.
7 Albert Soiland, William E. Costolow, Orville N. Meland, and Ludwig Lindberg, "Our Concept of the Management of Cancer Patients by Modern Therapeutic Methods," *International Congress of Scientific and Social Campaign Against Cancer* (1936): 326–338.
8 Los Angeles Tumor Institute brochure, 1407 South Hope Street, Los Angeles, 1939.
9 Albert Soiland, "The Therapeutic Aspect of Short Wave X-rays," *California State Journal of Medicine* 21 (1923): 415–417.
10 "ACR History Archive—Institution Chronology," http://www.acr.org/~/media/ACR/Documents/PDF/About%20Us/History/ACR%20History%20Institutional%20Chronology accessed November 3, 2013.
11 George R. Leopold, "The ABCs of Radiology," *Radiology* 198 (1996): 45A–47A.
12 William E. Costolow, "Radiation Therapy in Extensive Bladder Carcinoma," *California and Western Medicine* 56 (1942): 247–248.
13 Peter Galison, "Introduction: The Many Faces of Big Science," In Peter Galison and Bruce William Hevly, *Big Science: The Growth of Large-Scale Research* (Stanford, CA: Stanford University Press, 1992), 1–20.
14 Robert W. Seidel, "Technology Choice in Early High-Energy Physics," *History and Technology* 9 (1992): 175–187.

15 J. L. Heilbron and Robert W. Seidel, *Lawrence and His Laboratory: A History of the Lawrence Berkeley Laboratory* Vol. 1 (Berkeley, CA: University of California Press, 1989), 104, 106, 107, 113.
16 David C. Mowery, Richard R. Nelson, Bhaven N. Sampat, and Arvids A. Ziedonis, *Ivory Tower and Industrial Innovation: University–Industry Technology Transfer Before and After the Bayh-Dole Act* (Stanford, CA: Stanford University Press, 2004), 60.
17 "Medicine: Mobilizing for Cancer," *Time* September 29, 1930.
18 C. G. Ramsay to Ernest O. Lawrence, March 9, 1938. Ernest O. Lawrence papers, BANC FILM 2248. The Bancroft Library, University of California, Berkeley, CA.
19 Patrick J. McGrath, *Scientists, Business, and the State, 1890–1960* (Chapel Hill: University of North Carolina Press, 2002), 35.
20 J. L. Heilbron and Robert W. Seidel, *Lawrence and His Laboratory: A History of the Lawrence Berkeley Laboratory,* Vol. 1, (Berkeley, CA: University of California Press, 1989), 119–121.
21 William D. Coolidge to Ernest O. Lawrence, August 24, 1932; Ernest O. Lawrence to William D. Coolidge, September 3, 1932. Ernest O. Lawrence papers, BANC FILM 2248. Bancroft Library, University of California, Berkeley.
22 J. L. Heilbron and Robert W. Seidel, *Lawrence and His Laboratory: A History of the Lawrence Berkeley Laboratory,* Vol. 1, (Berkeley, CA: University of California Press, 1989), 121.
23 Herbert Childs, *An American Genius: The Life of Ernest Orlando Lawrence* (New York: E. P. Dutton, 1968), 192.
24 Howard E. Ruggles, "A Year's Experience with 800 kv Roentgen Rays," *American Journal of Roentgenology and Radium Therapy* 36 (1936): 366–367.
25 Robert S. Stone and J. Maurice Robinson, "Skin Reactions Produced by 200 kv and 1000 kv Radiations: A Comparison," *California and Western Medicine* 55 (1941): 11–14.
26 Gregg Herken, *Brotherhood of the Bomb* (New York: Henry Holt, 2002), 20.
27 Charles B. Ward, John E. Wirth, and John E. Rose, "One and One Half-Years' Experience with Supervoltage Roentgen Rays," *American Journal of Roentgenology and Radium Therapy* 36 (1936): 368–380. Carter Wood in discussion.
28 J. L. Heilbron and Robert W. Seidel, *Lawrence and his Laboratory: A History of the Lawrence Berkeley Laboratory,* Vol. 1 (Berkeley, CA: University of California Press, 1989), 122.
29 John E. Lodge, "Science's Siege Guns in War on Disease," *Popular Science Monthly* April 1937, 27.
30 "U.S. Science Wars Against an Unknown Enemy: Cancer," *Life* March 1, 1937, 11.
31 "Expert on Cancer Lauds Giant X-ray," *New York Times* June 12, 1937.
32 "700,000-Volt X-ray Found Cancer Foe," *New York Times* March 2, 1939.
33 J. L. Heilbron and Robert W. Seidel, *Lawrence and His Laboratory: A History of the Lawrence Berkeley Laboratory,* Vol. 1 (Berkeley, CA: University of California Press, 1989), 126.
34 Herbert Childs, *An American Genius: The Life of Ernest Orlando Lawrence* (New York: E. P. Dutton, 1968), 214.
35 American Institute of Physics, "The Rad Lab." www.aip.org/history/lawrence/radlab.htm accessed December 10, 2010.
36 Ruth Brecher and Edward Brecher, *The Rays: A History of Radiology in the United States and Canada* (Baltimore: Williams and Wilkins, 1969), 364; "Cyclotron for Cancer," *Time* November 28, 1938.
37 United States Public Health Service, Press Release, November 14, 1938. Ernest O. Lawrence Papers, BANC FILM 2248. Bancroft Library, University of California, Berkeley.
38 K. G. Scott, "Robert Spencer Stone (1895–1966)," *Radiation Research* 33 (1968): 675–676.

39 Ernest O. Lawrence to Professor Compton, September 19, 1938. Ernest O. Lawrence Papers, BANC FILM 2248. Bancroft Library, University of California, Berkeley.
40 Compton, Report to National Advisory Cancer Council, October 3, 1938. Ernest O. Lawrence Papers, BANC FILM 2248. Bancroft Library, University of California, Berkeley.
41 Ludvig Hektoen to Ernest O. Lawrence, January 13, 1939; Ernest O. Lawrence to Ludvig Hektoen, January 16, 1939. Ernest O. Lawrence Papers, BANC FILM 2248. Bancroft Library, University of California, Berkeley.
42 David S. Jones and Robert L. Martensen, "Human Radiation Experiments and the Formation of Medical Physics at the University of California, San Francisco and Berkeley, 1937–1962" In Jordan Goodman, Anthony McElligott, and Lara Marks, eds., *Useful Bodies: Humans in the Service of Medical Science in the Twentieth Century* (Baltimore: Johns Hopkins University Press, 2003), 81–108.
43 Gregg Herken, *Brotherhood of the Bomb* (New York: Henry Holt, 2002), 20, 22.
44 J. L. Heilbron and Robert W. Seidel, *Lawrence and His Laboratory: A History of the Lawrence Berkeley Laboratory,* Vol. 1, (Berkeley, CA: University of California Press, 1989), 391.
45 Ernest O. Lawrence to Ludvig Hektoen, June 4, 1940. Ernest O. Lawrence papers, BANC FILM 2248. Bancroft Library, University of California, Berkeley.
46 Ernest O. Lawrence to William Bell, June 21, 1940; William Bell to Ernest O. Lawrence, Aug 2, 1940; Helen Griggs to Ernest O. Lawrence, December 24, 1940. Ernest O. Lawrence papers, BANC FILM 2248. Bancroft Library, University of California, Berkeley.
47 Philip D. Reed to Ernest O. Lawrence, October 1, 1940. Ernest O. Lawrence papers, BANC FILM 2248. Bancroft Library, University of California, Berkeley.
48 Ernest O. Lawrence, "Nuclear Physics and Biology," In Hugh Stott Taylor, Ernest O. Lawrence and Irving Langmuir, *Molecular Films, The Cyclotron, and the New Biology* (New Brunswick: Rutgers University Press, 1942), 63–91.
49 Robert Stone, "Neutron Therapy and Specific Ionization," *American Journal of Roentgenology and Radiation Therapy* 59 (1948): 771–785.
50 Ruth Brecher and Edward Brecher, *The Rays: A History of Radiology in the United States and Canada* (Baltimore: Williams and Wilkins, 1969), 358.
51 Roger L. Geiger, *To Advance Knowledge: The Growth of American Research Universities, 1900–1940* (New York: Oxford University Press, 1986), 177; Edward B. Roberts, *Entrepreneurs in High Technology: Lessons from MIT and Beyond* (New York: Oxford University Press, 1991); Henry Etzkowitz, *MIT and the Rise of Entrepreneurial Science* (New York: Routledge, 2002), 2.
52 Elliot A. Fishman, "MIT Patent Policy, 1932–1946: Historical Precedents in University–Industry Technology Transfer," PhD diss., University of Pennsylvania, 1996, 31.
53 George Wise and Willis R. Whitney, *General Electric, and the Origins of U.S. Industrial Research* (New York: Columbia University Press, 1985). 274; Robert Kargon and Elizabeth Hodes, "Karl Compton, Isaiah Bowman, and the Politics of Science in the Great Depression," *Isis* 76 (1985): 300–318.
54 Christophe Lécuyer, "The Making of a Science Based Technological University: Karl Compton, James Killian, and the Reform of MIT, 1930–1957," *Historical Studies in the Physical and Biological Sciences* 23 (1992): 153–180.
55 "Science: 7,000,000 volts," *Time* December 11, 1933.
56 E. Alfred Burrill, "Van de Graaff Accelerators for Radiation Research and Applications," In A. Charlesby, ed., *Radiation Sources* (New York: Macmillan/ Pergamon, 1964), 85–127.
57 Robert J. Van de Graaff to John H. Chiles, November 27, 1959. High Voltage Engineering Corporation Records, MC 153, Box 2. Massachusetts Institute of Technology. Institute Archives and Special Collections, MIT Libraries, Cambridge, MA.
58 John G. Trump, "Megavolt X-rays and Electrons for Cancer Therapy at the Massachusetts Institute of Technology," October 15, 1964. John G. Trump papers,

MC 223, Box 2. Massachusetts Institute of Technology. Institute Archives and Special Collections, MIT Libraries, Cambridge, MA.

59 Otha W. Linton, *Radiology at Massachusetts General Hospital: 1896–2000* (Boston: The General Hospital Corporation, 2001), 100–101.

60 John Trump, "Generation and Maintenance of 1000-Kilovolt Electrostatic X-ray Generator," no date, John G. Trump Papers, MC 223, Box 7. Massachusetts Institute of Technology. Institute Archives and Special Collections, MIT Libraries, Cambridge, MA.

61 Collis P. Huntington Memorial Hospital, *Twenty-third Annual Report of the Collis P. Huntington Memorial Hospital, Year Ending June 30, 1935.* Publications from the Collis P. Huntington Memorial Hospital, 1913–1952, HUF 260.875. Harvard University Archives, Harvard University, Cambridge, MA.

62 Christophe Lécuyer, "Patrons and a Plan," In David Kaiser, ed., *Becoming MIT* (Cambridge: MIT Press, 2010), 59–80.

63 "The Production of High Voltage X-rays," Trump talk. High Voltage Engineering Corporation Records, MC 153, Box 9. Massachusetts Institute of Technology, Institute Archives and Special Collections, MIT Libraries, Cambridge, MA. Herman D. Suit and Jay S. Loeffler say it was April, 1937 in *Evolution of Radiation Oncology at Massachusetts General Hospital* (New York: Springer, 2011), 22.

64 Richard Dresser and Jack Spencer, "Physical and Clinical Observations on the Use of Million-Volt X-rays," *New England Journal of Medicine* 218 (1938): 415–417.

65 Milford D. Schulz, "The Supervoltage Story," *American Journal of Roentgenology, Radium Therapy, and Nuclear Medicine* 124 (1975): 541–559.

66 Richard Dresser, "Report of the Department of Roentgenology," In Collis P. Huntington Memorial Hospital, *Twenty-fifth Annual Report of the Collis P. Huntington Memorial Hospital, Year Ending June 30, 1937.* Publications from the Collis P. Huntington Memorial Hospital, 1913–1952, HUF 260.875. Harvard University Archives, Harvard University, Cambridge, MA.

67 J. G. Trump and R. J. Van de Graaff, "Proposed Development of a Million-Volt Pressure-Insulated X-ray Generator for Cancer Treatment and Research," September 1, 1937. John G. Trump Papers, MC 223, Box 7. Massachusetts Institute of Technology. Institute Archives and Special Collections, MIT Libraries, Cambridge, MA.

68 Proposed Development of High-Energy X-rays and Cathode Rays for Cancer Treatment and Research," no date, approximately 1939. John G. Trump Papers, MC 223, Box 7. Massachusetts Institute of Technology. Institute Archives and Special Collections, MIT Libraries, Cambridge, MA.

69 Massachusetts Institute of Technology, *President's Report 1938*. libraries.mit.edu/archives/mithistory/presidents-reports/1938.pdf accessed June 30, 2010.

70 George W. Holmes and Milford D. Schulz, "Supervoltage Radiation: A Review of the Cases Treated During an Eight Year Period (1937–1944) Inclusive," *American Journal of Roentgenology and Radium Therapy* 60 (1946): 533–554.

71 John G. Trump and Robert J. Van de Graaff, "Proposed Development of High-Energy X-rays and Cathode Rays for Cancer Treatment and Research February, 1939." John G. Trump Papers, MC 223, Box 7. Massachusetts Institute of Technology. Institute Archives and Special Collections, MIT Libraries, Cambridge, MA.

72 Ilana Löwy, *A Woman's Disease: The History of Cervical Cancer* (Oxford: Oxford University Press, 2011), 41, 47, 51, 58.

73 D. Y. Keith, "The Present Status of Radiation Therapy," *Kentucky Medical Journal* June, 1922, 411–418.

74 Janet E. Lane-Claypon, *Cancer of the Uterus: A Statistical Inquiry into the Results of Treatment, Being an Analysis of the Existing Literature* London: Ministry of Health, Reports on Public Health and Medical Subjects, no. 40, 1927, 5, 24.

75 William P. Healy, "Radiation Therapy in Cancer of the Cervix," *Canadian Medical Association Journal* 32 (1935): 647–651.

76 Hugh H. Trout and C. H. Peterson, "Cancer of the Breast: Use of Radium and Roentgen Therapy in Conjunction with the Radical Operation," *Journal of the American Medical Association* 95 (1930): 1307–1310; F. E. Adair, "The Results of Treatment of Mammary Carcinoma by Surgical and Irradiation Methods at the Memorial Hospital, New York City, during the Decade 1916 to 1926," *Annals of Surgery* 95 (1932): 410–424.
77 Fred M. Hodges, "The Section on Radiology," *Journal of the American Medical Association* 95(1930): 833–834.
78 Ira I. Kaplan, "Radiotherapeutics: A Foreword and an Editorial," In Charles A. Waters and Ira I. Kaplan, eds., *The 1932 Year Book of Radiology* (Chicago: Year Book Medical Publishers, 1932), 345–349.
79 Michael M. Davis and Mary C. Jarrett, *A Health Inventory of New York City* (New York: Welfare Council of New York City, 1929), 248.
80 William P. Healy, "Radiation Therapy in Cancer of the Cervix," *Canadian Medical Association Journal* 32 (1935), 647–651.
81 Burton J. Lee, "The Therapeutic Value of Irradiation in the Treatment of Mammary Cancer: A Survey of Five-Year Results in 355 Cases Treated at the Memorial Hospital of New York," *Annals of Surgery* 88 (1928): 26–47.
82 James Ewing, "Early Experiences in Radiation Therapy," *American Journal of Roentgenology and Radium Therapy* 31 (1934): 153–63.
83 Waldemar Kaempffert, "X-rays and Cancer," *New York Times* January 8, 1939, 55.
84 William L. Laurence, "Says Cancer Cure Depends on Funds," *New York Times* January 9, 1938, 112.
85 Charles DeForest Lucas, "The Therapeutic and Economic Indications for Teleradium and the Supervoltage X-ray Machine," *Radiology* 34 (1940) 193–199.

Part II

Competitive Megavoltage, World War II to the 1970s

"The public relations impact of these gadgets is enormous."
— Milton Friedman, New York University radiologist

Part II investigates impacts of the wartime and postwar economic and technological booms on radiation therapy. Medicine, academia, and business continued to work together to build competing radiation devices exceeding a million volts. Boosting institutional pride and medical price, each new device venture took clinical and financial risks. The radiation therapy profession further engaged in political activities that protected its trade and augmented the growth of its services.

Political and Economic Environment

The massive industrial growth that was mobilized for World War II and extended through the Korean and Cold War economies energized three decades of economic growth. The United States expanded the technological explosion by (partially) shifting military production to the mass production of consumer appliances. In the biggest economic boom in American history before or since, the total output of goods and services (gross domestic product) doubled, an employed populace eagerly consumed them—and *economic growth* became the new American value.[1]

Government took over much of the role that foundations and other sources of private wealth had previously played in technology growth. Public funding contributed substantially to the economic boom and remodeled education and health care in the process. Government projects advanced the research university as the dominant institution in higher education, and in return, university-based scientific research became an economic growth engine. Military research contributed to medical technology growth by funding high-powered radiotherapy devices based on microwaves developed for radar and elements made artificially radioactive in nuclear reactors built for the atomic bomb.

Government programs also supported the growth of institutions that purchased the new medical technologies. The 1947 *Hospital Survey and Construction*

Act (also known as the Hill–Burton program) expanded institutions in size, technological equipment, and specialty services. Private monies further augmented their growth. Three years after the father of a Ford Foundation president traveled across the country to receive the latest in megavoltage treatment (described in Chapter 5), the foundation inaugurated a hospital grant program. Ford's rules for using the grants meant that much of the program's $200 million passed through to the 3,000 US firms manufacturing hospital equipment. Radiology departments proudly captured the highest number of Ford grants.[2]

Simultaneous growth in health insurance supported consumer demand for the expanding supply of medical services and equipment. Private health-insurance coverage, usually linked to employment, shot up from less than 10 percent of the population in 1940 to more than 50 percent by 1950.[3] Insurance companies and banks expanded their roles further when the Hill–Burton program shifted from grant payments to guaranteed loans.[4] In 1965, the public Medicare and Medicaid programs provided a significant measure of health care security for most older, and some poorer, populations. At the same time, the public programs offered greater investment security by significantly reducing the likelihood that hospitals would default on their commercial loans.

The public–private insurance system integrated medical care into the circulation of capital in the wider economy. It provided the economic stability that hospitals needed and capital markets required to finance increasingly costly specialty services and technologies. Debt financing of hospital construction grew from less than 25 percent prior to 1950 to nearly 40 percent by 1968 and to 70 percent by 1977.[5] This meant that hospital administrators could charge their high-tech purchases and pay later when the technologies produced revenues. Fee-for-service insurance payments that factored in the cost of debt (interest and fees) fueled a spiral of inflationary growth in medical care, in its technologies, and in its specialties.[6]

Radiology got a bonus (after three decades of organized effort) when it successfully lobbied Medicare to free it from hospital employee status. Medicare granted radiologists the same entrepreneurial standing (along with anesthesiologists and pathologists) of owning their practices and billing for their services as colleagues in other specialties.[7] It did not take long after that for radiologists and radiotherapists to plan elaborate freestanding, revenue-generating diagnosis and treatment facilities.[8] The radiology specialty would come to perceive Medicare as a "cash cow" for constructing high-tech procedure units both inside and outside of hospitals.[9]

As technology-based specialists, radiologists attained professional leadership and status by developing and using new devices. In 1950, the world's leading radiologists, radiation physicists, and equipment manufacturers had congregated in London for the Sixth International Congress of Radiology. General Electric (GE), High Voltage Engineering, and many other companies promoted their products at its exhibition. The congress further arranged a field trip to the Metropolitan-Vickers company to view its betatron, linear accelerator, and resonance transformer.[10]

US participants at the congress may have feared that radiotherapy in their country lagged internationally. A British Empire Cancer Campaign delegation visiting in 1948 had concluded that the lack of practice standards and service coordination meant that US radiotherapy did not match the professional levels seen in Britain.[11] German and Swiss speakers at the 1950 congress talked about their betatrons, and British speakers informed the meeting of their synchrotron, betatron, and linear accelerators under development. Roy Errington, sales manager of the Canadian firm Eldorado Mining and Refining, Ltd., brought a model of his company's cobalt-60 teletherapy device to the London exhibition. He got the publicity he came for when he demonstrated his model to Britain's queen. (Errington and other participants would have known that Gilbert Fletcher had announced the forthcoming University of Texas/General Electric cobalt device one week earlier at the International Congress of Cancer in Paris.)

Other North American presenters at the London Congress included John Trump and Hugh Hare speaking on the Massachusetts Institute of Technology's 2 MeV Van de Graaff X-ray generator; Roger Harvey and University of Saskatchewan investigators Harold Johns and T. A. Watson speaking on their use of the Illinois betatron; and John Lawrence's team talking about testing protons and alpha particles at the University of California.[12] Henry Kaplan, who would help develop Stanford's linear accelerator, had to make do with a paper on barium enemas. These men would become major radiation therapy leaders in the United States and Canada, and their stories appear in the chapters to follow. They would all integrate their medical research and treatment with industry to build powerful medical technologies along with powerful university and hospital departments.

Megavoltage attained iconic status when the May 5, 1958 cover of *Life* magazine (Figure II.1) featured a 2 MeV device (probably GE's).[13] While appearing on coffee tables across America and contributing to popular acceptance of radiation treatment, *Life*'s one-shot publicity missed the larger question of how much patients benefited from their superpowered treatments. But the machine and its (masculine) power is the subject of the photograph, not the patient. It was not so widely broadcast that the woman it was aiming at died from cervical cancer shortly after her publicized treatment.[14]

One wonders what the patient was thinking as she gazed up at the monster machine hovering over her. Did she expect it to cure her? Could she have imagined becoming a symbol of medical progress despite her own demise? Decades later, when patients were asked what they "see" when treated with radiation, they reported frightening images of lightning, bombs, and fire.[15]

The studies in Part II illustrate various ways in which academic and industrial engineers worked with radiologists to attract funding to build new devices, collaborated with or established companies to manufacture them, worked with or operated clinical services to test and use them, and publicized their accomplishments. Each project sought to build a technology that would boom financially and medically—and, of course, improve patient outcomes. Would they achieve their goals?

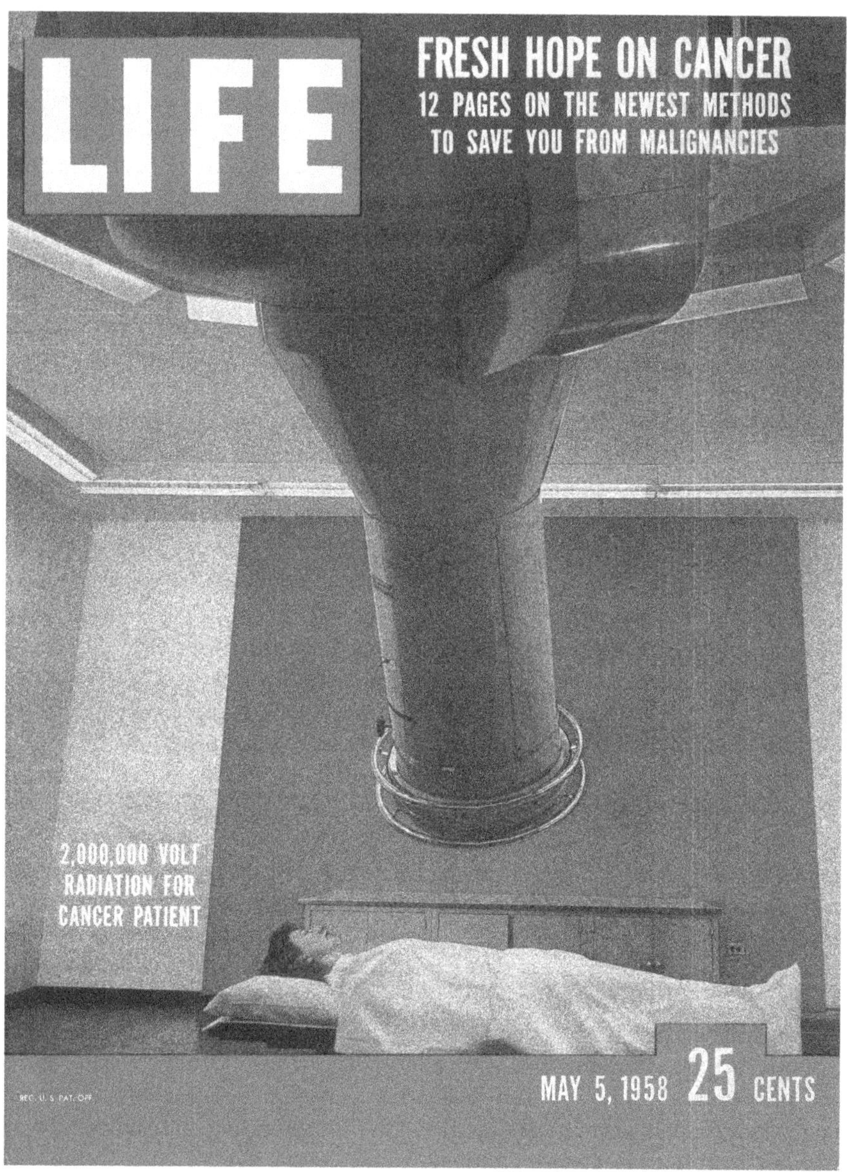

Figure II.1 Megavoltage Achieves Iconic Status.

Source: *Life*, May 5, 1958.
Photographer: Esther Bubley. Courtesy Getty Images

Notes

1 Robert Heilbroner and Aaron Singer, *The Economic Transformation of America: 1600 to the Present* (Fort Worth: Harcourt Brace, 1994), 323–326.
2 *General Electric X-ray News* February 1956; *General Electric X-ray News* April 1956. The Ford program amounted to approximately one-third of the Hill–Burton authorization in its first decade.
3 Ronald Andersen and John F. Newman, "Societal and Individual Determinants of Medical Care Utilization in the United States," *Milbank Quarterly* 83 (2005): 1–28.
4 Judith R. Lave and Lester B. Lave, *The Hospital Construction Act: An Evaluation of the Hill-Burton Program, 1948–1973* (Washington: American Enterprise Institute for Public Policy Research, 1974).
5 US Department of Health and Human Services, *Health Capital Is$ues* (Washington: 1981), 6–8.
6 Beth Mintz and Michael Schwartz, "Capital Formation and the United States Health Care System: The Relationship between the Private and the Public Sector," *Research in the Sociology of Health Care* 18 (2000): 229–248.
7 Otha W. Linton, *The American College of Radiology: The First 75 Years* (Reston, VA: American College of Radiology, 1997), 73–78.
8 Gerald F. Pyle, *Heart Disease, Cancer and Stroke in Chicago: A Geographical Analysis with Facilities, Plans for 1980* University of Chicago Department of Geography Research Paper No. 134 (Chicago: University of Chicago, 1971), 164.
9 Otha W. Linton, *The World of Stanford Radiology: 1901–2006* (Palo Alto: The Departments of Radiology and Radiation Oncology, Stanford University, 2006), 106.
10 Sixth International Congress of Radiology, *Preliminary Programme* (London: The Congress, 1950), 26.
11 Elizabeth Toon, "Does Bigger Mean Better? British Perspectives on American Cancer Treatment and Research, 1948," *Journal of Clinical Oncology* 25 (2007): 5831–5834.
12 Sixth International Congress of Radiology, *Abstracts of Papers* (London: The Congress, 1950).
13 "Cancer—On Brink of Breakthroughs," *Life* 44 (1958): 102–112.
14 Devra Davis, *The Secret History of the War on Cancer* (New York: Basic Books, 2007), 108.
15 Brittany Ashcroft, "Public Perceptions about Radiation Oncology," *ASTRO News* Spring 2014, 15.https://www.astro.org/uploadedFiles/Main_Site/News_and_Media/ASTROnews/Spring_2014/Spring2014issue.pdf accessed May 28, 2015.

5 Megavoltage Competition in Academia and Industry

Most of the participants in the megavoltage race before World War II resumed it afterwards. The Massachusetts Institute of Technology (MIT) held a stronger position than the University of California (UC) in pioneering not only a new technology but also a university–industry amalgamation to manufacture the technology and a new way of financing it. With its fingers in every supervoltage pie, the General Electric Company (GE) might have taken the prize.

General Electric Tries Everything

General Electric's medical X-ray development lagged during the war as the company devoted its research to military production. Its newsletter reassured medical customers, however, that company sales and service offices would remain open during the war, even if representatives could not drop by as often as they previously had.[1] GE designed a 1 MeV resonance transformer for general military use during the war and installed one for radiation therapy in the army's Walter Reed Hospital. Praising its capabilities at professional meetings, Walter Reed radiologist (not University of Chicago economist) Milton Friedman claimed in 1944 that "whatever high voltage (200 kv) can accomplish, supervoltage (1000 kv) can do much better."[2] He would come to doubt that belief.

Investigators using GE's 1 MeV device at New York's Memorial Hospital found—discouragingly—that most of the first 300 patients treated on the machine were dead 5 years later.[3] Many of the cancers were advanced to begin with, but the radiotherapists had hoped that their new high-powered machine would benefit that very population. Another Memorial Hospital study observed that megavoltage X-ray treatments played a significant palliative role for some cancers but concluded that "so far this study does not lend encouragement to the hope that million volt roentgen therapy may lead to a high percentage of five year survivals."[4]

Whether or not the company was disappointed in the performance of its resonance transformer, GE cultivated relationships with universities that were building a range of other megavoltage devices. Soon after collaborating with University of Illinois physicist Donald Kerst on his betatron, the company announced it would be marketing a 50 MeV betatron for medical treatment. Patent wars with the European Siemens and Brown-Boveri companies, however, may have discouraged GE betatron efforts.[5] General Electric also built a cobalt-60 irradiator for the University of Texas M.D. Anderson Hospital, adapted its 70 MeV synchrotron for the University of California, and held options on MIT's Van de Graaff patents. Finally, it signed an agreement with Stanford to build a medical linear accelerator and announced in 1954 that the device should be on the market within a few years.[6] But the company did not bring any of these machines to commercial fruition. As a huge, multiproduct corporation, GE could afford to hold claims on a range of products while waiting for the one that would dominate the market—and, in the meantime, profitably sell other appliances.

General Electric continued to build its product line in the lower X-ray voltages. Every important hospital, its newspaper advised, required a superficial X-ray machine, along with a 250 kv and a 400 kv device; even small community hospitals, the paper advised, deserved 250 kilovolts.[7] GE's competitive upgrading of its machines contributed to the competitive upgrading of radiology procedure units. The company also promoted the cancer center strategy that required complete collections of available equipment. The University of Buffalo's Roswell Park Cancer Institute, for instance, boasted GE megavoltage plus nine other devices ranging from 45 to 400 kv.[8]

Boosting its resonance transformer to 2 MeV in the 1950s, GE placed two devices in New York City—one at the city's Frances Delafield cancer hospital and the other at the Hospital for Joint Diseases. The radiologists in these hospitals worked with GE staff to study the clinical performance of their new machines, and the company (again) announced that studies demonstrated that megavoltage was "definitely superior" to kilovoltage.[9] The company conceded, however, that not all radiologists agreed with this assessment. It cited one therapist who claimed that recent developments in X-ray therapy had "added only about 5 percent salvage in spite of a very considerable degree of damage to the skin and adjacent tissues."[10] But GE forecast "real benefit" in terms of therapeutic, as well as professional and economic, gain.

Perceiving hospitals as "big business," GE's newspaper continued to instruct their administrators in management. Hospitals should enhance medical productivity, the paper advised, by applying methods of scientific management to clinical care and by purchasing equipment on the basis of projected revenues.[11] The company also pumped up popular advertising in order to increase demand for radiology's expanding supply.

GE designed a series of advertisements for the mass-market *Newsweek* magazine. The American College of Radiology–approved ads aimed at community "thought leaders"—identified as physicians, business executives, clergymen, lawyers, and engineers—dramatized the "indispensable role" of radiology in modern medicine.[12] The first such ad portrayed a sentimental greeting card–type scene of a grandmother and two grandchildren in a comfortable living room. Captioned "Death Took a Holiday," the ad emphasized that grandma would not be in the picture but for the radiologist who found her cancer, the radiologist who "attacked the cancer with a carefully planned sequence of X-ray treatments," and the surgeon who removed it.[13] The ad was patently designed to promote (paying) patient demand for X-ray examinations and treatments at a time when the medical profession prohibited provider-specific advertising.

Medical centers purchasing GE devices also engaged in publicizing the devices along with their own services. Hollywood's photogenic Ronald Reagan (third from right in Figure 5.1), employed by General Electric to soothe community as well as labor relations,[14] arrived in 1953 to celebrate Baylor University Medical School's new 2 MeV resonance transformer. University radiologists appreciated that Reagan's appearance conferred star power on their department, which went on to claim national prominence in radiology based on its high-powered therapeutic equipment.[15] Reagan's hosting of GE's popular television show, *General Electric Theater*, conferred on him national prominence that he would later parlay into a political career that would—among other things—lobby against socialized medicine and dismantle regulatory attempts to curtail excessive technology growth in hospitals.

Despite the star power of Hollywood and the radiologists using GE machines, the company did not maintain the dominant position in medical radiation it had enjoyed before the war. While US X-ray sales (diagnostic and therapeutic) quintupled from 1929 to 1947, GE's market share dropped from half to less than a third.[16] Staking claims on virtually the entire range of postwar radiation therapy devices, the company seemed to be searching for a breakthrough that—like its 1913 and 1920 Coolidge tubes—would recover its market monopoly. It undoubtedly hoped that its resonance transformer could accomplish the task, but the company would, in the end, sell only 31 of them.[17] Meanwhile, the High Voltage Engineering Corporation threatened to capture the market.

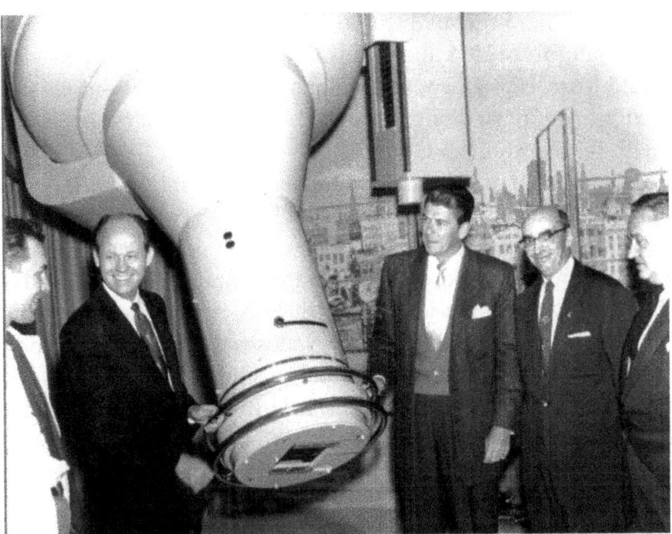

Figure 5.1 A Movie Star Advertises GE Radiation Therapy.

Courtesy Baylor University Medical Center.

High Voltage and Venture Capital at MIT

Fortune magazine was not surprised that the General Electric Company had extended its tentacles into every aspect of medical radiation. How then, it wondered in 1950, could a small start-up company surpass the mighty GE?[18] The High Voltage Engineering Corporation (HVEC) boasted only one technology, the magazine noted, the Massachusetts Institute of Technology's Van de Graaff electrostatic X-ray generator, while GE was developing the entire spectrum of radiation machines. But, at a little over half of GE's price, HVEC's 2 MeV Van de Graaff was outselling GE's 2 MeV resonance transformer.

Having arranged for his MIT engineering lab to continue its X-ray work while he was away during the war, John Trump jumped back in immediately afterwards. Trump founded HVEC after several abortive attempts to get existing companies interested in manufacturing his technology. General Electric had tried to license Van de Graaff patents in the 1930s, but MIT would not accept the company's exclusive licensing demands.[19] On its own terms, the Institute awarded GE a two-year option, which the company allowed to lapse. Subsequently, MIT dropped a contractual agreement with Picker X-ray, and Westinghouse dropped an agreement with MIT. Whether or not he had desired these efforts to succeed, Trump was able to fulfill his wartime dream of building a company to produce commercial Van de Graaff accelerators for medical treatment.[20] By June 1946, he had decided the company's name and sent its prospectus to a select group of people.

"Dear Mom," Trump wrote (making a carbon copy for posterity), his dream of the High Voltage Engineering Corporation was about to become reality. He had found the right building and the "right people" to finance the new company.[21] The right people were Karl Compton, MIT president; Merrill Griswold, chairman of the trustees of Massachusetts Investors Trust; and Ralph Flanders, engineer, industrialist, president of the Federal Reserve Bank of Boston, and soon-to-become Republican senator from Vermont. This group had an idea for a new kind of business that would finance commercial development of university-originated technological inventions and, in so doing, generate new investment channels and new sources of wealth for investor capital.

In creating the American Research & Development Corporation (ARD), the Boston-based group helped invent the venture capital industry. The "increasing degree to which the liquid wealth of the nation is tending to concentrate in fiduciary hands," ARD's brochure explained, was impeding the financing of innovative companies.[22] ARD would free up the idle capital held by insurance companies and educational institutions and invest it in new industrial growth. In the process, it would expand investment outlets for local businesses and institutions. Massachusetts Investors Trust and John Hancock Life Insurance invested in the new company, as did several universities, including MIT.[23] This was the beginning of a productive relationship in which high-tech medicine and the venture capital industry reinforced each other.

Karl Compton's ARD involvement complemented MIT's long dedication to advancing regional industrial development by capitalizing its own scientific work.[24] As institute president, he consciously extended his wartime duties of coordinating governmental, educational, and industrial research to postwar technology development. Compton and other MIT personnel became deeply engaged in ARD's mission; Compton served on its board, MIT's treasurer served as ARD treasurer, MIT department heads comprised ARD's scientific advisory board, and MIT initially housed some of the ARD-funded companies.[25] Not surprisingly, ARD's first investments were MIT spin-offs: Tracerlab for radioactive isotopes and HVEC for the Van de Graaff generator. Trump accommodated MIT patent policies to ARD terms, and the institute granted HVEC a 10-year exclusive license on Van de Graaff patents.[26]

The American Research & Development Corporation intentionally selected companies that held critical patents—or other specialized knowledge that would lead to competitive advantage—and took equity positions in them.[27] ARD held 60 percent of HVEC's stock, and Trump and Van de Graaff each held 13 percent.[28] ARD actively managed the companies it financed, placing its own board members on their boards. ARD president Georges Doriot served on HVEC's board of directors along with Compton and closely monitored the company's economic performance. Initially considered a high-risk investment, HVEC shares were the major contributor to a 200 percent leap in ARD's net assets in its first 3 years.[29] HVEC's radiation therapy business not only owed its own existence to venture capital, it reinforced the development of the venture-capital industry, which provided a new conduit for capital flow to medical care.

Trump worked simultaneously for MIT and HVEC, which were themselves closely interwoven. He had expected to serve as full-time president of the company in addition to his duties as full-time MIT professor, but ARD vetoed that option.[30] Nonetheless, Trump "doubled as the very active Technical Director and Chairman of the Board of the new company, and continued his full time duties and development work as professor at MIT," as HVEC president Denis Robinson later appreciated.[31] Trump would appear on company books for half-time work and receive payments equivalent to three-quarters of Robinson's salary in addition to his MIT salary.[32] Trump's dual roles and their inherent potential conflict of interest did not escape rival General Electric.

In a 1951 letter to James Killian, MIT's new president, a GE vice-president contended that Trump's endorsement as MIT faculty member of a product with which he was commercially involved constituted unethical behavior.[33] Killian responded that the institute did not restrict faculty members' business activities or board memberships, but he strenuously—if disingenuously—asserted that "MIT has no interest in the commercial product or the company making this commercial product." He further objected to the accusation that Trump "improperly used his status as a consultant to influence the purchase of a piece of equipment in which [Trump] has a special interest."[34] Because Trump did, or at least would in the future, influence purchases of equipment in which he had both professional and financial interests, the argument may have hinged on the perception of *improper*. Trump's standard procedure when radiologists and hospital administrators contacted him at MIT's High Voltage Research Laboratory (HVRL) for advice on purchasing radiation therapy equipment would be to refer them to HVEC, which would send follow-up reports back to the MIT lab.[35] When Killian fought back, however, GE backed down and apologized for any unintended impropriety.[36]

Trump's High Voltage Research Laboratory continued to conduct research congruent with the interests of the High Voltage Engineering Corporation. The company depended on the lab for product assessment and new ideas, and the lab's *raison d'être* became technical support for the company as well as for the field of radiotherapy in general. Trump built up the lab as a research and consultation center for radiation physics and radiation treatment planning. Supported by government and foundation-funded research grants, the lab would gain national and international repute for the therapeutic procedures it studied, used, and taught. Lab staff investigated biological reactions of living tissue to high-voltage X-rays, measured dose distribution, advised doctors on the use of X-ray machines, and developed accessories for those machines. As Trump would pronounce in one of its progress reports, the High Voltage Research Laboratory was a "forerunner in the use of megavolt X-rays and electrons for the control of malignant disease."[37] MIT's development and use of a medical technology exemplified a tightly-knit collaboration of education, finance, and manufacturing. But (after the earlier brief connection with the Massachusetts General Hospital), the lab was missing an essential ingredient—medical delivery. The lab turned to Boston's Lahey Clinic for collaboration in developing the medical radiation program planned in its 1939 grant report.

In 1949, Trump contacted Hugh Hare, Lahey's radiology chief, and invited members of Hare's department over to MIT to view his lab's facilities and machines.[38] Lahey started sending patients across the river for treatments at MIT shortly thereafter. As MIT saw it, Lahey radiologists supervised the clinical care, and lab engineers supervised the radiation treatments. The exchange was mutually advantageous; MIT provided Lahey megavoltage capacity, and Lahey provided MIT medical legitimacy—and patients.

Trump co-authored medical journal articles with Lahey radiologists, and Denis Robinson would come to boast that the "top radiologists" in the world accepted Trump as an "expert with them in super-voltage therapy" (although some clearly did not, as seen below).[39] Trump's purpose in establishing the joint clinical program was to expedite the "evaluation, acceptance, and effective use of [Van de Graaff] supervoltage therapy technique in the shortest possible time."[40] The MIT–Lahey connection clearly benefitted HVEC.

Robinson assured ARD's Doriot that the High Voltage Engineering Corporation (HVEC) was "closely associated" with the Lahey–High Voltage Research Laboratory clinic.[41] The high voltage company appreciated technical feedback from the clinic along with suggestions of improvements and commercially viable accessories for its equipment.[42] HVEC utilized the laboratory's research and its clinical connections with Lahey to persuade potential purchasers to choose the Van de Graaff over its competitors.[43] But HVEC had to report to Doriot in 1952 that its sales to the medical market were low and that the company would work to improve the situation.[44]

Trump and Hare actively publicized their technology and their treatments in the popular media, marketing their medical therapy directly to the American public. Glibly calling Trump's method of rotating the patient an "X-ray barbecue," *Life* magazine vaguely asserted that most of the people so treated in the previous six months had "substantially benefited."[45] *Newsweek* similarly credited Trump with "spectacular progress in the field of radiation." Van de Graaff X-rays "pin-pointed on the cancer target," it contended, "leaving the healthy tissues untouched."[46] Promoters of each new technology would reiterate this theoretical claim again and again over the next 60 years. While the fanfare of publicity about Trump and his 2 MeV device in *Fortune*, *Life*, *Newsweek*, and *Business Week* advanced medical marketing, it also generated professional backlash.

Massachusetts General Hospital radiology chief Laurence Robbins fired off a letter to Trump complaining about the *Newsweek* article. As president of the New England Roentgen Ray Society, Robbins wrote, it was his duty to report the situation to the society's Committee on Ethics and Hospital–Physician Relations. Not only did the article raise "unfounded hope for many incurable patients," he charged, but even "more important," the article falsely associated Trump with the Massachusetts General Hospital.[47] Robbins further reprimanded Trump for reporting medical results, acidly reminding him that he was not a physician. Trump responded that it was *Newsweek* that had associated him with Mass General (although it hadn't, literally), and he wearily reminded Robbins that they had already hashed out the "reporting of medical results" issue.[48]

The American College of Radiology (ACR) weighed in when it asked University of California radiologist Henry Garland—of all people—to respond to the issue. Garland had already accused Hugh Hare of overselling megavoltage and, what's more, of stealing patients from the university. There was no need for patients to go all the way to Boston for megavoltage, he had charged, when perfectly good [kilovoltage] treatment was in San Francisco.[49] Although ACR may not have known of this dispute conducted via private correspondence, Garland was known for a feisty hostility to supervoltage. Living up to his reputation, Garland queried "New Hope or New Hoax?" in ACR's August 1954 newsletter. He accused fund-raising organizations like the American Cancer Society of "over-optimistic, journalistic 'cures'" and charged that a "'sales approach' has been substituted for the judicious skepticism of science."[50] He cited scientific reports finding that 5-year cancer cures following megavoltage treatments were not substantially different from those following kilovoltage treatments, and he quoted a condemnation of "fiendish torture" inflicted on cancer patients that had appeared in the 1953 *Year Book of Radiology*.

Magnus Smedal, Hare's successor at Lahey, complained to the ACR about its "Hoax" article. Although he did not contest the over-optimism, Smedal deplored that the college had not seen fit to contact the Lahey–MIT program before publishing Garland's diatribe. He challenged the allegation that physicists controlled the program by insisting that radiologists were more involved in patient treatments at MIT than they were in most hospitals. "How many people in this country doing therapy," he inquired in a draft (but deleted in the final letter), "have the same degree of control over their patients?"[51]

Lahey's connection with MIT, while enhancing the lab's reputation, did not boost sales of its radiotherapy device. The High Voltage Engineering Corporation found a more profitable market for its machines in physics labs conducting Cold War research. Some of its investors and managers still deemed HVEC's sales figures to be insufficient, however, and they urged the company to diversify its single-product business. An internal financial memo recommended that the company get into the promising linear accelerator business.[52]

HVEC contracted to build a Stanford-type linear accelerator for the Argonne Cancer Research Hospital, the Chicago-area facility built and lavishly equipped under the Atoms for Peace program. The company widely proclaimed the deal: "With the successful completion of this pioneering effort," it announced in 1954, High Voltage Engineering Corporation "can now add linear accelerator technique to its already broad engineering ability in the design and construction of atom-smashers for medicine, research, and industry."[53] The *Wall Street Journal* picked up HVEC's announcement that it was ready to manufacture a commercial linear accelerator, and the proposed venture boosted the company's initial stock offering.[54]

Boston's C. E. Unterberg, Towbin Co. investment bank took High Voltage Engineering Corporation public nine months after its linear-accelerator announcement. The bank's prospectus for the company acclaimed the clinical and engineering expertise of HVEC staff and its MIT advisors and proclaimed that the HVEC Argonne accelerator would "prove a valuable extension of the company's leadership in therapy equipment."[55] Belmont Towbin played conflicting—if common—multiple roles in the process: he served as HVEC director, his company sold HVEC stock, and he advised newspaper readers to purchase the stock. Its public offering meant that HVEC had to meet the demands of its own stockholders as well as those of ARD, both of which expected expanding growth and profits. By this time, ARD's initial investment in HVEC had multiplied nine-fold.[56] But HVEC would not enter the linear accelerator business, and Wall Street pressured it to sell more Van de Graaff devices.

HVEC stockholders did not get the growth they had hoped for. The Donner Foundation accounted for a significant portion of the company's medical sales by funding the 1956 purchase of 12 Van de Graaffs for installation in teaching hospitals across the country.[57] The Donner installations did not catalyze further hospital sales, however, and Trump embellished his efforts to sell High Voltage Engineering Corporation products and High Voltage Research Laboratory services to the medical community. He achieved greater success with the services. He attained sponsorship from the New England Roentgen Ray Society to train radiology residents in radiation physics, and he invited radiologists to participate in his MIT course on "Engineering and Medical Innovation."[58] Even as its device did not become a major clinical success, HVEC and HVRL led the way in marketing radiation therapy and making it a collaborative production of industry, academia, and medical care.

Trump wore multiple hats in the process. He concurrently represented the high-voltage laboratory and the high-voltage corporation—as Robinson had acclaimed and General Electric had accused. When the administrator of Monmouth Medical Center in New Jersey wrote him at the lab requesting consultation on purchasing a machine that could best expand the medical center's patient volume in radiation therapy,[59] Trump made a personal visit to the hospital. He advised the administrator that a 2 MeV X-ray machine—which at the time had to mean an HVEC Van de Graaff or a GE resonance transformer—would best meet the hospital's needs, and he invited the hospital's radiotherapist to visit his lab at MIT.[60] Lab staff escorted the Monmouth visitor to the High Voltage Engineering Corporation, where he admitted he was there only to please his hospital board and that what he really wanted was a betatron, which he felt would be more prestigious and draw more patients.[61] But when HVEC staff showed him its Van de Graaff and the Peter Bent Brigham Hospital's linear accelerator, he changed his view. Monmouth hospital purchased a Van de Graaff for the short term and planned to buy a linear accelerator after the Van de Graaff machine had attracted a sufficient patient load to support the more costly device.[62] Monmouth, like many radiologists, hospitals, and clinics, was using high-powered radiation therapy to enhance its status and revenues.

Lacking a medical facility, MIT had built a freestanding radiation therapy clinic connected to its lab on campus. The success of the first treatment center and its affiliation with Lahey allowed Trump to build a larger cancer research laboratory and treatment center in 1965.[63] The Lahey Clinic Foundation contributed substantially to the new building, its medical treatment costs, and its operational expenses.[64] Radiology residents rotated in from Boston-area hospitals, and radiation physicists from the High Voltage Research Lab staffed the new high-voltage facility, built to treat 45 patients a day.

Despite the MIT–Lahey showcase for its product, however, HVEC continued to struggle with low medical sales and low stock prices. Attempting to quell jitters in the capital markets, President Robinson reassured the New York Society of Security Analysts in 1964 that none of the company's 16 competitors came close to HVEC's 50 percent share of the total particle acceleration market.[65] Conceding the company's recent decline and volatility in its stock, Merrill Lynch financial management attempted to revive HVEC stock by issuing a wire flash that projected significant HVEC recovery and long-range growth.[66]

American Research & Development Corporation president Georges Doriot also monitored HVEC's position in the stock market and tried to impose managerial methods to boost sales. Research needed to translate into equipment orders, he harangued Robinson; he needed to develop new ways to apply radiation.[67] Doriot also reminded the company's board of directors that listing on the New York Stock Exchange required measuring achievement in terms of profitability.[68] Finally, he accused HVEC of relying too much on the government as a customer.[69]

But a whole new era of government funding opened up in the same year, and the company expected to gain from it. A 1965 HVEC marketing memo suggested that the new Medicare and Medicaid programs would help the company sell more machines.[70] Trump convened a special meeting of the company's R&D Policy Committee to consider (once again) commercial development of a 3 MeV Van de

Graaff device. He argued that the anticipated expansion of hospital facilities and paying patients in addition to rising cancer incidence would support continuing growth in radiation therapy.[71] He even suggested that the upgraded Van de Graaff might replace existing cobalt installations and capture a significant share of the radiation therapy market.[72] But, although the policy committee approved the customary procedure in which HVEC would construct a prototype, the High Voltage Research Laboratory would improve upon it, and the MIT–Lahey program would test it clinically, the company did not market a 3 MeV device.

The government programs did pay for significant laboratory and clinic growth, however, and the MIT–Lahey clinical facility would come to provide a large portion of the High Voltage Research Laboratory's budget.[73] The Lahey Clinic left the joint venture, which had treated more than 15,000 patients over the course of 25 years, only when it built a new hospital complex of its own in the mid-1970s. As chairman of the Lahey Clinic Foundation Board of Trustees at that time, Trump raised funds for a new clinic and 200-bed hospital on a 40-acre site on Massachusetts' high-tech Route 128 corridor, conveniently across the road from High Voltage Engineering Corporation—if not so conveniently for patients.

The first building in Lahey's new complex housed a clinic and a radiation therapy center named for Trump. The Trump center was equipped with the Van de Graaff device used at MIT plus a new linear accelerator. Lahey's financial feasibility studies, certified by accounting firm Price Waterhouse, projected that income from radiation therapy alone would cover most of the costs of building a whole new hospital.[74] Lahey expected MIT staff to continue to "assist, advise, admonish and monitor" its radiation therapy service.[75] Presumably expecting to benefit from Lahey's new proximity itself, HVEC donated $100,000 to the new facility.[76]

Trump made a career out of developing, testing, and promoting the Van de Graaff accelerator for X-ray treatment of cancer. He dedicated his research laboratory to formulating clinical techniques using the device, collaborated with a medical specialty to test and promote it, spun off a company to manufacture it, helped build the venture-capital industry to fund technological innovation, taught hospital administrators and radiologists how to use the new high-powered technology and the public to accept it, and helped build a new medical center for its major champion. These interlocking interests built a medical–industrial complex in itself. MIT also demonstrated the financial feasibility of a freestanding radiation therapy procedure unit with relatively loose medical connections. Despite the fact that its own device underachieved in the market, MIT provided a model for future developments in radiation therapy.

Ultimately, the High Voltage Engineering Corporation did not measure up to *Fortune* magazine's expectations. Total medical installations of the Van de Graaff barely exceeded those of the competing 2 MeV device, the GE resonance transformer. Many radiologists and hospital administrators thought that the technology was too large, clunky, and technologically unsophisticated. But (together with the GE device) the Van de Graaff set a multimillion-volt benchmark in radiation therapy. The synchrotron was the biggest of them all.

The Most Powerful of All at California

The University of California appreciated that, having headed radiation safety for the Manhattan project, its radiology chief was "well placed" to channel federal funding to its medical school in San Francisco. The Atomic Energy Commission and the National Institutes of Health joined the American Cancer Society in funding Robert Stone's new radiological laboratory as part of the university's project to build a "great medical school by the Golden Gate."[77]

Having already led the clinical use of neutrons from the Lawrence cyclotron and supervoltage X-rays from the Sloan device, Stone chose the most powerful of all: a 70 MeV synchrotron. Other machines in other radiology departments occupied energy niches up to 30 MeV, he noted, reasoning that an even higher level was the best way to retain a position of professional leadership.[78] His choice was ironic in light of his earlier vigorous refutation of the claim that higher voltages led to better treatments and more cancer cures.[79] But the Soviet Union, the country's Cold War nemesis, was building a medical synchrotron, and General Electric had the technology available. GE built California's medical synchrotron using Lawrence Laboratory technologies and a wartime machine it had built for the Office of Naval Research, and it announced its delivery in 1952.[80] It took 5 more years to make the machine clinically operational, however, and in the meantime Stone had to read reports of synchrotron use in the United Kingdom and publicity about US radiotherapists who were outleading him.

Besides proving his leadership by experimenting with ultra-high voltage, Stone felt he needed it to retain patients—important ones in particular. When radiologist Hugh Hare moved from the MIT–Lahey Clinic program to the Los Angeles Tumor Institute in 1953, he applied to the California division of the American Cancer Society (ACS) for a grant to purchase a 2 MeV Van de Graaff device. Unfortunately for Hare, Stone received the request as the appropriate California ACS official. Stone first straightforwardly informed Hare that grants of that size were available only from the national society or from the National Institutes of Health. His resentment about previous events then spewed forth and, "speaking as an individual," he accused Hare of stealing patients.

After first arranging treatment at UC, Stone charged, an influential patient with advanced cancer had traveled across the country to receive treatments at MIT. Reiterating Henry Garland's complaints, Stone charged that—in the absence of 5- and 10-year outcome data—Hare could not possibly justify telling patients that traveling to Boston for multimillion-volt therapy was their "only hope of cure."[81] The purloined patient's son, president of the Ford Foundation, weighed in and brought up patient choice, acidly informing Stone that he and his father had chosen to go to the prestigious MIT– Lahey Clinic program.[82] This episode must have strengthened Stone's resolve to get his own multi-megavoltage machine in working order. He might also have been justified in believing that the highest-level technology was necessary in retaining the highest-level patients.

Stone reacted vehemently against what he saw as advertising and deceptive publicity about the MIT program and its Van de Graaff device. The *San Francisco*

Examiner published an article that "made me spill so much adrenalin," Stone complained to the American Cancer Society's Charles Cameron, that he'd better cool off before sounding off.[83] The opening sentence of the article that had hyperstimulated his adrenal glands proclaimed that "The American Cancer Society reports today that a mighty new X-ray cannon is mowing down tumors with an efficiency beyond scientists' dreams." The article featured Hare, Trump, MIT, and their multimillion-volt Van de Graaff generator. Stone accused Cameron of damaging ACS's reputation with overblown publicity and advertising a particular machine at a particular institution.

Stone—or Cameron—attached to Cameron's response another newspaper clipping that credited Van de Graaff X-ray treatments with saving "hopeless cancer victims from the grave." "Two million-volt X-ray treatments abolished all signs of cancer in 5 of 23 patients whose lung cancers were too extensive for surgery," the article claimed.[84] Articles like these, Stone told Cameron, made patients receiving therapy in ordinary hospitals on ordinary machines (like the ones he had at the time) "feel as if they are being cheated out of something." Stone again stressed that longer survival studies were necessary to justify such a confident outlook. After 5 or 10 years, he predicted, "you will have difficulty showing that a single additional case has been cured by this machine who might not have been cured by standard 200 or 250 kv x-rays."[85] This was a curious acknowledgment coming from the radiologist working so hard to put a 70 MeV synchrotron into clinical use—although it was in accord with much professional thought at the time. Cameron conceded in response that the newspaper articles generated from ACS publicity could be construed as advertising, but he rationalized that he would not want to be accused of withholding information.[86] This example of MIT–Van de Graaff advertising (seen from Stone's point of view) illustrates how engineers and radiotherapists publicized their services and used their cancer guns to battle over patients.

After some delay, Stone expressed condolences to the Ford Foundation president regarding his father's death. Stone even refrained from pointing out that the father seemed to have died from acute complications of the treatments he had received at MIT (or at least, Henry Garland so thought).[87] Stone also ostensibly sent Hare an apology for inserting personal opinions into his "semi-official" ACS letter, but then once again carried on with his grudgments. A "hopeless incurable patient was put to the inconvenience of going across the continent for treatments," he charged. He further phrased as an ethical principle that a "doctor must not entice patients from his colleagues."[88] Stone accused Hare of (1) advertising his services, (2) making false claims of therapeutic efficacy, and (3) taking over "another doctor's patient while the original physician is still in charge of the case and has neither relinquished the case nor been dismissed by the patient" (having learned his lesson about patient choice, it seems). Stone also noted that the medical profession needed to review the issue.

Stone made good on his threat and wrote the Los Angeles County Medical Association to challenge the fanfare of publicity that had accompanied Hare's move from the Lahey Clinic to the Los Angeles Tumor Institute. This kind of publicity, he suggested, constituted advertising that Hare himself could have instigated.[89] Stone further accused that Hare's appearance on a Los Angeles television program served as "very thinly veiled advertising" for high-voltage Van de Graaff therapy at the Los Angeles Tumor Institute.

Stone's vendetta continued in a letter written to the Rosenstiel Foundation in New York City. He accused its director of recommending that another of his department's patients travel from San Francisco to Los Angeles for the "Hare Trump method of treatment" on the Tumor Institute's new 2 MeV Van de Graaff machine.[90] "You might wonder what business it is of mine to write you at all," Stone conceded, but, as professor of radiology and former member of the National Advisory Cancer Council, he claimed a responsibility to those who "might be influenced by the name of a prominent foundation." He advised the foundation director that there was no professional consensus on the superiority of the megavoltage Van de Graaff treatments and that she was encroaching on medical prerogatives. In response, the director pulled out all the East Coast prestige and rank stops on the Californian, attributing her recommendations to a "most distinguished and high ranking member of the medical profession … chief of an important service in one of the highest ranking and esteemed hospitals, and clinical professor in one of the highest ranking medical schools in the country."[91] Both sides, it seems, weighed medical treatment on the scales of academic rank and authority.

While some of the publicity was clearly over the top, hype about curing cancer and beating death was (and still is) not uncommon in medicine, and it contributed to popular and professional acceptance of radiation therapy. Stone might not have been so outraged at the Van de Graaff/Hare publicity if he'd had megavoltage of his own at the time. Stone finally did get his publicity in May 1958—and did not seem to object to the advertising. The *Life* issue with the cover photo of a 2 MeV device (Figure II.1) included a large photo of Stone's GE synchrotron along with the flamboyant claim that "science forges stupendous arsenal of new weapons."[92] At the same time, the article rather puzzlingly suggested that the megavoltage it so prominently pictured may have reached the limits of its capabilities. Although not evident from the cover and its photograph, the putative "fresh hope" the magazine identified was chemotherapy.

San Francisco investigators obtained a series of publications out of their new synchrotron, but they did not obtain improved outcomes, and they decommissioned their costly machine after only a few years.[93] The answer to their research question, they advised, was that ultra-high voltage did not raise curative outcomes or palliative benefits for cancer patients.

The widespread photography and photogenicity of the synchrotron and other high-voltage devices, however, enhanced radiation therapy's appeal as the image of medical modernity. Each of the three megavoltage devices discussed in this chapter underachieved both clinically and economically. But each got its "15 minutes of fame," identified leaders, attracted grants, and taught the field more about how to market its products and services.

It was another contender, coming along around the same time, that would shatter the market. Sales of cobalt-60 teletherapy would eclipse those of the resonance transformer, the Van de Graaff, and the synchrotron put together. Its leaders would claim that its phenomenal economic success was due to a demonstrable increase in clinical effectiveness. Was it? The following chapter examines the rise of this technology.

Notes

1 *Victor News* March 1943.
2 Milton Friedman, "Supervoltage (One Million Volt) Roentgen Therapy at Walter Reed General Hospital," *Surgical Clinics of North America* 24 (1944): 1424–1432.
3 Alfred F. Hocker and Ruth J. Guttman, "Three and One Half Years' Experience with the 1,000 Kilovolt Roentgen Therapy Unit at Memorial Hospital," *American Journal of Roentgenology and Radium Therapy* 51 (1944): 83–94.
4 William L. Watson and Jerome Urban, "Million Volt Roentgen Therapy for Intrathoracic Cancer: Palliative Effects in a Series of Sixty-three Cases," *American Journal of Roentgenology and Radium Therapy* 49 (1943): 299–306.
5 Pedro Waloschek, "Box 7: The War of the Patents," *Life and Work of Rolf Wider e.* http://www-library.desy.de/elbooks/wideroe/WiE-CONT.htm accessed Jan 23, 2011.
6 *General Electric X-ray News* January 1954.
7 *Victor News* August 1946.
8 *Victor News* February 1947.
9 *General Electric X-ray News* February 1954.
10 Joseph H. Marks, "New England Deaconess Hospital Enlarges Program of Basic, Applied Cancer Research. High-Voltage X-ray Therapy," *General Electric X-ray News* September 1954.
11 "Industry Urges Methods to Cut Hospital Costs," *General Electric X-ray News* March 1954; "Hospital Methods Engineering Advocated for Increasing Efficiency and Economy," *General Electric X-ray News* November 1954.
12 *General Electric X-ray News* February 1955.
13 "Death Took a Holiday," *Newsweek* April 14, 1955, 11.
14 Thomas W. Evans, *The Education of Ronald Reagan: The General Electric Years and the Untold Story of his Conversion to Conservatism* (New York: Columbia University Press, 2006), 57.
15 Herbert L. Steinbach, "History of the Department of Radiology at Baylor University Medical Center," *Baylor University Medical Center Proceedings* 17 (2004): 425–431.
16 Kendall Birr, *Pioneering in Industrial Research; the Story of the General Electric Research Laboratory* (Washington: Public Affairs Press: 1957), 153.
17 Milford D. Schulz, "The Supervoltage Story," *American Journal of Roentgenology Radium Therapy and Nuclear Medicine* 124 (1975): 541–559.
18 "Supervoltage Machines," *Fortune* April 1, 1950, 113–118, 120, 124.
19 Elliot A. Fishman, "MIT Patent Policy, 1932–1946: Historical Precedents in University–Industry Technology Transfer," PhD diss., University of Pennsylvania, 1996, 159–160.
20 John Trump to Mr. and Mrs. Donald Asquith, May 16, 1946. John G. Trump papers, MC 223, Box 12. Massachusetts Institute of Technology. Institute Archives and Special Collections, MIT Libraries, Cambridge, MA.
21 John Trump letter, "Dear Mom," September 4, 1946. John G. Trump papers, MC 223, Box 12. Massachusetts Institute of Technology. Institute Archives and Special Collections, MIT Libraries, Cambridge, MA.
22 American Research and Development Corporation, Brochure, January 1, 1947. American Research and Development Corporation, MC 495, Box 1. Massachusetts Institute of Technology. Institute Archives and Special Collections, MIT Libraries, Cambridge, MA.

23 Robert Teitelman, *Profits of Science: The American Marriage of Business and Technology* (New York: Basic Books, 1994), 84, 88–89.
24 Henry Etzkowitz, *M.I.T. and the Rise of Entrepreneurial Science* (New York: Routledge, 2002), 1–2.
25 Edward B. Roberts, *Entrepreneurs in High Technology: Lessons from M.I.T. and Beyond* (New York: Oxford University Press, 1991), 34, 132–134.
26 American Research and Development Corporation, Prospectus, March 15, 1950. American Research and Development Corporation, MC 495, Box 1. Massachusetts Institute of Technology. Institute Archives and Special Collections, MIT Libraries, Cambridge, MA; Elliot A. Fishman, "M.I.T. Patent Policy, 1932–1946: Historical Precedents in University–Industry Technology Transfer," PhD diss. University of Pennsylvania, 1996, 28, 173.
27 American Research and Development Corporation, Brochure, January 1, 1947. American Research and Development Corporation, MC 495, Box 1. Massachusetts Institute of Technology. Institute Archives and Special Collections, MIT Libraries, Cambridge, MA.
28 "Supervoltage Machines," *Fortune* April 1, 1950, 113–118, 120, 124.
29 Spencer E. Ante, *Creative Capital: Georges Doriot and the Birth of Venture Capital* (Boston: Harvard Business Press, 2008), 143.
30 Elliot A. Fishman, "M.I.T. Patent Policy, 1932–1946: Historical Precedents in University–Industry Technology Transfer," PhD diss., University of Pennsylvania, 1996, 168.
31 Denis Robinson, "Men, Atoms and Enterprise in a Favorable Economic Climate," address at Newcomen Society in North America, May 1, 1962. John G. Trump papers, MC 223, Box 3. Massachusetts Institute of Technology. Institute Archives and Special Collections, MIT Libraries, Cambridge, MA.
32 "Agreements of Employment," Board of Directors Meeting, January 1, 1967. William W. Buechner Papers. MC 229, Box 1. Massachusetts Institute of Technology. Institute Archives and Special Collections, MIT Libraries, Cambridge, MA.
33 Ralph M. Darrin to James R. Killian Jr., August 27, 1951. John G. Trump papers, MC 223, Box 12. Massachusetts Institute of Technology. Institute Archives and Special Collections, MIT Libraries, Cambridge, MA.
34 James R. Killian to Ralph M. Darrin, August 29, 1951. John G. Trump papers, MC 223, Box 12. Massachusetts Institute of Technology. Institute Archives and Special Collections, MIT Libraries, Cambridge, MA.
35 Eric F. Walker to George J. Bartel, December 30, 1963. John G. Trump papers, MC 223, Box 7. Massachusetts Institute of Technology. Institute Archives and Special Collections, MIT Libraries, Cambridge, MA.
36 Ralph M. Darrin to James R. Killian, August 30, 1951. John G. Trump papers, MC 223, Box 12. Massachusetts Institute of Technology. Institute Archives and Special Collections, MIT Libraries, Cambridge, MA.
37 MIT High Voltage Research Laboratory, "Progress Report," June 1965. John G. Trump papers, MC 223, Box 9. Massachusetts Institute of Technology. Institute Archives and Special Collections, MIT Libraries, Cambridge, MA.
38 Magnus I. Smedal, "Lahey Clinic—M.I.T. Relationship," January 9, 1963. John G. Trump papers, MC 223, Box 7. Massachusetts Institute of Technology. Institute Archives and Special Collections, MIT Libraries, Cambridge, MA.
39 Denis Robinson to William F. Burt, October 30, 1959. John G. Trump papers, MC 223, Box 3. Massachusetts Institute of Technology. Institute Archives and Special Collections, MIT Libraries, Cambridge, MA.
40 John G. Trump, "High Voltage Research Laboratory: Building 28 Program," June 15, 1950. John G. Trump papers, MC 223, Box 4. Massachusetts Institute of Technology. Institute Archives and Special Collections, MIT Libraries, Cambridge, MA.

41 Denis Robinson to Georges F. Doriot, December 9, 1952. John G. Trump papers, MC 223, Box 3. Massachusetts Institute of Technology. Institute Archives and Special Collections, MIT Libraries, Cambridge, MA.
42 Kenneth A. Wright to James Bly, January 11, 1957. John G. Trump papers, MC 223, Box 3. Massachusetts Institute of Technology. Institute Archives and Special Collections, MIT Libraries, Cambridge, MA.
43 High Voltage Engineering Corporation, "Financial Summary," no date, figures cover data through 1952. John G. Trump papers, MC 223, Box 3. Massachusetts Institute of Technology. Institute Archives and Special Collections, MIT Libraries, Cambridge, MA.
44 Denis Robinson to Georges F. Doriot, December 9, 1952. John G. Trump papers, MC 223, Box 3. Massachusetts Institute of Technology. Institute Archives and Special Collections, MIT Libraries, Cambridge, MA.
45 "X-ray Barbecue," *Life* April 17, 1950, 87-88.
46 "Cancer: New Methods—and Drugs—Hold High Hope," *Newsweek* May 17, 1954, 58, 60–61.
47 Laurence L. Robbins to John G. Trump, May 14, 1954. John G. Trump papers, MC 223, Box 7. Massachusetts Institute of Technology. Institute Archives and Special Collections, MIT Libraries, Cambridge, MA.
48 John G. Trump to Laurence L. Robbins, May 20, 1954. John G. Trump papers, MC 223, Box 7. Massachusetts Institute of Technology. Institute Archives and Special Collections, MIT Libraries, Cambridge, MA.
49 L. Henry Garland to Hugh Hare, March 17, 1953. Robert S. Stone papers, BANC MSS 80/80 c., correspondence. The Bancroft Library, University of California, Berkeley, CA.
50 L. Henry Garland, "Cancer Treatment Claims: What Are They: New Hope or New Hoax?" in American College of Radiology, *Monthly Newsletter* August 1954. John G. Trump papers, MC 223, Box 7. Massachusetts Institute of Technology. Institute Archives and Special Collections, MIT Libraries, Cambridge, MA.
51 Magnus I. Smedal to Editor, *ACR Monthly Newsletter* November 12, 1954, draft and final version. John G. Trump papers, MC 223, Box 8. Massachusetts Institute of Technology. Institute Archives and Special Collections, MIT Libraries, Cambridge, MA.
52 High Voltage Engineering Corporation, "Financial Summary," not dated, figures run through 1952. John G. Trump papers, MC 223, Box 3. Massachusetts Institute of Technology. Institute Archives and Special Collections, MIT Libraries, Cambridge, MA.
53 "News Release," February 18, 1954. John G. Trump papers, MC 223, Box 3. Massachusetts Institute of Technology. Institute Archives and Special Collections, MIT Libraries, Cambridge, MA.
54 "New Atom Smasher for Medicine. Industry Fires 7 Million Volts," *Wall Street Journal* January 7, 1955, 5.
55 C. E. Unterberg, Towbin Co. Investments, "High Voltage Engineering Corporation, Organization," November 12, 1954. John G. Trump papers, MC 223, Box 3. Massachusetts Institute of Technology. Institute Archives and Special Collections, MIT Libraries, Cambridge, MA.
56 Paul A. Gompers, "The Rise and Fall of Venture Capital," *Business and Economic History* 23 (1994): 1–16.
57 Luther W. Brady, Simon Kramer, Seymour H. Levitt, R. G. Parker, and W. E. Powers, "Radiation Oncology: Contributions of the United States in the Last Years of the 20th Century," *Radiology* 219 (2001):1–5.
58 John G. Trump to F. A. Salzman and Robert Wise, October 20, 1960. John G. Trump papers, MC 223, Box 7. Massachusetts Institute of Technology. Institute Archives and Special Collections, MIT Libraries, Cambridge, MA; John G. Trump, "Summary of Active Research in the HVRL-24-090," March 22, 1965. John G. Trump papers, MC 223, Box 2. Massachusetts Institute of Technology. Institute Archives and Special Collections, MIT Libraries, Cambridge, MA.

59 Carlton R. Bradford, High Voltage Engineering Corporation memo, "Organization: Monmouth Medical Center, Subject: Supervoltage," April 17, 1964. John G. Trump papers, MC 223, Box 3. Massachusetts Institute of Technology. Institute Archives and Special Collections, MIT Libraries, Cambridge, MA.
60 John G. Trump to George J. Bartel, April 24, 1964. John G. Trump papers, MC 223, Box 7. Massachusetts Institute of Technology. Institute Archives and Special Collections, MIT Libraries, Cambridge, MA.
61 Memorandum, High Voltage Engineering Corporation, "Organization: Monmouth Medical Center, Subject: Supervoltage," May 1, 1964. John G. Trump papers, MC 223, Box 7. Massachusetts Institute of Technology. Institute Archives and Special Collections, MIT Libraries, Cambridge, MA.
62 Stewart Weiss to John Trump, June 26, 1964. John G. Trump papers, MC 223, Box 7. Massachusetts Institute of Technology. Institute Archives and Special Collections, MIT Libraries, Cambridge, MA.
63 John G. Trump, "M.I.T. High Voltage Research Laboratory, Progress Report," June 1965. John G. Trump papers, MC 223, Box 9. Massachusetts Institute of Technology. Institute Archives and Special Collections, MIT Libraries, Cambridge, MA.
64 John G. Trump to Herbert D. Adams, June 4, 1964. John G. Trump papers, MC 223, Box 7. Massachusetts Institute of Technology. Institute Archives and Special Collections, MIT Libraries, Cambridge, MA.
65 Denis M. Robinson, "A Review of High Voltage Engineering Corporation," Presented Before the New York Society of Security Analysts, August 10, 1964. High Voltage Engineering Corporation Records, MC 153, Box 1. Massachusetts Institute of Technology, Institute Archives and Special Collections, MIT Libraries, Cambridge, MA.
66 Merrill Lynch Wire Flash, "High Voltage Engineering/HVE," August 10, 1964. High Voltage Engineering Corporation Records, MC 153, Box 2. Massachusetts Institute of Technology, Institute Archives and Special Collections, MIT Libraries, Cambridge, MA.
67 Georges F. Doriot to Denis Robinson, August 13, 1965. High Voltage Engineering Corporation Records, MC 153, Box 2. Massachusetts Institute of Technology, Institute Archives and Special Collections, MIT Libraries, Cambridge, MA; Georges F. Doriot to Denis Robinson, September 13, 1965. High Voltage Engineering Corporation Records, MC 153, Box 2. Massachusetts Institute of Technology, Institute Archives and Special Collections, MIT Libraries, Cambridge, MA.
68 High Voltage Engineering Corporation, "One Hundred and Forty-Fifth Meeting of the Board of Directors," August 24, 1965. High Voltage Engineering Corporation Records, MC 153, Box 1. Massachusetts Institute of Technology, Institute Archives and Special Collections, MIT Libraries, Cambridge, MA.
69 Denis Robinson to The Executive Committee, October 21, 1965. High Voltage Engineering Corporation Records, MC 153, Box 1. Massachusetts Institute of Technology, Institute Archives and Special Collections, MIT Libraries, Cambridge, MA.
70 E. Alfred Burrill to Denis M. Robinson, April 4, 1965. High Voltage Engineering Corporation Records, MC 153, Box 1. Massachusetts Institute of Technology, Institute Archives and Special Collections, MIT Libraries, Cambridge, MA.
71 R&D Planning Committee, "A New 3-MV X-ray Generator for Therapy," May 27, 1966. High Voltage Engineering Corporation Records, MC 153, Box 1. Massachusetts Institute of Technology, Institute Archives and Special Collections, MIT Libraries, Cambridge, MA.
72 "Minutes of the R&D Policy Committee–Medical," October 28, 1966. High Voltage Engineering Corporation Records, MC 153, Box 1. Massachusetts Institute of Technology, Institute Archives and Special Collections, MIT Libraries, Cambridge, MA.
73 "A Statement to the Alexander and Margaret Stewart Trust Proposing Support for the Development of Two Techniques for the Treatment of Cancer Patients at the

Massachusetts Institute of Technology's High Voltage Research Laboratory," May, 1974. John G. Trump papers, MC 223, Box 3. Massachusetts Institute of Technology. Institute Archives and Special Collections, MIT Libraries, Cambridge, MA. It accounted for two-thirds of the budget in 1974.

74 Draft letter John G. Trump to Herbert C. Englert, June 23, 1975. John G. Trump papers, MC 223, Box 2. Massachusetts Institute of Technology. Institute Archives and Special Collections, MIT Libraries, Cambridge, MA.

75 F. A. Salzman, "Remarks at Opening Ceremonies of Primary Care Clinic and Radiotherapy Center," September 25, 1976. John G. Trump papers, MC 223, Box 2. Massachusetts Institute of Technology. Institute Archives and Special Collections, MIT Libraries, Cambridge, MA.

76 John G. Trump to D. Robinson, April 11, 1974. John G. Trump papers, MC 223, Box 2. Massachusetts Institute of Technology. Institute Archives and Special Collections, MIT Libraries, Cambridge, MA.

77 "History of UCSF, Chapter Four: Building a Great Medical School by the Golden Gate: 1928–1958." http://history.library.ucsf.eduaccessed May 31, 2007. Stanford's medical school at the time was closer to downtown.

78 Robert S. Stone and Rose V. Louie, "The Use of a 70-Mev Synchrotron in Cancer Therapy: II Clinical Aspects," *Radiology* 83 (1964): 797–806.

79 Ruth Brecher and Edward Brecher, *The Rays: A History of Radiology in the United States and Canada* (Baltimore: Williams and Wilkins, 1969): 358.

80 James Stokley, "Atomic Artillery," *General Electric Review* June, 1947, 9–19; "Research: Synchrotron Helps Fight Cancer," *General Electric Review* January, 1952, 8.

81 Robert S. Stone to Hugh F. Hare, June 18, 1953. Robert S. Stone papers, BANC MSS 80/80 c., correspondence. The Bancroft Library, University of California, Berkeley, CA.

82 H. Rowan Gaither, Jr. to Robert S. Stone, July 20, 1953. Robert S. Stone papers, BANC MSS 80/80 c., correspondence. The Bancroft Library, University of California, Berkeley, CA.

83 Robert S. Stone to Charles S. Cameron, October 22, 1953. Robert S. Stone papers, BANC MSS 80/80 c., correspondence. The Bancroft Library, University of California, Berkeley, CA.

84 Unidentified newspaper clipping, November 5, 1953. Robert S. Stone papers, BANC MSS 80/80 c., correspondence. The Bancroft Library, University of California, Berkeley, CA.

85 Robert S. Stone to Charles S. Cameron, October 22, 1953. Robert S. Stone papers, BANC MSS 80/80 c., correspondence. The Bancroft Library, University of California, Berkeley, CA.

86 Charles S. Cameron to Robert S. Stone, November 12, 1953. Robert S. Stone papers, BANC MSS 80/80 c., correspondence. The Bancroft Library, University of California, Berkeley, CA.

87 L. Henry Garland to Hugh Hare, March 17, 1953; Robert S. Stone to H. Rowan Gaither, November 16, 1953. Robert S. Stone papers, BANC MSS 80/80 c., correspondence. The Bancroft Library, University of California, Berkeley, CA. The purloined patient may have been Garland's, which may have contributed to his allegation.

88 Robert S. Stone to Hugh F. Hare, November 17, 1953. Robert S. Stone papers, BANC MSS 80/80 c., correspondence. The Bancroft Library, University of California, Berkeley, CA. It is not clear how many patients were involved.

89 Robert S. Stone to Ewing L. Turner, January 7, 1954. Robert S. Stone papers, BANC MSS 80/80 c., correspondence. The Bancroft Library, University of California, Berkeley, CA.

90 Robert S. Stone to Estelle S. Frankfurts, November 27, 1954. Robert S. Stone papers, BANC MSS 80/80 c., correspondence. The Bancroft Library, University of California, Berkeley, CA.

91 Estelle S. Frankfurts to Robert S. Stone, December 1, 1954. Robert S. Stone papers, BANC MSS 80/80 c., correspondence. The Bancroft Library, University of California, Berkeley, CA.

92 "Cancer—On Brink of Breakthroughs," *Life* 44 (1958): 102–112.

93 Robert S. Stone and Rose V. Louie, "The Use of a 70-Mev Synchrotron in Cancer Therapy. II. Clinical Aspects," *Radiology* 83 (1964): 797–806.

6 Medicine's Nuclear Arms Race

Time magazine called it medicine's "peacetime bomb."[1] Using fragments of metallic cobalt made artificially radioactive in nuclear reactors invented for the atomic bomb, the cobalt-60 bomb became the first teletherapy device since kilovoltage to achieve a mass market. Its sales boom was not due to higher demonstrated effectiveness. "We have been working with some of the products of the atomic pile for the past 12 years," Berkeley's John Lawrence told the South Dakota medical association in 1947, "and I can assure you that the cancer problem is not going to be suddenly solved with their aid."[2] But cancer treatment using the radioactive cobalt-60 isotope embodied the Atoms for Peace politics that strengthened (government-financed) national enterprise and helped make nuclear power socially acceptable.[3]

Initially established to promote as well as regulate nuclear industries (including nuclear weapons), the US Atomic Energy Commission joined forces with an ambitious medical center and a giant manufacturer to build the new medical technology. The massive postwar expansion of hospitals, health insurance, and research funding fueled its boom. But it was Canada that built and used the first cobalt-60 device—and the second. Provincial cancer programs, entrepreneurial ambitions, and Cold War politics led to a race between two Canadian provinces.

Ontario versus Saskatchewan

Eldorado Mining and Refining, Ltd., the Canadian radium producer of the 1930s, had prospered by supplying uranium to the Manhattan project.[4] After the war, the company acquired exclusive distribution rights of the cobalt-60 created in the Chalk River reactor of Canada's National Research Council (NRC). Company sales manager Roy Errington searched for ways to apply the new product commercially. After reading British physicist W. V. Mayneord's suggestion that cobalt-60 be used in teletherapy, Errington called it "the only presently obvious source of substantial revenue in the isotopes field."[5] Errington initiated a connection with physician Ivan Smith, and together they lobbied the NRC and the Ontario Cancer Treatment and Research Foundation for funding to build a medical cobalt-60 device. After working with the NRC and university physicists on design, Errington contracted with the Canadian Vickers company to build the machine. It was the model of this device that he took to the 1950 International Congress of Radiology (as mentioned in the section "Political and Economic Environment" in the introduction to Part II). Errington was well aware of the public-relations value of publicity generated by first use of a new technology—not to mention the progress of a cobalt device in another Canadian province.

Saskatchewan had initiated its Cancer Commission in 1932, and by 1944 the province was providing free cancer care for all of its residents. After the war, Premier T. C. Douglas initiated the plan that put Canada on the road to its province-based comprehensive health insurance system. Also a physician, Douglas had high hopes for radiotherapy, and he funded the University of Saskatchewan to become the first institution to use the University of Illinois/Allis-Chalmers betatron for medical treatment. The province then funded university physicist Harold Johns to work with physician T. A. Watson to design a cobalt-60 teletherapy device and commissioned the local Acme Machine and Electric Company to build it.[6]

Making discs of metallic cobalt sufficiently radioactive took several years in the reactor, and it happened that the Americans' set was delayed. Chalk River released radioactive discs to the two Canadian teams in 1951, and "the cobalt race was on!" as Saskatchewan physicist Sylvia Fedoruk retrospectively announced it. With their set still "cooking" in the reactor, the Americans were "left in the starting gate and the Canadians ran for the roses—Saskatoon jumped into an early lead," busily calibrating its machine after receiving the first release of radioactive cobalt. But, Fedoruk noted, the Eldorado company was anxious to generate publicity, and Ontario "passed [Saskatchewan] in the stretch," treating its first patient in October 1951, days after installing its new device.[7] Known to be terminal at the time of his widely publicized treatment, the patient died a few weeks later—but history had been made. Ontario and Eldorado claimed the trophy for the first worldwide clinical use of cobalt-60 teletherapy. The Ontario cobalt clinic made its official opening a media event.

Twelve days after Ontario's first treatment, Saskatchewan took second place and resented it ever after. Ontario had won by not taking time to calibrate its machine, Saskatchewan charged, claiming for itself the first "calibrated" use of the technology, as well as the first "non-commercial" device. Ontario rebutted that the National Research Council had calibrated its machine prior to delivery. The "cobalt bomb war" was fought largely in the media. Fedoruk credited *MacLean's* magazine article, "The Atom Bomb That Saves Lives," with contributing substantially to the device's popular acceptance, which built its market. Probably related more to patient selection than to machine calibration, Saskatchewan would be able to document that its first patient to complete a full course of treatment survived to report, 37 years later, "all's well so far."[8]

Eldorado's Roy Errington patented modifications of the Vickers prototype and took Eldorado into production. He purposely designed the Eldorado A to be (relatively) small, compact, and simple to operate in order to sell it to a broad range of medical providers.[9] With no complex electronics, it was cheaper and (arguably) more reliable than megavoltage machines. Errington made the rounds of radiology conferences with his device and published papers on its design. Splitting

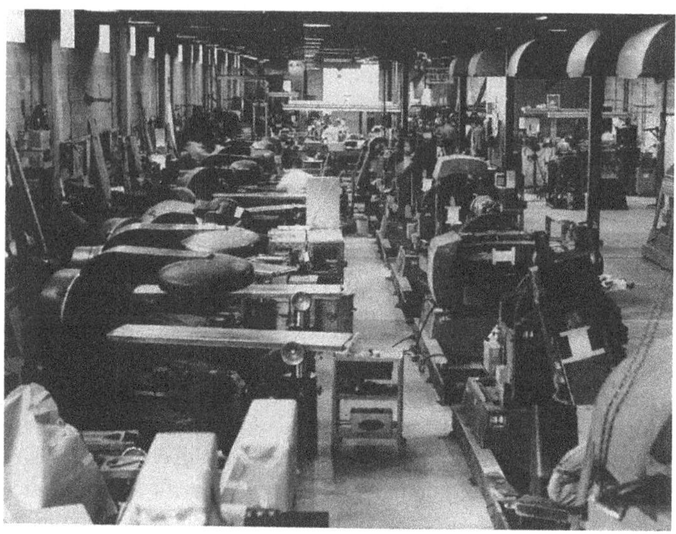

Figure 6.1 Batch Cobalt Device Production at AECL.
Reprinted with permission, Nordion Communications.

off the Eldorado division building the device, he partnered with the Canadian government to form Atomic Energy of Canada, Ltd. (AECL), which would become the world's largest seller of cobalt-60 teletherapy devices.

Competition from other manufacturers and pressure from its distributor/partner in the United States (General Electric) impelled AECL to offer a product line of cobalt devices. The company designed standardized products and adapted industrial mass-production techniques to produce and market large numbers of them, as illustrated in Figure 6.1.

Meanwhile, south of the border, the Picker X-ray Corporation bought the rights to Saskatchewan's machine and would become AECL's only major competitor in North America. It was neither Picker nor AECL, however, but General Electric that contracted with the federal government and an aspiring new medical center to build the first cobalt-60 teletherapy device in the United States.

The Rise of the Texas Medical Center

The US Atomic Energy Commission established the Oak Ridge Institute for Nuclear Studies (ORINS), a consortium of southern universities, to advise it on peacetime uses of nuclear products. ORINS's brief was to release the Manhattan project's "huge stockpile of experience and information" to industry—and its stockpile of radioactive elements.[10] The industries it helped build spread new radioactive elements throughout the world. ORINS's Medical Division held a series of conferences that brought together academic researchers and manufacturers seeking medical applications of radioactive products. ORINS, General Electric, and the new M. D. Anderson Hospital for Cancer Research of the University of Texas reinforced each other's ambitions.

The hospital was a specialized cancer center from its beginning in 1941, when the Texas legislature established it but did not appropriate sufficient funds to build it. Seeking to employ a fortune from cotton and banking, the M. D. Anderson Foundation came to the rescue with the means to develop 134 acres of Houston real estate. Hill–Burton and US Public Health Service research construction grants further contributed to the new center. Adulating its "ultramodern" technologies as well as its rose-colored marble facade, *Time* magazine called the sumptuous new hospital a "Pink Palace of Healing."[11] In a reversal of most academic medical center development, the specialty hospital invited Baylor Medical School and the University of Texas to join its endeavor, and the Texas Medical Center—which would become the largest of its kind in the world—was born. Houston's Chamber of Commerce saw it as a major asset for the city's businesses, and within two decades, the hospital would portray itself as a "world-renowned cancer center."[12]

It was the job of former Army Air Force surgeon R. Lee Clark to raise the funds necessary for the hospital to achieve its aspirations. The hospital director proposed fee-charging clinical services and funded research as its major sources of revenue.[13] Appreciating medical technology as a means of advancing both, Clark stocked the hospital with a heavily-equipped radiation therapy unit, which included the first US cobalt-60 teletherapy device.

To achieve rapid entry into radiotherapy, Clark had sent Gilbert Fletcher, his newly trained radiology chief, to inspect installations across the Atlantic. Fletcher recruited London physicist Leonard Grimmett, an expert in radium teletherapy, to design M. D. Anderson's cobalt-60 apparatus. As a member of its medical board, Clark turned to ORINS to fund Grimmett's device. ORINS accepted his design in principle and put out a call for proposals. As the specifications in the call matched those of Anderson's design, it was no surprise that, a few months later, ORINS chose it from a large group of submissions.[14]

There were no competitive bids when the Anderson–ORINS team allied with General Electric to manufacture the machine. Fletcher announced the forthcoming device at the July 1950 International Cancer Congress in Paris, the same month he signed the contract with GE. Fletcher's announcement, intended perhaps to be preemptive, was instead premature. Oak Ridge's reactor was fully committed to nuclear weapons production, and the Americans had to wait for Canada's Chalk River facility to release the third batch of radioactive cobalt discs.[15]

Intent on winning the Cold War nuclear arms race, it seems, the United States lost the medical nuclear arms race. Texas had to stand by and watch Canada grab the "firsts" in the field, as Fedoruk gloated. To add insult to injury, the small but feisty Los Angeles Tumor Institute claimed that it also had beaten M. D. Anderson to the punch. Tumor Institute radiologists reported that they had replaced the radium in their radium bomb with an assortment of 108 pieces of radioactive cobalt acquired from Oak Ridge and first used it to treat a patient in 1952.[16] Their published paper neither provided details nor elucidated how the institute had obtained the pieces from Oak Ridge. It would be two more years before Anderson's cobalt-60 device irradiated its first patient, but its use would add to the Texas Medical Center's renown.

Entrepreneurship in Practice and Research

Accruing funds to purchase, use, and research a wide spectrum of devices, M. D. Anderson Hospital amassed the largest collection of radiation therapy devices in the world. Its "radiotherapeutic armamentarium," the hospital boasted in the mid-1960s, comprised radium, an assortment of lower-kilovoltage units, an 800 kv device, two AECL cobalt irradiators, one Allis-Chalmers betatron, and one Siemens betatron.[17] Anderson added a cesium-137 irradiator to fill in the range of study—and, in the process, help the Atomic Energy Commission investigate how it might usefully employ the massive amounts of the radioactive waste product created in its reactors. Anderson's collection did not include a 2 MeV device (Van de Graaff or GE), as Fletcher held that there was "no fundamental difference" between the 2 MeV devices and cobalt-60.[18] Anderson used its well-stocked radiotherapy department to treat 40 percent of the hospital's cancer patients in its first 15 years with radiation (alone or with other treatments).[19] The hospital also used its wide range of devices to formulate radiation therapy practice standards and research agendas. Although the National Institutes of Health (NIH) funded him to "determine which type of radiotherapy offers the patient with a specific type of tumor the greatest benefit,"[20] Fletcher's published studies did not so report.

M. D. Anderson was experimenting on patients as it tested its wide armamentarium. Fletcher advised that his machines were complementary in function—implying that a full-fledged radiation therapy department required a broad set of them. At the very least, Fletcher's 1966 textbook advocated, radiotherapy centers should have one cobalt-60 unit, a 20 MeV photon beam, and electron beam capacity.[21] That recommendation required multiple megavoltage devices (both cobalt and a betatron) but not necessarily a linear accelerator.

With perhaps some antipathy toward Stanford, whose persistence in retaining the linear accelerator as its sole megavoltage technology flouted Fletcher's multidevice standards, M. D. Anderson delayed acquiring that technology. Linear accelerators required more maintenance and were less predictable than cobalt, Fletcher argued, maintaining that cobalt devices operating at the longer source-to-skin distances were equivalent to 4 and 6 MeV linear accelerators—"provided the beam is collimated to minimize the penumbra."[22] When Anderson did decide to acquire a linear accelerator in 1970, it commissioned a specially built 25 MeV unit from the Raytheon Company rather than purchase one of the 4 or 6 MeV Stanford/Varian devices on the market.[23] After its Raytheon purchase, the hospital upped its radiotherapy standards, advocating that a 25 MeV machine was now necessary for an "optimally equipped" department.[24] Anderson's standards set *de facto* professional policy that reinforced institutional hierarchy. Hospitals that could not achieve the advised technological level, according to the standards, should not treat cancer patients—or at least not beyond palliation.

Gilbert Fletcher enforced a professional hierarchy within his department as well as among hospitals. He had an increasingly acrimonious relationship with Leonard Grimmett, who died of a heart attack at age 49 shortly before the cobalt-60 irradiator he designed became operational.[25] "Mercurial and feisty," as historian James Olson described Fletcher, he "could at once terrorize staff and residents and then shrink obsequiously in front of [his boss, R. Lee] Clark, like a puppy in the presence of an alpha male."[26] Although far from uncommon in academic medical departments, such a hierarchy was clearly not conducive to junior staff members questioning their supervisors' research projects, choice of devices, or clinical practices.

For financial reasons, M. D. Anderson administrators expected its radiotherapy department to run at full capacity. To assure a sufficient case load, the hospital designed a regionalization program that defined the whole state of Texas as its market area and trained physicians in selecting patients to refer to Anderson's supervoltage machines.[27] But it did not take long for radiologists at community hospitals to proclaim that cobalt-60 teletherapy had graduated from a research tool to a practice standard that they all needed to offer. The cobalt boom was under way.

Cobalt Treatment Booms

The International Atomic Energy Agency counted 22 worldwide manufacturers of cobalt-60 teletherapy machines by 1959.[28] The following year, the United States and Canada accounted for 288 installed cobalt devices (out of 326 in the Americas), Europe for 137, and Asia for 218 (200 of which were in Japan).[29] These figures compared to a worldwide total of 32 resonance transformers, 31 Van de Graaffs, 32 betatrons, 3 synchrotrons, and 17 linear accelerators.

Benefiting from their head start, the Canadian AECL and the US Picker companies had supplied over 80 percent of cobalt instruments sold in the United States in the 1960s.[30] General Electric chose not to remain in the game as a manufacturer; the company's crystal ball was apparently cloudy as it foresaw sales of only 10 devices in the first decade.[31] GE entered the market as distributor, announcing in 1954 that it had joined forces with AECL; it would sell, install, and service AECL cobalt devices in the United States and work with AECL engineers on upgrades.[32] The distributorship agreement provided a profitable business in itself as the cobalt market exploded.

Cobalt-60 teletherapy boomed for two decades in the United States, peaking at around 1,000 installations in the mid-1970s. Most hospitals leapt into megavoltage with cobalt, bypassing the GE resonance transformer, the Van de Graaff accelerator, and the betatron. Cobalt's low price and relative simplicity even enabled radiologists to continue the tradition of installing devices in their private offices, especially when banks became willing to loan them money to do so.[33] Doctors' offices accounted for 25 percent of megavoltage services in New York State in 1968 and 40 percent of those in Florida.[34]

Cobalt's strong growth was not a function of higher energy; the Van de Graaff and the resonance transformer matched the power of cobalt-60, and the betatrons vastly exceeded it. Nor was its growth due to strong evidence of (or even strong belief in) greater effectiveness of its treatments compared to other supervoltage instruments. Even as it promoted the product, General Electric noted that "the hope for more cures with cobalt-60 may be dim."[35] Laboratory researchers pointed out that the biological effects of gamma-ray photons emitted by cobalt-60 were very like those of megavoltage X-ray photons.

Nonetheless, radiologists were eager to use the new device, and patients were apparently eager to be treated with it. Immediately after taking first place in the cobalt race, the Ontario team launched into 18-hour work days to treat as many patients as possible on the grounds that it was unwilling to deny cobalt treatment to anyone.[36] After 5 years of its use, however, Ivan Smith reluctantly concluded that cobalt-60 had "not revolutionized the treatment of cancer."[37]

Effectiveness Research

Other Ontario Cancer Foundation researchers were encouraged to find 1-year survival rates among lung cancer patients rising from 14 percent of those treated earlier with kilovoltage to 27 percent of those treated with cobalt, and they attributed the gain to the new technology.[38] But they would see a 5-year lung cancer survival rate of only 4 percent. Another report from Ontario concluded that there had been little gain in 5-year lung cancer survival between 1930 and 1957, "despite the introduction of supervoltage and Co-60 gamma therapy."[39] Cervical cancer outcomes were mixed. A third Ontario team found cervical cancer survival rates using cobalt-60 equivalent to those achieved after treatment with 400 kv, and it concluded that adding radium brachytherapy to the mix was necessary for achieving optimal radiation results. Their study found survival rates following betatron treatment to be higher than those after cobalt, but it also found greater bowel damage—which sometimes killed the patient.[40] Ivan Smith continued to find cobalt disappointing.[41]

Nor did the Texans experience an effectiveness revolution, as Gilbert Fletcher conceded. While M. D. Anderson Hospital annual reports took credit for curing a small number of cancers with supervoltage radiation, they acknowledged that there was little correlation between the often remarkable tumor regressions and longer-term local control, let alone control of metastases. Like other radiotherapists, Fletcher noted that supervoltage incurred less skin burn and bone necrosis and thus protected patients from certain harms that earlier radiation treatments had inflicted.[42] But, reflecting his early training in physics and engineering, Fletcher's professional papers tended to focus on the technologies themselves and on instructing radiologists how to use them rather than on patient outcomes.[43] Spreading treatment across its large collection of devices meant that Fletcher's team selected only a few cancer types for cobalt-60 treatment. These cancers included lymphomas and head, neck, and lung as well as breast tumors—the latter nearly always in conjunction with radical mastectomy.[44] For cervical cancer, Fletcher used betatrons to irradiate the entire pelvis.[45]

Reports from other centers concurred with Fletcher in finding (only) incremental improvements under certain conditions using cobalt-60 and megavoltage devices on selected cancers.[46] It is not usually possible to use their reports to tease out the contribution of specific radiotherapy devices. Fletcher's studies reflected his belief that cobalt, betatrons, 2 MeV devices, and linear accelerators were clinically equivalent, and his papers generally did not report which devices were used on which patients. Although cobalt-60 developers had high hopes for their technology, their own findings did not support a retrospective claim that "cobalt-60 treatments proved to be one of the most successful and practical anti-cancer therapies of its time," at least not in terms of clinical success.[47] Cobalt teletherapy did advance the success of the radiology specialty and played a major role in elevating its therapeutic subspecialty to full specialty status.

Economic and professional factors drove the cobalt-60 boom more than science did. While nearly all mid-sized hospitals had offered some form of radiation therapy in the early 1960s, cobalt initially priced many of them out of the market and offered competitive advantage to wealthier hospitals. Consequently, AECL and GE engineers worked on cheaper machines that could expand the market to smaller hospitals.[48] They offered a competitive price: one-half that of the Allis-Chalmers betatron and one-quarter that of the ARCO linear accelerator on the market by then. Calling cobalt-60 less technologically demanding than megavoltage devices, some radiotherapists deemed cobalt suitable only for the "unsophisticated environment" of community hospitals.[49] (The reciprocal of this argument was, of course, that hospitals defining themselves as sophisticated had to opt for the more costly machines.) Cobalt became known as "poor man's supervoltage."[50] Fletcher held that the "relative merits" of the different machines were "a matter of economics only."[51] He would credit the linear accelerator's growing dominance to manufacturers' spurious claims and a "keeping up with the Jones' complex" in the competitive medical economy.[52] Nonetheless, the Stanford/Varian linear accelerator would soon replace cobalt-60 as the latest mass-market device.

Notes

1 "Medicine: Peacetime Bomb," *Time* November 19, 1951.

2 John Lawrence, talk to South Dakota Medical Association, 1947: Ernest O. Lawrence papers, BANC FILM 2248. The Bancroft Library, University of California, Berkeley, CA.

3 Ellen Leopold, *Under the Radar: Cancer and the Cold War* (New Brunswick: Rutgers University Press, 2009), 18, 34.

4 J. E. Arsenault, "The Eldorado Radium Silver Express," *CNS Bulletin* 26 (2005). https://cns-snc.ca/media/history/fifty_years/fedoruk.html accessed September 10, 2010.

5 Paul Litt, *Isotopes and Innovation: MDS Nordion's First Fifty Years, 1946–1996* (Montreal: Published for MDS Nordion by McGill-Queen's University Press, 2000), 23, 48, 53, 55, 65, 71, 73.

6 C. Stuart Houston, *Steps on the Road to Medicare: Why Saskatchewan Led the Way* (Montreal: McGill-Queens University Press, 2002), 5–6.

7 Sylvia Fedoruk, "The Growth of Nuclear Medicine," talk to 1989 Annual Conference of the Canadian Nuclear Association and the Canadian Nuclear Society. http://www.snc.ca/history/fifty_years/fedoruk.html accessed May 31, 2007. Fedoruk would go on to serve as Lieutenant-Governor of Saskatchewan and be inducted into the Canadian Curling Hall of Fame as well as the Canadian Medical Hall of Fame. In the United

Kingdom, University College Hospital, London was reported to have installed a cobalt-60 teletherapy device in 1951. Caroline Claire Scanlon Murphy, "A History of Radiotherapy to 1950: Cancer and Radiotherapy in Britain 1830–1950," PhD thesis, University of Manchester, 1986, Chapter 8.

8 Sylvia Fedoruk, "The Growth of Nuclear Medicine," talk to 1989 Annual Conference of the Canadian Nuclear Association and the Canadian Nuclear Society. http://www.cns-snc.ca/history/fifty_years/fedoruk.html accessed May 31, 2007.

9 D. T. Green and R. F. Errington, "1000 Curie Cobalt Units for Radiation Therapy. III. Design of a Cobalt 60 Beam Therapy Unit," *British Journal of Radiology* 25 (1952): 309–313.

10 Milton Friedman, Marshall Brucer, and Elizabeth Anderson, eds., *Roentgens, Rads, and Riddles, A Symposium on Supervoltage Radiation Therapy* (Oak Ridge: Oak Ridge Institute of Nuclear Studies, 1956), 426.

11 "Medicine: Pink Palace of Healing," *Time* December 13, 1954.

12 M. D. Anderson Foundation, University of Texas, Houston, *Proceedings at the Dedication of the M. D. Anderson Hospital for Cancer Research* Houston, February 17, 1944, 17–19, 119–120; C. J. Sutro, "The University of Texas M.D. Anderson Hospital and Tumor Institute: The Southwest's World-renowned Cancer Center," *CA: A Cancer Journal for Clinicians* 14 (1964): 236–243.

13 M. D Anderson Hospital and Tumor Institute, *The First Twenty Years of the University of Texas M. D. Anderson Hospital and Tumor Institute* (Houston: University of Texas, 1964), 215–216, 429.

14 Ellen Leopold, *Under the Radar: Cancer and the Cold War* (New Brunswick: Rutgers University Press, 2009), 66–67.

15 Roger F. Robison, "The Race for Megavoltage: X-rays versus Telegamma," *Acta Oncologica* 34 (1995): 1055–1074. There are other versions of the discs story. Johns and Watson held that the third set was originally intended for W. V. Mayneord in London, England, and that Fletcher got it after Mayneord declined it. H. E. Johns and T. A.Watson, "The Cobalt-60 Story" *Cancer in Ontario* (1982): 20–24. I would like to thank Jessica Pontone of Cancer Care Ontario for sending me a copy of this article. Angela Creager held that the Chalk River reactor's use in the Korean War delayed the Texas discs. Angela N. H. Creager, *Life Atomic: A History of Radioisotopes in Science and Medicine* (Chicago: University of Chicago Press, 2013), 320.

16 Russell H. Neil, William E. Costolow, and Orville N. Meland, "Design and Construction of a Simple Applicator for 1,000 Curies of Cobalt 60," *Radiology* 61 (1953):408–410.

17 M. D. Anderson Hospital and Tumor Institute, *General Report 1961–1964* Houston: University of Texas, 1964, 15.

18 Gilbert Fletcher, "Supervoltage Roentgentherapy: Clinical Evaluation Based on 2,000 Cases," *Texas State Journal of Medicine* 55 (1959): 676–683.

19 M. D Anderson Hospital and Tumor Institute, *The First Twenty Years of the University of Texas M. D. Anderson Hospital and Tumor Institute* (Houston: University of Texas, 1964), 375.

20 *Newsletter*, M. D. Anderson Hospital and Tumor Institute, Houston: University of Texas, July 1963.

21 Gilbert H. Fletcher, *Textbook of Radiotherapy* (Philadelphia: Lea & Febiger, 1966), 109–10.

22 Gilbert H. Fletcher, "Supervoltage Roentgentherapy: Clinical Evaluation Based on 2,000 Cases," *Texas State Journal of Medicine* 55 (1959): 676–683; Lloyd Reaume, Interview of Gilbert Fletcher and Walter Rider, "Cobalt 60 vs. Linear Accelerator: Cobalt is Still the Answer," Veterinary Tumor Institute, no date. http://veterinarytumor-institute.com/id1.html accessed May 24, 2008.

23 M. D. Anderson Hospital and Tumor Institute, *General Report 1968–1970* Houston: University of Texas, 1970, 36.

24 R. Lee Clark and Clifton D. Howe, *Cancer Patient Care at M.D. Anderson Hospital and Tumor Institute* (Chicago: Year Book Medical Publishers, 1976), 15.
25 Peter R. Almond, *Cobalt Blues: The Story of Leonard Grimmett, the Man Behind the First Cobalt-60 Unit in the United States* (New York: Springer, 2013), 70–72, 90–95.
26 James S. Olson, *Making Cancer History: Disease and Discovery at the University of Texas M. D. Anderson Cancer Center* (Baltimore: Johns Hopkins University Press, 2009), 51.
27 M. D. Anderson Hospital and Tumor Institute, *Annual Report 1953–1954* Houston: University of Texas, 1954, 70, 184.
28 International Atomic Energy Agency, *Radioisotope Teletherapy Equipment: International Directory* (Vienna: IAEA, 1959), 117–118.
29 International Atomic Energy Agency, *Use of Radioisotopes and Supervoltage Radiation in Radioteletherapy* (Vienna: IAEA, 1960), 24–25.
30 Calculated from data in International Atomic Energy Agency, *Directory of High-Energy Radiotherapy Centres* (Vienna: IAEA, 1968).
31 Roger F. Robison, "The Race for Megavoltage: X-rays versus Telegamma," *Acta Oncologica* 34 (1995): 1055–1074.
32 "New Rotational, Stationary Co60 Units Offered by GE," *General Electric X-Ray News* March 1954; *General Electric X-ray News* October 1957; *General Electric X-Ray News* February 1954.
33 Wendell G. Scott, *Planning Guide for Radiologic Installations* (Chicago: Year Book Publishers, 1966, 2nd ed.), 181.
34 International Atomic Energy Agency, *Directory of High-Energy Radiotherapy Centres* (Vienna: IAEA, 1968), 25–27, 44–50.
35 "Group Discussions Indicate Trend to Cobalt Treatment," *General Electric X-Ray News* November, 1957.
36 S. M. Busby, "The Cobalt Bomb in the Treatment of Bladder Tumours," *Canadian Medical Association Journal* 73 (1955): 872–875.
37 Ivan H. Smith, "Cobalt-60 Beam Therapy: Some Impressions after Five Years," *Canadian Medical Association Journal* 77 (1957): 289–297.
38 R. C. Burr, E. N. MacKay, and A. H. Sellers, "Radiation Therapy in Treatment of Carcinoma of Lung," *Canadian Medical Association Journal* 88 (1963): 1181–1184.
39 W. R. Bruce and C. L. Ash, "Survival of Patients Treated for Cancer of the Breast, Cervix, Lung, and Upper Respiratory Tract at the Ontario-Cancer-Institute (Toronto) from 1930 to 1957," *Radiology* 81 (1963): 861–870.
40 W. E. C. Allt, "Supervoltage Radiation Treatment in Advanced Cancer of the Uterine Cervix," *Canadian Medical Association Journal* 100 (1969):792–797.
41 Ivan H. Smith, J. C. H. Fetterly, J. S. Lott, J. C. F. MacDonald, Lois M. Myers, P. M. Pfalzner, and D. H. Thomson, *Cobalt-60 Teletherapy: A Handbook for the Radiation Therapist and Physicist* (New York: Harper and Row, Hoeber Medical Division, 1964), 173.
42 Gilbert H. Fletcher, "Supervoltage Roentgentherapy: Clinical Evaluation Based on 2,000 Cases," *Texas State Journal of Medicine* 55 (1959): 676–683.
43 Gilbert H. Fletcher, "Present Status of Cobalt-60 Teletherapy in the Management of the Cancer Patient," *Journal of the American Medical Association* 164 (1957): 244–248.
44 M. D. Anderson Hospital and Tumor Institute, *The First Twenty Years of the University of Texas M. D. Anderson Hospital and Tumor Institute* (Houston: University of Texas, 1964), 434; Gilbert H. Fletcher and Edgar C. White, "Possibilities of Supervoltage Roentgenotherapy in the Management of Cancer of the Breast," *Southern Medical Journal* 52 (1959): 805–812.
45 Gilbert H. Fletcher and Felix N. Rutledge, "Over-all Results in Radiotherapy for Carcinoma of the Cervix," *Clinical Obstetrics and Gynecology* 10 (1967) 958–964; M. F. Strockbine, J. E. Hancock, and G. H. Fletcher, "Complications in 831 Patients

with Squamous Cell Carcinoma of the Intact Uterine Cervix Treated with 3,000 Rads or More Whole Pelvis Irradiation," *American Journal of Roentgenology Radium Therapy and Nuclear Medicine* 108 (1970): 293–304.

46 Paul Mercado and Jose M. Sala, "Comparison of Conventional and Supervoltage Radiation in the Management of Cancer of the Cervix," *Radiology* 90 (1968): 967–970; Richard D. Marks, "Fourteen Years' Experience with Cobalt-60 Radiation Therapy in the Treatment of Early Cancer of the True Vocal Cords," *Cancer* 28 (1971): 571–576; M. Stuart Strong, Charles W. Vaughan, Herbert L. Kayne, I. M. Aral, A Ucmakli, M. Feldman, and G. B. Healy, "A Randomized Trial of Preoperative Radiotherapy in Cancer of the Oropharynx and Hypopharynx," *American Journal of Surgery* 136 (1978): 494–500; E. D. Montague and G. H. Fletcher, "Curative Value of Irradiation in the Treatment of Nondisseminated Breast Cancer," *Cancer* 46, supplement S4 (1980): 995–998.

47 Peter R. Almond, *Cobalt Blues: The Story of Leonard Grimmett, The Man Behind the First Cobalt-60 Unit in the United States* (New York: Springer, 2013), 110.

48 "AECL-G.E. Design Eases Use of Cobalt by More Hospitals," *General Electric X-ray News* October, 1957.

49 H. E. Johns and T. A. Watson, "The Cobalt-60 Story," *Cancer in Ontario* 1982, 20–24.

50 Howard J. Barnhard, "Supervoltage Therapy Comes of Age: A Report for the Practicing Physician," *New England Journal of Medicine* 258 (1958): 275–277.

51 Gilbert H. Fletcher, "Cobalt-60 in Management of Cancer," *Journal of the American Medical Association* 183 (1963): 103–108.

52 Lloyd Reaume, "Cobalt 60 vs. Linear Accelerator: Cobalt is Still the Answer," Interview of Gilbert Fletcher and Walter Rider, Veterinary Tumor Institute, undated. http://veterinarytumorinstitute.com/id1.html accessed May 24, 2008.

7 An Economic Success Story at Stanford

Compared to cobalt-60's surge from the beginning, sales of the Stanford/Varian linear accelerator got off to a slow start. Most hospital radiology departments purchased the cheaper cobalt device first and waited until its depreciation period ended and it had generated sufficient revenues to cover the more costly machine. But the *linac*, as it was nicknamed, would come to surpass all other devices in professional and commercial success. The rise in linac installations crossed the decline in new cobalt installations around 1980 and continued to skyrocket.

Did the rise of the linear accelerator signify that the definitive technology had finally been achieved? Some historians as well as physicians have thought so, claiming that they had finally attained "science-based medicine."[1] But all radiotherapy devices are science based, and that alone does not make their clinical use scientific. The rise of the linac was an economic success story. Two enterprising engineers, a motivated radiation therapist, an ambitious research university, and an innovative company put it all together.

Higher Education: A Highly Competitive Business

Stanford University supported technological entrepreneurship as early as 1909, when its then president, David Starr Jordan, invested in the Federal Telegraph Company and engineering faculty consulted for it.[2] As a junior member of the engineering faculty two decades later, Frederick Terman (unsuccessfully) offered Federal Telegraph the opportunity to put him on retainer as consultant.[3] As he would later ask conferees at a business meeting, where else besides universities could industry get "men with top scientific qualifications to work for the pay of a college professor?"[4]

Despite his initial snub from Federal Telegraph, Terman emulated his Massachusetts Institute of Technology mentors and went on to develop close working relationships with a wide range of manufacturers. Repudiating charges that Stanford became a "captive of industry funding," a history professor later emphasized the extent to which his employer was government funded and proactively collaborated with industry.[5] The university was not so much *captive* of industry, it seems, as *part of* it. Research universities like Stanford—and the Massachusetts Institute of Technology (MIT) and the California Institute of

Technology (Caltech) and California and Texas (and, eventually, Harvard)—built an education–industry–government nexus that restructured all three. Following his own maxim that "higher education is a highly competitive business,"[6] Terman rose to positions that enabled him to help make Stanford University competitive and a business.

As chair of the electrical engineering department in the 1930s, dean of engineering in the 1940s, and university provost in the 1950s, Terman worked with successive Stanford presidents to build a flourishing research university. He recruited faculty members who could accrue funding to develop technologies that generated revenues in the forms of product royalties and more research grants. Terman encouraged the financial industry to partner in the process, pointing out the high returns on capital investment in technology research. The purpose of a research university, he advised bankers in 1947, was to train industrial leaders to turn scientific discoveries into products that expanded economic growth.[7] Terman played an active role in the lucrative—if initially serendipitous for Stanford—activities that built a new vacuum tube and parlayed it into a successful medical industry.

A Technology, a Company, and an Industrial Park

Stanford gained financially and learned a constructive business lesson when brothers Russell (Rus) and Sigurd (Sig) Varian invented the klystron tube in 1937. Rus Varian enjoyed getting together with William Hansen, a young physics professor, to discuss Hansen's new rhumbatron tube and his interest in generating high-voltage X-rays. Rus had an idea for a new vacuum tube based on the rhumbatron but, having been rejected as a continuing graduate student in Stanford's physics department, he had no means of developing it.

With Sig Varian, the intrepid pilot, navigating, the brothers approached Hansen and David Webster (the department chair who had rejected Rus), asking solely for "access to the physics department equipment and the right to consult with Bill Hansen and others" to work on Rus's vision.[8] Hansen may have foreseen that the proposed invention could help him build a supervoltage X-ray. Having failed to acquire funding for a supervoltage X-ray generator of his own,[9] Webster may have foreseen an alternate route. In any case, Hansen and Webster agreed to the Varians' request.

When the proposal reached the desk of Stanford president Ray Lyman Wilbur, the canny physician offered the Varians a contract providing them with $100 and use of the physics department's equipment (and brains) in exchange for all ensuing patent rights and 50 percent of any royalties. Within months, Rus had designed and Sig had built a tube that amplified microwaves, and Stanford University held a promissory note for a fortune. The new klystron tube would fulfill the Varians' hope of developing radar and Hansen's hope of generating supervoltage X-rays. Not parenthetically, it also enhanced Stanford's appreciation of the patent process; the board of trustees subsequently claimed university ownership of all patents related to a faculty member's research or teaching.[10]

An exclusive contract with the Sperry Gyroscope Company brought in money and personnel to develop the klystron. Terman recruited Edward Ginzton to work on the Sperry contract as a graduate student. Ginzton, who would become the second important engineer in this story, would later credit the "$100 Idea" with validating the coupling of university science to the market.[11] Building klystrons at Sperry during the war, the Varians, Ginzton, and Hansen dreamed of establishing their own company and making products their own way.[12] They pooled their resources after the war and incorporated Varian Associates, with Russell Varian as president and Ginzton, Hansen, Terman, and Leonard Schiff, Stanford's new physics chairman, serving on its board of directors.

Although Rus had wanted Ginzton to manage the new company,[13] Ginzton initially chose to become assistant director of Hansen's newly-funded Microwave Research Laboratory—which owed its existence to the klystron. It did not take Hansen long to demonstrate the technical feasibility of a microwave-based linear electron acceleration technique he had been thinking about, and it did not take Varian Associates long to start manufacturing it. Varian's move onto Stanford property, Terman announced in a 1951 company pep talk, would strengthen connections between university and industry.[14] The university was in the process of building the Stanford Industrial Park (later tactically re-named Stanford Research Park), and Varian would be the first company to move in.

Capitalizing a chunk of its increasingly valuable real estate, the university established the park as a venue for an "emerging electronics industry tied closely to a prominent electronics department at Stanford," as an official Stanford history described it.[15] It helped collect the "'cream of the crop' from all over the entire country," Terman advised, and "funnel them into local industry."[16] In a typical arrangement, Stanford faculty, graduate students, and staff worked with company researchers to develop commercial applications of Stanford research patents. Some ventures further blurred boundaries between academia and business as the university hired "entire teams of scientists from industry as Stanford faculty heading up their own teaching and research programs."[17]

In recruiting General Electric (GE) to the park, for example, Stanford offered to build its facility, help it select scientific staff, and "in its discretion give faculty appointments" to GE staff.[18] GE, in return, offered retainer contracts to six Stanford faculty and staff, including Terman.[19] Terman contracted for $4,200 a year—a considerable augmentation of faculty salaries—in exchange for rights to his inventions.[20] An added perk for GE (not in the contract) was that Terman would sponsor the facility's manager for membership in the Los Altos Golf and Country Club.[21]

Country clubs and other elite watering holes were more than playgrounds for the wealthy; they were work sites where men made contacts, wrote contracts, and circulated capital. Clubs catalyzed dynamic interactions between manufacturers searching for capital and financiers searching for remunerative investments. San Francisco's Bohemian Club and its bucolic Grove, for example, intermingled corporate executives with well-heeled academicians (of the right sex, color, and religion).[22] Terman advised his Bohemian comrades that electronic devices like Stanford's linear accelerator portended a new industrial revolution.[23]

At the same time Stanford was building its industrial park, Terman was working with Stanford President J. E. Wallace Sterling to move the university's medical school from San Francisco to Palo Alto and to revamp it in the process.

Technology Development at a Self-Financing Medical School

Stanford selected Henry Kaplan, its young and recently-hired radiology department executive, to chair the medical school's Committee on Future Plans. The committee's 1952 report proposed a self-supporting medical school that would use revenues from research grants and clinical services to become financially independent of the university. Combining San Francisco clinical departments with Palo Alto basic and applied science departments on one campus, the future plans report held, would link clinical care to research and make medical practice more scientific.[24] The process would also permit Stanford to follow the practice of leading medical schools in using research grants to pay staff salaries and overhead costs. Harvard's medical school dean, for example, would acknowledge the following decade that ability to attract research funding was a primary consideration in faculty recruitment.[25]

The future plans committee further endorsed a full-time faculty practice plan that, located in the wealthier Palo Alto community, would accrue practice revenues and at the same time relieve the school of its San Francisco charity care burden. The two strategies together would bring in considerable revenue: research would come to generate nearly one-half and clinical services nearly one-quarter of the medical school's budget in the early 2000s.[26] The radiology department excelled in both revenue sources.

Henry Kaplan was in a position to know that other universities were reaping fame and funding with supervoltage technologies. Hearing their reports at the 1950 International Congress of Radiology, he would have been all too aware that his barium enema paper did not place his department in their ranks. Kaplan later reminisced (and historians have oft repeated) that he'd heard rumors of Hansen's linear accelerator at Stanford cocktail parties and set up a meeting with Terman, Ginzton, and Schiff in the fall of 1951 to discuss its potential application in medicine.[27]

But Kaplan was already clearly familiar with the linear accelerator and did not need to rely on cocktail-party lore. While working at the National Cancer Institute, he had attended (and may have helped organize) a 1947 National Advisory Cancer Council "Conference on Multimillion Volt Radiations and Their Use in Cancer Research and Therapy," which had discussed the Van de Graaff, betatrons, synchrotrons, proton beams from synchrocyclotrons, and linear accelerators—all technologies that would come to add to the radiotherapy repertoire.[28] A university press release would later attribute Kaplan's move to Stanford in part to his interest in working with its physicists on a medical linear accelerator.[29]

Kaplan and Ginzton's *Joint Statement about the Medical Application of the Linear Electron Accelerator* was ready by February 1951.[30] Written apparently for fundraising purposes, the statement acknowledged—but disparaged—existing technologies. It called Sloan devices unreliable, betatrons inflexible, synchrotrons massive, and cobalt-60 teletherapy "as yet unborn" (although its gestation was notably advanced at the time). A linear accelerator offered a "striking contrast" to these drawbacks and a serious challenge to the competition, the statement affirmed. Stanford was the natural place to develop such a device, the statement maintained, because of its strong research capabilities in both physics and radiology. At the same time, it noted that clinical outcomes from megavoltage treatment were "not dramatic," a conclusion that Kaplan would reiterate in professional articles.[31] Nonetheless, they forged ahead.

Taking the lead organizational role, Ginzton outlined the Stanford proposal at a National Cancer Institute (NCI) meeting in July 1951.[32] President Sterling helped raise funds from the NCI as well as from the Office of Naval Research, the American Cancer Society, the James Irvine Foundation, General Electric, and Varian Associates. The university announced in a 1952 press release that it was building a high-powered linear accelerator that every major hospital in the country would want to buy.[33] Stanford had to work fast to establish position, however, because hospitals and companies in the United Kingdom were leading the race. As it turned out, Stanford would not be the first (or even the second) to use its linear accelerator technology in medical treatment in the United States. The Massachusetts Institute of Technology (MIT) built the Argonne device in 1954, and—with technical assistance from Stanford—Chicago's Michael Reese Hospital built a 45 MeV linear accelerator for experimental electron beam treatments in 1955.

The following year—three years after the UK Mullard and Metropolitan-Vickers companies installed medical linear accelerators in London and Manchester—Stanford was finally able to announce its new "cancer gun"[34] (Figure 7.1). Ginzton's staff and graduate students had built the 6 MeV X-ray irradiator and—the medical school not yet having moved into its new campus—installed it in the Stanford Hospital in San Francisco, Stanford's private hospital next door to its Lane Hospital for indigent patients. The device's physical location in the private hospital and the separate budgets of the two hospitals suggested that the linear accelerator was expected from the beginning to make money treating private patients.[35] Ginzton had assured donors that the machine would not require operational funding after installation, since patient payment for treatments would support it.[36]

The new device embodied the medical school's incipient image of itself as the place to go for sophisticated technologies. Three years later, publicity for the opening of the Palo Alto–Stanford Hospital Center prominently featured the "atom smashing linear accelerator in X-ray therapy."[37]

Ginzton and Kaplan together built a large radiation research program at Ginzton's lab in close proximity to Kaplan's new radiology department. Kaplan's prior employment at the National Institutes of Health (NIH) and his continuing membership on its advisory councils would have augmented his grantsmanship—although he later asserted that an MIT professor and stockholder in the High

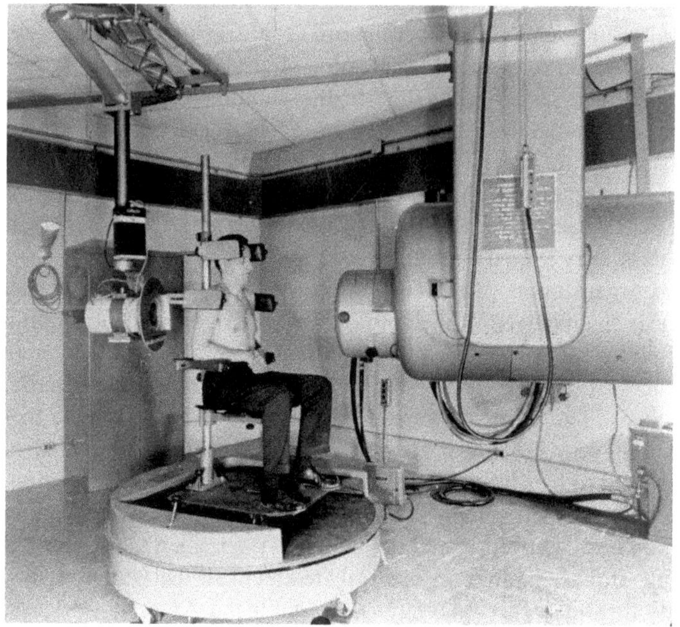

Figure 7.1 Stanford's "Cancer Gun."

Courtesy Stanford University Department of Radiation Oncology.

Voltage Engineering Company [presumably John Trump] had delayed linear accelerator development by manipulating rejection of Stanford grant applications.[38] Kaplan's research using the linear accelerator contributed to its clinical acceptance and commercial development, as did Ginzton's energetic entrepreneurial activities.

Commercializing the Medical Linear Accelerator

Edward Ginzton and Russell Varian saw the linear accelerator as a potentially profitable venture from the start,[39] although they may initially have expected to license the technology to a large corporation. Stanford signed a 1953 agreement with General Electric permitting the company to develop the Stanford accelerator. GE would send staff to Palo Alto, the contract detailed, and Stanford would provide "complete research, design, technical and manufacturing information and material, including drawings, photographs, data, descriptive matter and any other material" on an ongoing basis, in return for financial payments and a percentage of the net selling price of each Stanford–GE linac sold (which would be zero).[40]

Shortly after Stanford signed the nonexclusive agreement with GE, Ginzton informed Terman that the university had signed a similar one with Varian

Associates.[41] Terman reflected that Ginzton's commercial activities might constitute a conflict of interest with his Stanford employment, but he rationalized that although Ginzton's ties with Varian rendered it inappropriate for him to *consult* with other companies, as a Stanford faculty member, he could *educate* them.[42] Education being a two-way street, working with GE may have taught Ginzton that Varian could outcompete it in linear acceleration. In any case, the Stanford–GE arrangement petered out, and *Varian Associates* magazine announced in 1956 that the company was in the linear accelerator business.[43]

As the participants knew all too well, Varian was a relatively late entrant in the competitive megavoltage market. A physics department memo pointed out to Ginzton and Kaplan that commercially available, high-powered teletherapy devices already included the Van de Graaff, cobalt-60, two British linear accelerators, and three betatrons, one of which was under development at the University of Illinois. The memo seemed to be suggesting that medicine did not need another megavoltage device. But, it enthused, having a commercial product of its own significantly enhanced university prestige and that of its physicists and radiologists.[44]

Ginzton and Kaplan divided the labor required to develop the project. Ginzton's laboratory improved the Varian machine technically, and Kaplan's studied biological reactions, recommended improvements, expanded avenues for clinical use, and developed standards of care using the device.[45] Combined, their government-funded labs conducted the necessary research and development (R&D) for commercializing the linear accelerator. But Varian also required capital to manufacture and market the machine.

Although company founders had envisioned a cooperative—hence the name Varian *Associates*—keeping its stockholding internal significantly curtailed the company's access to capital and capacity for growth. Varian turned to the financial industry for help in funding its linear accelerator. Wall Street was increasing its appreciation of the wealth potential of the electronics industry, and X-ray would soon account for over 70 percent of the emerging medical electronics market.[46] In its prospectus for Varian's 1956 initial public offering, Dean Witter Investment Bankers trumpeted Varian's leadership in the expanding electronics industry together with its close Stanford connections.[47] It optimistically—if self-servingly—prophesied a continuation of Varian's "phenomenal growth."

With Wall Street financing in Varian coffers, Ginzton took a sabbatical leave from Stanford to assess the global market for another medical linear accelerator. With German and Swiss companies in production, Europe was "pretty much dominated by the betatrons," Ginzton reported back—although the Siemens company feared its betatron would not be financially competitive with cobalt-60 and had hinted at collaborating with Stanford on linear acceleration.[48]

Ginzton was particularly impressed with the engineering of the Metropolitan-Vickers linear accelerator installed four years earlier in Manchester's Christie Hospital—and with Christie's system of managing a steady flow of patients through its radiotherapy department.[49] The linear accelerator could outcompete cobalt-60 despite its substantially higher cost, Metropolitan-Vickers managers advised Ginzton, because its higher-energy radiation combined with efficient patient processing allowed it to treat between two and three times the number of patients per day.[50] Stanford seems to have paid attention to Christie's patient processing; its own radiology department acquired the reputation of herding patients like "2-legged cattle."[51]

Ginzton was witnessing a characteristic alliance of government, universities, and high-tech industries in the United Kingdom.[52] Its Medical Research Council sponsored university physicists working with the Metropolitan-Vickers and Mullard companies in developing linear accelerators for medical use. The nascent National Health Service, providing publicly funded medical care for the entire population, purchased five of the new accelerators to distribute to major hospitals around the country.[53]

The radiotherapists he spoke with did not try to convince Ginzton that their new supervoltage instruments were clinically more effective than their older machines. It was "virtually impossible to say," a Hammersmith Hospital radiologist advised, "whether there has or has not been an improvement in the total survival picture."[54] Therapists at a Zurich hospital also confirmed that megavoltage had not improved their cancer outcomes over kilovoltage. Some physicians exaggerated favorable results, they suggested, in order to attract more patients and keep up with the Joneses.[55] Despite these beliefs, Ginzton reported, supervoltage was becoming "universally accepted" in Europe.[56]

As his barrage of reports implied, one of Ginzton's hardest marketing jobs was to sell its own machine to top management at Varian—at least until he became top management himself. Ginzton stated his credo plainly: supervoltage would take hold in the United States, and Varian Associates held a competitive advantage in the field due to its microwave experience.[57] But Varian had no time to spare, Ginzton warned its president; other companies were gearing up to enter the linear accelerator business. Varian should plan an "immediate advertising campaign announcing availability of medical linear accelerators." Of all the radiotherapy technologies, Ginzton argued, echoing Metropolitan-Vickers, only cobalt-60 would remain competitive with linear acceleration—and it was not going to be "defeated easily." Most US hospitals would still initially purchase cobalt because of its lower price, he predicted, but they would turn to linear accelerators to attain higher productivity levels because cobalt-60's relatively low radiation dose rate meant that it could not rapidly process large numbers of patients. The game would be won and cobalt defeated, Ginzton held, on economic grounds.

Ginzton's internal lobbying took root. Varian's annual report that year drew attention to potential medical applications of the linear accelerator it was already marketing for food irradiation, weapons inspection, and physics research.[58] Its accelerator was more flexible than cobalt, the report advised, cheaper than reactors, and (like the Van de Graaff and betatrons, which it didn't mention), could generate high-energy electron beams as well as X-rays for medical treatment.

Varian built its prototype upon Ginzton's return from Europe and gave it to Kaplan's department for testing and refining. In reporting the gift to Terman, Ginzton noted the "value of close cooperation between Stanford and Varian."[59] He appreciated that Varian would benefit from having its machine prominently installed in the University Hospital and from financial payments when the unit generated clinical income. In accepting the Varian instrument, Kaplan welcomed the "tangible evidence of the close collaborative spirit that has long prevailed between Stanford and Varian Associates." Acknowledging the economic imperative of fully utilizing costly equipment, Kaplan saw no difficulty in paying Varian Associates out of clinical revenues "if and when the clinical load reaches a level adequate to keep the machine busy."[60] Kaplan would develop clinical programs that kept the machine busy.

When Russell Varian died suddenly in 1959, Ginzton stepped into the positions of chairman of the board and chief executive officer of Varian Associates, while maintaining close ties with Stanford. Ginzton's service on all the company's policy-making committees, many felt (including Sig Varian), made him the obvious choice.[61] Ginzton now went to the other side of campus to his job. Varian Associates plunged into medical linear accelerator production under Ginzton's direction, knowing that with 200 US units already installed, cobalt-60 held a significant head start, and that marketing would be critical.

The company covered its gawky X-ray-generating machinery with a sleek, award-winning casing obviously designed to appeal to radiologists, hospital administrators, and patients as the ultimate in medical modernity. With the nickname *linac* already in use, the cleverly named Clinac® made the two terms nearly synonymous. Radiologists would come to use them interchangeably when lobbying their hospital administrators for new machines. Product design was only one business lesson Ginzton had to learn in producing products for the medical market—finance was another.

As the High Voltage Engineering Corporation had already discovered, Varian Associates found that listing on the stock exchange subjected the company to the power of Wall Street. Despite the self-proclaimed socialist leanings that had led the Varians and Ginzton to prefer worker ownership,[62] Varian executives learned that turning to the stock market for capital meant that shareholders owned the company and the financial industry managed it. The financiers pressured Varian to develop products not on the basis of scientific interest, skilled engineering, or social usefulness, as founders had originally planned, but on the basis of market position, return on investment, and profit. This was the tack Ginzton took when he reported in to the New York Society of Security Analysts in 1966. Although Varian was not yet turning a profit, Ginzton assured the analysts that it soon would.[63] The company subsequently designed a compact Clinac 4 in order to open up a "whole new market in medium-to-small size hospitals and treatment centers."[64] In this way, Wall Street played a significant role in the widespread diffusion of megavoltage technology.

Despite the mass-market Clinac 4, financiers still criticized Varian's attention to quality engineering that produced financially unsuccessful "custom" linear accelerators.[65] The financial industry demanded mass production to match the mass marketing. Ginzton assured the security analysts in 1969 that the company would no longer build custom machines and that it was in the process of retooling for mass production.[66] He turned to business consulting firms for guidance on fulfilling this promise—although they had little new to say. Recapitulating the criticism from the security analysts, Loeb, Rhoades & Co. advised him that Varian still placed too high a value on "technical achievement at the expense of return on investment," recommending "more hard-headed business-oriented decision making."[67] Walter B. Delafield & Co. gave similar advice.[68] The finance industry's version of a command economy shaped radiation therapy development through such advice. Varian brought out a product line of standardized models with different power levels and features.[69] Varian advertisements in clinical journals applied Ginzton's appreciation of the value of rapid throughput of large numbers of patients. Ads noted in 1970 that "Clinac® 4 speeds the procedure" and in 1972 that the Clinac® 18 could treat 40–60 patients a day.[70]

By developing a product and publicizing it within their professions, Stanford's radiology, engineering, and physics departments played vital roles in the commercialization of Varian's linear accelerator. Ginzton appreciated that the radiology department trained specialists who would want linear accelerators of their own when they took positions in other hospitals.[71] Kaplan appreciated that the linear accelerator conferred income and power on the Stanford radiology department.

Money and Power in the Radiology Department

The radiology department's comparatively large budget, supported by outside funding, made Henry Kaplan a powerful political force in the university. Stanford found itself in the increasingly common situation whereby research-funded departments became personal fiefdoms. Departmental tails wagged the medical-school dogs—or at least that's how the deans saw it.

The conflict at Stanford was partly due, ironically, to the success of Terman's "steeples of excellence" tactic of creating strong departments that brought renown and revenue to the university. When President Sterling established the position of provost and appointed Terman to it, he directed Terman to restructure all university departments as self-supporting entities (preferably with self-supporting faculty members), as Terman had done in engineering.[72] The radiology department more than fulfilled this assignment. But self-supporting did not mean self-governing, and Kaplan would come to resent Sterling's and Terman's efforts to centralize administration and reduce departmental autonomy.

The discord came to a crisis when the medical school moved to Palo Alto, built a new hospital, and (once again) resolved to implement its proposed full-time faculty practice plan. The existing clinical system, medical school dean Robert Alway contended in 1961, operated like an "emporium for the private practice of medicine."[73] Although Kaplan probably agreed with Alway and had ostensibly supported the full-time system as chair of the Committee on Future Plans, he took umbrage when its implementation infringed on his own authority. He objected vehemently when the board of directors of the new Stanford–Palo Alto Hospital took managerial oversight of activities in his department.[74] Sterling supported the hospital administrators, driving Kaplan to what Terman called in one of his telegraphic-style memos to himself "paranoid attacks … in staff and in public."[75]

Siding with Kaplan and chanting a common medical refrain, a radiology colleague defined the issue in terms of "fundamental problems of interference with professional control of the quality of medical care."[76] Terman defined the issue more simply: "Henry wants all on his terms."[77] The hospital would like to control the radiology department, Terman noted, but couldn't finance it by itself.

The dispute was not just a matter of personality conflicts—although those were in abundance. Terman was himself difficult to get along with and tried to micromanage staff reporting to him.[78] In the larger picture, however, it was a struggle over who would control money and practice in the academic medical center. "Sooner or later," Alway advised Sterling, "the Medical School, and I believe you as well, will have to decide just how far we wish to adapt ourselves to Henry's ways." Kaplan's "rather violent intransigence," Alway warned, jeopardized the full-time plan and set up a "potentially disastrous" financial situation.[79]

Despite Kaplan's intransigence, Stanford launched its full time revenue-generating service plan in September 1962. The plan put a ceiling on medical-faculty salaries—which were generous relative to salaries in other university departments. Many faculty members objected to the plan because they wanted to continue their lucrative private practices courtesy of Stanford, although this was not Kaplan's issue. As executive of one of the wealthiest departments, he wanted to control its budget and keep its revenues internal.

Terman would have been well aware that the National Institutes of Health funded three-quarters of the radiology department's budget at the time, primarily via research grants.[80] He credited radiology as one of the medical school's three prestigious steeples of excellence and Kaplan as its star.[81] Whatever the university did to adapt to his ways, Kaplan sat on the 1964 search committee for a new medical school dean—not a new radiology chairman. Kaplan was a dedicated and decorated, if difficult, radiology leader, and Stanford did not want to lose him.

In addition to his clinical and administrative work, Henry Kaplan was an accomplished laboratory scientist who sought to uncover causes of cancer. He engaged deeply in research, acquiring grants to lead some major research trends and follow others. Some radiologists feared that so much laboratory work denigrated medical experience and intuition. Milton Friedman, for example, snidely wondered why certain radiologists worked so hard to eradicate cancer from the "society of rats and mice."[82] Although Kaplan's basic research found that radiation caused leukemias and lymphomas in mice,[83] it is not clear whether he thought the same might happen to patients.

The report on clinical outcomes for the linear accelerator's first year of operation was positive, but Kaplan conceded that his team had intentionally selected patients with good prognoses in order to demonstrate good results.[84] The team had chosen a small boy with retinoblastoma of the eye, a cancer that was known to respond to radiation, as an early linear accelerator patient. The boy would become a poster child for the device, and Stanford radiologists would maintain that his survival with some useful vision demonstrated the value of the linear accelerator. They recognized, however, that conventional radiation devices led to equivalent results.[85] After several years of linear accelerator use, Kaplan announced that they stood "at the threshold of a new scientific era in radiotherapy" (a threshold he would again proclaim two decades later). At the same time, he conceded that the new device had not yielded superior outcomes for the most part and that the situation was ... complicated.[86] Kaplan turned to another cancer known to respond to radiation. Alongside of battling university administrators, Kaplan embarked on a program to battle Hodgkin's Lymphoma.

Kaplan Takes On Hodgkin's

As Kaplan told the story, after witnessing the eradication of a tumor that had been treated at the University of Illinois, he decided to apply radical treatment practices used at the time on patients with extensive Hodgkin's Lymphoma to patients with localized disease.[87] Kaplan defined *radical* as high-dosage radiation used with curative (rather than palliative) intent. His Hodgkin's program implied an acceptance of other contemporary medical definitions of radical. Milton Friedman defined it as going beyond scientific evidence with an "individualized, aggressive attack on each tumor."[88] Such an approach, Friedman recognized, caused greater damage to patients' normal tissues as a trade-off for greater damage to their cancerous ones. Gilbert Fletcher's view that radical radiotherapy "closely approaches maximum tolerance" also tolerated significant patient damage.[89]

Kaplan's approach to Hodgkin's Lymphoma was based on treatment processes reported by Toronto radiotherapist Vera Peters—whom he was not eager to credit. In the process of building up Stanford's program, Kaplan would obstruct Peters' professional activities and invite her to get out of the Hodgkin's field.[90] (She did.) Radiotherapy was already the primary Hodgkin's treatment at the time, as Peters' and other reports noted; over 40 percent of California Hodgkin's patients in the 1940s were treated with radiation.[91] But Peters astonished the specialty in 1950 when she reported a 51 percent 5-year survival rate of Hodgkin's patients treated with radiation at the Ontario Institute of Radiotherapy between 1924 and 1942.[92] Under the direction of Gordon Richards, her unit had applied high doses of radiation to diseased lymph nodes plus "prophylactic" irradiation of surrounding nodes. Radiotherapists at the time—including Peters—attributed some of Ontario's success not only to the radical treatments but also to a predominance of early-stage cases in the first group of treated patients.[93]

Stanford also was irradiating patients with Hodgkin's, combining it with total body irradiation or nitrogen mustard chemotherapy in patients with disseminated disease.[94] Kaplan's new program specifically applied radical treatments to early-stage disease. It raised radiation doses to "tumoricidal" levels, irradiated wide fields of what appeared to be healthy lymph nodes, and used nitrogen mustard from the beginning. Kaplan also ordered routine removal of patients' spleens as well as liver, lymph node, and bone marrow biopsies for purposes of disease staging and planning radiation treatments of every involved area. While a useful research tool yielding information on Hodgkin's disease progression, the staging surgery was dangerous in itself; it carried 12 percent morbidity and 4 percent major complication rates, and its use would decline.[95]

Kaplan had known from the start that his high-dose and wide-field treatments could seriously damage patients, many of whom were children and young adults. "It was entirely conceivable," he acknowledged in the *New England Journal of Medicine* a few years after starting the project, that "radical treatment might well kill more patients than it cured."[96] Kaplan's biographer, Stanford radiation oncologist Charlotte DeCroes Jacobs, has starkly portrayed agonizing patient suffering and death resulting directly from the high-intensity treatments. Hodgkin's patients at Stanford accumulated so much physical damage that a medical resident called one young boy a "walking textbook of radiation morbidity."[97] Kaplan's team would report severe radiation damage to patients' lungs, livers, kidneys, hearts, brains, and gastrointestinal tracts.[98] The severity of damage correlated with radiation dose, providing strong evidence that radiation itself (rather than the disease) was the major culprit. Some of the inflicted damage took longer than the standard 5 years to reveal itself. It would turn out that nearly 20 percent of Stanford's first treatment cohort developed secondary leukemias and lymphomas—an outcome that, ironically, Kaplan's mouse experiments had portended.[99]

Kaplan and Stanford oncologist Saul Rosenberg called themselves (and their patients) "courageous" in their willingness to experiment with methods "often criticized by informed colleagues."[100] But Rosenberg's advocacy of controlled trials threatened Kaplan and his mode of "attack with all barrels blasting," as DeCroes Jacobs put it, and Kaplan withdrew from their collaboration.[101] Herself sometimes devastatingly critical of his methods, his biographer ascribed Kaplan's aggressive clinical treatments to a "remarkable self-confidence, bordering on a sense of his own infallibility."

Despite my reporting criticism of some of his clinical practices, it is not my purpose to single out Henry Kaplan for censure. His aggressive practices and aggressive personality did not distinguish him very much from the personality and practices of Howard Kelly, Hugh Hare, Robert Stone, Henry Garland, and Gilbert Fletcher, among other radiotherapy leaders, as previously discussed. Their collective practice is the important issue. It was common at the time to use cancer patients with advanced disease to test "almost every kind of speculative, and often toxic, therapy."[102] Collectively, the practices raise questions concerning whether conformity to common practice ethically justifies treatment and the extent to which improving outcomes for future patients justifies damaging present patients.

Alongside of patient damage, Kaplan's treatments were reporting longer remissions and longer survival times for Hodgkin's patients. Although his studies did not compare his results with survival of Stanford patients prior to the beginning of his program, nor did they use controls or compare his treatments with other protocols, Kaplan reported that 5-year survival rates of Stanford Hodgkin's patients treated with radiation and/or chemotherapy increased from 67 percent for the 1961–65 patient cohort, to 79 percent for the 1966–70 cohort, and to 84 percent for the 1971–75 one (and that 5-year relapse-free survival rates rose from 49 percent, to 62 percent, to 69 percent, respectively).[103] Kaplan compared these figures to reports in the literature of 30–35 percent 5-year survival of Hodgkin's patients in the time of kilovoltage and implied that voltage increase was the primary factor in the measured survival gain.[104]

But factors other than voltage increases were also involved. Earlier diagnosis, more accurate staging, and patient selection could also have contributed to the gains in Hodgkin's survival. With a prestigious clinical research program paying for patient care, primary-care physicians may have referred patients earlier in their disease, which in and of itself would have improved the measured 5-year survival rates. More accurate staging permitted Kaplan to claim improved cure rates for early-stage disease by eliminating more advanced cases from the calculations. Furthermore, it is not possible to tease out the role of radiotherapy in the survival gains. While Kaplan's reports tended to credit radiation, his combined use of radio- and chemotherapy meant that the relative contribution of each remained murky. Contemporary studies suggested that chemotherapy and radiotherapy both had to be used in order to achieve best results in late-stage Hodgkin's patients.[105]

Around the same time, National Cancer Institute director Vincent DeVita credited his own Hodgkin's successes entirely to chemotherapy—although he had included radiation in his first combination chemotherapy protocol. When DeVita reported cures from his second-generation chemotherapy protocol, which had eliminated radiation, he concluded that radiation was not necessary for patients with early-stage Hodgkin's. DeVita later reported that this advice did not please radiotherapists. He accused them of refusing to cooperate in trials unless radiation was included in both study arms (which would assure continuing use of radiation and rule out possible measures of comparative effectiveness of the two treatment modalities).[106]

Whatever the cause(s), Hodgkin's survival gains became one of the few success stories in cancer treatment. By 2015, the US 5-year Hodgkin's survival rate reported in at 85 percent and the 10-year rate at 80 percent.[107] Although an oncologist noted that Kaplan's treatment of Hodgkin's became "the guiding paradigm for modern oncology,"[108] it is not scientifically valid to generalize to all cancers the experience with a single disease representing less than 1 percent of them. While Hodgkin's outcomes offer hope, every cancer is a separate disease. Many patients with other cancers have undergone similarly radical treatments without similarly positive results. Kaplan himself recognized that Hodgkin's outcomes surpassed those of other cancers. At best, he summarized in 1965, megavoltage improved results over kilovoltage only for a select group of tumors, which, in addition to Hodgkin's, he named as cancers of the cervix, bladder, oral cavity, and testis.[109]

Ongoing reports of Hodgkin's success contributed significantly to widespread adoption of megavoltage radiotherapy.[110] Although both Ontario and Stanford had initiated their Hodgkin's treatments with kilovoltage, Peters moved to cobalt-60 when it became available to her in 1953.[111] Fletcher and his colleagues at M. D. Anderson also chose cobalt when they initiated radical treatment of Hodgkin's and other lymphomas.[112] Kaplan shifted from kilovoltage to his linear accelerator when it opened in 1956. The media enhanced popular and professional enthusiasm for the linac; *Time* magazine's "Hope for Hodgkin's" featured Kaplan and his machine.[113]

Kaplan's treatment of Hodgkin's showcased himself, Stanford, Varian, and the linear accelerator. Despite other investigators' use of cobalt, Kaplan's textbook, *Hodgkin's Disease*, pictured Varian's 6 MeV Clinac® and advised that such a machine was particularly desirable for intensive treatment of the disease. Kaplan and his team often paid tribute to their linear accelerator in the titles of their papers, and Ginzton reciprocally credited Kaplan's work on Hodgkin's with providing the knowledge base for developing the Clinac product line.[114] At the same time, Kaplan conceded that radical irradiation for Hodgkin's and other cancers could be equally achieved with the betatron or cobalt-60 devices that operated at source-to-skin distances of 80 cm or more.[115] There was "nothing magic about a linear accelerator," he explained, except in its ease of use—the same advantage that Gilbert Fletcher claimed for cobalt.[116]

The linear accelerator boom was not a case of finally building the right gun, and it was not based on evidence from scientific studies of significantly improved clinical outcomes over other megavoltage devices (more on this in Chapter 8). Nor did Kaplan believe the linac to be the best radiotherapy technology that could be achieved. If only he could get the right beam, energy level, dose, delivery schedule, and masking technique, he held, radiation therapy would work better,[117] and Kaplan continued the search for a better device.

Kaplan also worked with Stanford's engineering team on another teletherapy device—a hospital-based pi-meson (pion) irradiator.[118] The project foundered, however, when NIH turned down his development grant application to build a huge pion center. Theoretically, researchers enthused, referring to beam characteristics and presaging arguments for protons, pions' dose localization properties made them ideal radiotherapy agents.[119] The Los Alamos Meson Physics Facility, with equipment and expertise left over from the atomic bomb, started treating patients on its pion-generating machine in 1974.[120] But a retrospective study of all 228 patients treated at Los Alamos found severe complications and high failure rates.[121] A later paper out of the Vancouver pion facility reported no local control or survival gains.[122] Pion devices did not come to threaten the linac's ascendency in the radiation therapy market.

As this chapter has shown, all the ingredients of a successful radiation-therapy industry came together at Stanford: an engineer at an entrepreneurial university, a well-financed manufacturer, a self-supporting hospital specialty department, and a self-confident radiologist on a quest to conquer cancer. The following chapter describes how the massive growth of radiation therapy devices at midcentury was sometimes at odds with professional opinions as well as available data concerning their effectiveness. Yet the specialty continued to play a strong political role in reinforcing growth in the field.

Notes

1 Takahiro Ueyama and Christophe Lécuyer, "Building Science-Based Medicine at Stanford: Henry Kaplan and the Medical Linear Accelerator, 1948–1975," In Carsten

Timmermann and Julie Anderson, eds., *Devices and Designs: Medical Technologies in Historical Perspective* (Basingstoke: Palgrave Macmillan, 2006), 137–155.

2 Martin Kenney and W. Richard Goe, "The Role of Social Embeddedness in Professorial Entrepreneurship: A Comparison of Electrical Engineering and Computer Science at UC Berkeley and Stanford," *Research Policy* (2004) 33: 691–707.

3 Frederick Terman to C. H. Suydam, April 10, 1928; Frederick Terman to Frederick A. Kolster, July 9, 1928. Frederick E. Terman Papers, SC160, Series 5, Box 5. Special Collections and University Archives, Stanford University Libraries.

4 Frederick Terman, "Why Do We Do Research?" Stanford Business Conference, July 22, 1958. Frederick E. Terman Papers, SC 160, Series 8, Box 2. Special Collections and University Archives, Stanford University Libraries.

5 Timothy Lenoir, "Draft: Myths about Stanford's Interactions with Industry," Department of History, Stanford University, 2004, 1. fsi-media.stanford.edu/evnts/4097/TLenoir_Myths_about_Stanford.pdf accessed Jan 3, 2007.

6 Frederick Terman, note on yellow paper, typed, not dated. In file dated 1969. Frederick E. Terman Papers, SC160, Series 3, Box 64. Special Collections and University Archives, Stanford University Libraries.

7 Frederick Terman, "Notes for "Electronics—a Basic Industry," 21st Regional Trust Conference, San Francisco, October 22–24, 1947. Frederick E. Terman Papers, SC160, Series 8, Box 1. Special Collections and University Archives, Stanford University Libraries.

8 Dorothy Varian, *The Inventor and the Pilot* (Palo Alto, CA: Pacific Books, 1983), 182.

9 Bruce Hevly, "Stanford's Supervoltage X-ray Tube," *Osiris* 9 (1994): 85–100.

10 C. Stewart Gillmor, *Fred Terman at Stanford: Building a Discipline, a University, and Silicon Valley* (Stanford, CA: Stanford University Press, 2004), 152–153.

11 E. E. Ginzton, "The $100 Idea," *IEEE Spectrum* 12 (1975): 30–39.

12 "A Brief History of Varian Associates," no date. Russell and Sigurd Varian Papers, SC 345, Varian Associates Series, Box 3. Special Collections and University Archives, Stanford University Libraries.

13 Dorothy Varian, *The Inventor and the Pilot* (Palo Alto, CA: Pacific Books, 1983), 231.

14 Frederick Terman, handwritten notes, "Varian Associates," December 3, 1951. Frederick E. Terman Papers, SC160, Series 8, Box 1. Special Collections and University Archives, Stanford University Libraries.

15 "Stanford Research Park." www.stanford.edu/home/stanford/history/marks?.html accessed Jan 3, 2007.

16 Frederick Terman, "Fundamental Research in University and College Laboratories," notes for talk at First Annual Northern California Research Conference, January 12, 1949. Frederick E. Terman Papers, SC160, Series 8, Box 1. Special Collections and University Archives, Stanford University Libraries.

17 Timothy Lenoir, "Myths about Stanford's Interactions with Industry," Department of History, Stanford University, 2004, 11. http://iis-db.stanford.edu/evnts/4097/TLenoir_Myths_about_Stanford.pdf accessed January 3, 2007.

18 Tube Department and Advanced Tube Development Laboratory Study Group, "Proposal for a General Electric Microwave Laboratory at Stanford University," April 12, 1954. Frederick E. Terman Papers, SC 160, Series 2, Box 18. Special Collections and University Archives, Stanford University Libraries.

19 H. R. Oldfield to F. Terman, July 14, 1954. Frederick E. Terman Papers, SC 160, Series 2, Box 18. Special Collections and University Archives, Stanford University Libraries.

20 R. L. Krapf to F. Terman, enclosing copies of proposed retainer agreement, May 13, 1955. Frederick E. Terman Papers, SC160, Series 5, Box 5. Special Collections and University Archives, Stanford University Libraries.

21 J. W. Brown to F. Terman, October 6, 1954; F. Terman to J. W. Brown, October 14, 1954. Frederick E. Terman Papers, SC 160, Series 2, Box 18, Special Collections and University Archives, Stanford University Libraries.

22 G. William Domhoff, *The Bohemian Grove and Other Retreats; A Study in Ruling-class Cohesiveness* (New York, NY: Harper & Row, 1974).

23 Frederick Terman, "Bohemian Grove," notes for talk, July 23, 1951. Frederick E. Terman Papers, SC160, Series 8, Box 1. Special Collections and University Archives, Stanford University Libraries.

24 Stanford University Committee on Future Plans, *Stanford Medical School Council Report* (Stanford, CA.: Stanford University, 1952); Stanford University Committee on Future Plans, *Reports, 1952–1953*. Special Collections and University Archives, Stanford University Libraries.

25 Robert H. Ebert, "The Role of the Medical School in Planning the Health-Care System," *The Journal of Medical Education* 42 (1967): 481–488.

26 Timothy Lenoir, "Myths about Stanford's Interactions with Industry," Department of History, Stanford University, 2004, 6. http://iis-db.stanford.edu/evnts/4097/TLenoir_Myths_about_Stanford.pdf accessed January 3, 2007.

27 "A Conversation with Henry S. Kaplan," December 7, 9, 14, 1983. Edward L. Ginzton Papers, SC 330, Box 13. Special Collections and University Archives, Stanford University Libraries.

28 Roger. F. Robison, "The Race for Megavoltage: X-rays Versus Telegamma," *Acta Oncologica* 34 (1995):1055–1074.

29 M. Baker, "Physician–Physicist Partnership Built First U.S. Medical Accelerator," *Stanford Report* May 18, 2005.

30 Henry Kaplan and Edward L. Ginzton, "Joint Statement about the Medical Application of the Linear Electron Accelerator," enclosure in letter from H. Kaplan to E. Ginzton, February 2, 1951. Edward L. Ginzton Papers, SC 330, Box 6. Special Collections and University Archives, Stanford University Libraries.

31 Henry S. Kaplan, "Recent Experimental Contributions to Radiotherapy," *American Journal of Roentgenology Radium Therapy and Nuclear Medicine* 80 (1958): 822–832.

32 Walter E. Meyerhof, "Comments upon a Proposal by Drs. Ginzton and Kaplan for a 6 MeV Linear Electron Accelerator to be Built for Clinical Use," November 12, 1951. Edward L. Ginzton Papers, SC 330, Box 6. Special Collections and University Archives, Stanford University Libraries.

33 "High-Power X-Rays Made at Low Cost: Stanford Rigs Atom Smasher to Put Cancer Treatment Within Reach," *New York Times* July 15, 1952, 23.

34 "Stanford University's Long-awaited 'Cancer Gun' Was Unveiled Today at Stanford Medical School," *Stanford University News*, April 27, 1956. http://med.stanford.edu/content/dam/Timeline/legacy_1956_hkaplan_A2.pdf accessed January 7, 2016; Stanford University, "High-Energy X-Ray 'Cancer Gun' Accelerator Now in Operation," *Stanford Today* August 15, 1956, 1–2. Edward L. Ginzton Papers, SC 330, Box 6. Special Collections and University Archives, Stanford University Libraries

35 "Budgets for the Year 1957–1958: Lane Hospital, Stanford Hospital, Out-Patient Clinics." Special Collections and University Archives, Stanford University Libraries.

36 "Development of a Medical Linear Electron Accelerator for High Energy Radiation Therapy," September 1, 1955. Frederick E. Terman Papers, SC 160, Series 2, Box 18. Special Collections and University Archives, Stanford University Libraries.

37 Palo Alto–Stanford Hospital Center, *News* Palo Alto, October, 1959. Special Collections and University Archives, Stanford University Libraries.

38 "A Conversation with Henry S. Kaplan," December 7, 9, 14, 1983. Edward L. Ginzton Papers, SC 330, Box 13. Special Collections and University Archives, Stanford University Libraries.

39 Russell Varian to "Sig and Winny," November 23, 1946, Edward L. Ginzton Papers, SC 330, Box 19. Special Collections and University Archives, Stanford University Libraries.

40 Martin A. Edwards to E. L. Ginzton, January 7, 1953, with enclosure: "Draft Agreement with GE." Frederick E. Terman Papers, SC 160, Series 2, Box 18. Special Collections and University Archives, Stanford University Libraries.

41 E. L. Ginzton to F. Terman, November 30, 1962. Frederick E. Terman Papers, Series 3, SC 160, Box 59. Special Collections and University Archives, Stanford University Libraries.

42 Memo to file, "Subject: Mr. William Brown of Raytheon," January 14, 1954. Frederick E. Terman Papers, Series 2, SC160, Box 16. Special Collections and University Archives. Stanford University Libraries.

43 *Varian Associates* June, 1956, 6. Varian, Inc. Records, SC 889, Box 38. Special Collections and University Archives, Stanford University Libraries.

44 M. Weissbluth to E. Ginzton and H. Kaplan, July 15, 1957. Edward L. Ginzton Papers, SC 330, Box 3. Special Collections and University Archives, Stanford University Libraries.

45 Microwave Laboratory and Department of Radiology, "Proposed [sic] for Biological and Medical Investigations with the Linear Electron Accelerator to be Installed in the New Microwave Laboratory Building Stanford University," April, 1954. Frederick E. Terman Papers, SC 160, Series 2, Box 18. Special Collections and University Archives, Stanford University Libraries; H. S. Kaplan to D. W. Seldin, December 6, 1954, Henry S. Kaplan Papers, SC 317, Box 11. Special Collections and University Archives, Stanford University Libraries.

46 Stanford Research Institute, *A Study of Small Business in the Electronics Industry* (Washington, DC: Small Business Administration, 1962), 79; Christophe Lécuyer, *Making Silicon Valley: Innovation and the Growth of High Tech, 1930–1970* (Cambridge: MIT Press, 2006), 92–94, 98, 123–124.

47 Dean Witter Investment Bankers, "Varian Associates: Report from Research Department," August 17, 1955; Dean Witter Investment Bankers, "Varian Associates: Report from Research Department," September, 1956. Russell and Sigurd Varian Papers, SC345, Varian Associates Series, Box 4. Special Collections and University Archives, Stanford University Libraries.

48 E. Ginzton to H. Kaplan, January 2, 1957. Henry S. Kaplan Papers, SC 317, Box 11, Special Collections and University Archives, Stanford University Libraries; E. L. Ginzton, "Visit to Siemens-Reiniger-Werke, AG," October 17, 1957. Henry S. Kaplan Papers, SC 317, Box 11. Special Collections and University Archives, Stanford University Libraries.

49 E. L. Ginzton, "Visit to Christie Hospital and Holt Radium Institute," December 6, 1957. Henry S. Kaplan Papers, SC 317, Box 11. Special Collections and University Archives, Stanford University Libraries.

50 E. L. Ginzton, "Visit to Metropolitan-Vickers Electrical Co, Ltd, Research Department," December 5, 1957. Henry S. Kaplan Papers, SC 317, Box 11. Stanford Special Collections and University Archives, Stanford University Libraries.

51 Frederick Terman note to self, "Alway," December 29, 1961. Frederick E. Terman Papers, Series 2, SC 160, Box 15. Special Collections and University Archives, Stanford University Libraries.

52 John V. Pickstone, *Ways of Knowing: A New History of Science, Technology, and Medicine* (Chicago, IL: University of Chicago Press, 2000), 173–186.

53 "Multi-Volt X-rays Held Aid in Cancer," *New York Times* July 28, 1950, 19.

54 E. L. Ginzton, "Visit to Radiotherapeutic Research Unit, Hammersmith Hospital," December 4, 1957. This remark is underlined by hand in the report Kaplan received, presumably by Kaplan himself. Henry S. Kaplan Papers, SC 317, Box 11. Special Collections and University Archives, Stanford University Libraries.

55 E. L. Ginzton, "Visit to Canton Hospital, Zurich," October 10, 1957. Henry S. Kaplan Papers, SC 317, Box 11. Special Collections and University Archives, Stanford University Libraries.

56 E. L. Ginzton, "Visit to Radiotherapeutic Research Unit, Hammersmith Hospital," December 4, 1957. Henry S. Kaplan Papers, SC 317, Box 11. Special Collections and University Archives, Stanford University Libraries.

57 E. L. Ginzton to Myrl Stearns, December 18, 1957. Russell and Sigurd Varian Papers, SC 345, Varian Associates Series, Box 2. Special Collections and University Archives, Stanford University Libraries.

58 Varian Associates, *Annual Report 1957*. Russell and Sigurd Varian Papers, SC 345, Varian Associates Series, Box 2. Special Collections and University Archives, Stanford University Archives.

59 E. L. Ginzton to F.E. Terman, "Development of Linear Electron Accelerator by Varian Associates," March 16, 1959. Frederick E. Terman Papers, Series 3, SC 160, Box 59.Special Collections and University Archives, Stanford University Libraries.

60 H. S. Kaplan to Emmet G. Cameron, March 5, 1959. Edward L. Ginzton Papers, SC 330, Box 6. Special Collections and University Archives, Stanford University Libraries.

61 "Sig's talk," September 19, 1959. Russell and Sigurd Varian Papers, SC 345, Varian Associates Series, Box 2. Special Collections and University Archives, Stanford University Libraries.

62 Christophe Lécuyer, *Making Silicon Valley: Innovation and the Growth of High Tech, 1930–1970* (Cambridge, MA: MIT Press, 2006), 94.

63 Edward Ginzton, "Address to the New York Society of Security Analysts," June 14, 1966. Russell and Sigurd Varian Papers, SC 345, Varian Associates series, Box 4. Special Collections and University Archives, Stanford University Libraries.

64 Varian Associates, *Annual Report 1968*. Russell and Sigurd Varian Papers, SC 345. Varian Associates series, Box 1. Special Collections and University Archives, Stanford University Libraries.

65 Varian Associates, *Annual Report 1968*. Russell and Sigurd Varian Papers, SC 345, Varian Associates series, Box 1. Special Collections and University Archives, Stanford University Libraries.

66 Edward Ginzton, "Address to the New York Society of Security Analysts," March 27, 1969. Russell and Sigurd Varian Papers, SC 345, Box 4. Varian Associates series. Special Collections and University Archives, Stanford University Libraries.

67 Loeb, Rhoades & Co., "Research Department Notes, Industry: Electronics, Varian Associates," January, 1970. Edward L. Ginzton Papers, SC 330, Box 4. Special Collections and Archives, Stanford University Libraries.

68 Walter B. Delafield & Company, "Performance Briefs," February 17, 1970. Edward L. Ginzton Papers, SC 330, Box 4. Special Collections and University Archives, Stanford University Libraries.

69 Varian Associates, *Annual Report 1971*. Russell and Sigurd Varian Papers, SC 345, Varian Associates series, Box 1. Special Collections and University Archives, Stanford University Libraries.

70 Varian Associates advertisements, *Radiology* 94 (February 1970), np; *Radiology* 103 (May, 1972), np.

71 Edward L. Ginzton and Craig S. Nunan, "History of Microwave Electron Linear Accelerators for Radiotherapy," *International Journal of Radiation Oncology Biology Physics* 11 (1985): 205–216.

72 Rebecca S. Lowen, *Creating the Cold War University: The Transformation of Stanford* (Berkeley, CA: University of California Press 1997), 149, 156–157.

73 Robert Alway, "Statement by Dr. Alway Regarding Medical Service Plan and Related Matters," October 20, 1961. Frederick E. Terman Papers, SC160, Series 3, Box 41. Special Collections and University Archives, Stanford University Libraries.

74 Henry S. Kaplan to Lowell Rantz, "Resolution of PASHC Board's Responsibility for Service Activities," December 12, 1960. Frederick E. Terman Papers, SC160, Series 3, Box 41. Special Collections and University Archives, Stanford University Libraries.

75 Frederick Terman, note to self, not dated, in with 1962 files. Frederick E. Terman Papers, SC 160, Series 3, Box 41. Special Collections and University Archives. Stanford University Libraries. Underline original.

76 Herbert L. Abrams to Robert H. Alway, "Hospital Interference with Professional Control of Medical Care; Standards of Consultative Radiology, and University Objectives in the Radiology Department," February 19, 1962. Frederick A. Terman Papers, Stanford University Special Collections and Archives. SC160, Series 3, Box 41.
77 Frederick Terman, note to self, "Alway," December 29, 1961. Frederick E. Terman Papers, SC160, Series 3, Box 41. Special Collections and University Archives, Stanford University Libraries.
78 Terman called one hapless dean at 11:30 one night to discuss budgets. Dinner guests heard the dean respond … *this really isn't a very convenient time to talk, Fred … it's really very late, Fred …* "Dammit, Fred, it's New Year's Eve!" C. Stewart Gillmor, *Fred Terman at Stanford: Building a Discipline, a University, and Silicon Valley* (Stanford, CA: Stanford University Press, 2004), 424.
79 Robert Alway to Wallace Sterling, "Dean's-Eye View of the School," July 13, 1962. Frederick E. Terman Papers, SC160, Series 3, Box 41. Special Collections and University Archives, Stanford University Libraries.
80 Takahiro Ueyama and Christophe Lécuyer, "Building Science-Based Medicine at Stanford: Henry Kaplan and the Medical Linear Accelerator, 1948–1975," In Carsten Timmermann and Julie Anderson, eds., *Devices and Designs: Medical Technologies in Historical Perspective* (Basingstoke, Hampshire: Palgrave Macmillan, 2006), 137–155.
81 Frederick Terman, note to self, October 18, 1962. Frederick E, Terman Papers, SC 160, Series 3, Box 41. Special Collections and University Archives, Stanford University Libraries. Terman named DNA research and Norman Shumway's cardiac surgery as the other two medical school steeples.
82 M. Friedman, "The Light is Better Here," *American Journal of Roentgenology Radium Therapy and Nuclear Medicine* 102 (1968): 3–7.
83 Henry S. Kaplan, "Early Microscopic Diagnosis of Lymphosarcoma in Situ in Thymus of Irradiated Mice," *Federation Proceedings* 19 (1960): 399.
84 Henry Kaplan, "Summary of Experience with Six MEV Linear Accelerator," enclosure in letter from E. L. Ginzton to Frederick Terman, January 29, 1957. Frederick E. Terman Papers, SC 160, Series 3, Box 41. Special Collections and University Archives, Stanford University Libraries.
85 Malcolm A. Bagshaw and Henry S. Kaplan, "Supervoltage Linear Accelerator Radiation Therapy VIII: Retinoblastoma," Radiology 86 (1966): 242–246.
86 Henry S. Kaplan, "New Horizons in Radiotherapy of Malignant Disease," *Journal of the American Medical Association* 171 (1959): 133–138.
87 Henry S. Kaplan "The Radical Radiotherapy of Regionally Localized Hodgkin's Disease," *Radiology* 78 (1962): 553–569.
88 Milton Friedman, "Concepts of Radical Irradiation Therapy," *CA: A Cancer Journal for Clinicians* 5 (1955): 20–28.
89 Gilbert H. Fletcher, *Textbook of Radiotherapy* (Philadelphia, PA: Lea & Febiger, 1966), 472.
90 Charlotte DeCroes Jacobs, *Henry Kaplan and the Story of Hodgkin's Disease* (Stanford, CA: Stanford University Press, 2010), 255.
91 California Tumor Registry, *Cancer Registration and Survival in California* (Berkeley: State of California Department of Public Health, 1963), 313.
92 M. Vera Peters, "A Study of Survivals in Hodgkin's Disease Treated Radiologically," *American Journal of Roentgenology and Radium Therapy* 63 (1950): 299–311.
93 Charles M. Nice and K. Wilhelm Stenstrom, "Irradiation Therapy on Hodgkin's Disease," *Radiology* 62 (1954): 641–653.
94 Frank A. Brown and Henry S. Kaplan, "Hodgkin's Disease: A Revised Clinical Classification and an Approach to the Treatment of its Localized Form," *Stanford Medical Bulletin* 15 (1957): 183–192.

95 Richard Slavin and Thomas S. Nelsen, "Complications from Staging Laparotomy for Hodgkin's Disease," *National Cancer Institute Monograph 36, International Symposium on Hodgkin's Disease* 1973, 457–459.
96 Henry S. Kaplan, "Clinical Evaluation and Radiotherapeutic Management of Hodgkin's Disease and the Malignant Lymphomas," *New England Journal of Medicine* 278 (1968): 892–899.
97 Charlotte DeCroes Jacobs, *Henry Kaplan and the Story of Hodgkin's Disease* (Stanford, CA: Stanford University Press, 2010), 151–158, 193, 295.
98 Henry S. Kaplan and J. Robert Stewart, "Complications of Intensive Megavoltage Radiotherapy for Hodgkin's Disease," *National Cancer Institute Monograph 36, International Symposium on Hodgkin's Disease* 1973, 439–444; Saul A. Rosenberg and Henry S. Kaplan, "The Evolution and Summary Results of the Stanford Randomized Clinical Trials of the Management of Hodgkin's Disease: 1962–1984," *International Journal of Radiation Oncology Biology Physics* 11 (1985): 5–22.
99 John D. Boice and Lois B. Travis, "Body Wars: Effect of Friendly Fire (Cancer Therapy)," *Journal of the National Cancer Institute* 87 (1995): 705–706; Anita Gustavson, Birgitta Osterman, and Eva Cavallin-Ståhl, "A Systematic Overview of Radiation Therapy Effects in Hodgkin's Lymphoma," *Acta Oncologica* 42 (2003): 589–604; Peter Borchmann, Dennis A. Eichenauer, and Andreas Engert, "State of the Art in the Treatment of Hodgkin Lymphoma," *Nature Reviews Clinical Oncology* 9 (2012): 450–459; Chris R. Kelsey, Anne W. Beaven, Louis F. Diehl, and Leonard R. Prosnitz, "Combined-Modality Therapy for Early-Stage Hodgkin Lymphoma: Maintaining High Cure Rates While Minimizing Risks," *Oncology—New York* 26 (2012): 1182–1193.
100 Saul A. Rosenberg and Henry S. Kaplan, "The Evolution and Summary Results of the Stanford Randomized Clinical Trials of the Management of Hodgkin's Disease: 1962–1984," *International Journal of Radiation Oncology Biology Physics* 11 (1985): 5–22.
101 Charlotte DeCroes Jacobs, *Henry Kaplan and the Story of Hodgkin's Disease* (Stanford, CA: Stanford University Press, 2010), 4, 156–157.
102 Gerald Kutcher, *Contested Medicine: Cancer Research and the Military* (Chicago, IL: University of Chicago Press, 2009), 5.
103 Henry S. Kaplan, *Hodgkin's Disease* 2nd ed., (Cambridge, MA: Harvard University Press, 1980), 367, 556.
104 Henry S. Kaplan, "Radiotherapeutic Advances in the Treatment of Neoplastic Disease," *Israel Journal of Medical Sciences* 13 (1977): 808–814.
105 Leonard R. Prosnitz, Rafael L. Montalvo, Diana B. Fischer, Allen B. Silberstein, and David S. Berger, "Treatment of Stage IIIA Hodgkin's Disease: Is Radiotherapy Alone Adequate?" *International Journal of Radiation Oncology Biology Physics* 4 (1978): 781–787.
106 Vincent T. DeVita and Elizabeth DeVita-Raeburn, *The Death of Cancer* (New York, NY: Farrar, Straus and Giroux, 2015), 106–107.
107 American Cancer Society, "What Are the Key Statistics about Hodgkin Disease?" http://www.cancer.org/cancer/hodgkindisease/detailedguide/hodgkin-disease-key-statistics accessed May 15, 2015.
108 Joseph M. Connors, "Henry Kaplan and the Story of Hodgkin's Disease. Book Review," *Journal of the History of Medicine and Allied Sciences* 67 (2012): 501–504.
109 Henry S. Kaplan, "Current Status of Radiotherapy for Neoplastic Disease," *DM Disease-a-Month* 11 (1965): 1–56.
110 Juan A. Del Regato, *Radiological Oncologists: The Unfolding of a Medical Specialty* (Reston, VA: Radiology Centennial, 1993), 246.
111 M. Vera Peters, "Prophylactic Treatment of Adjacent Areas in Hodgkin's Disease," *Cancer Research* 26 Part I (1966): 1232–1243.

112 Lillian M. Fuller and Gilbert H. Fletcher, "The Radiotherapeutic Management of the Lymphomatous Diseases," *American Journal of Roentgenology, Radium Therapy and Nuclear Medicine* 88 (1962): 909–923; Lillian M. Fuller, "Results of Large Volume Irradiation in the Management of Hodgkin's Disease and Malignant Lymphomas Originating in the Abdomen," *Radiology* 87 (1966): 1058–1064.

113 "Hope for Hodgkin's," *Time*, April 3, 1964.

114 Edward L. Ginzton and Craig S. Nunan, "History of Microwave Electron Linear Accelerators for Radiotherapy," *International Journal of Radiation Oncology Biology Physics* 11 (1985): 205–216.

115 Henry S. Kaplan, "Hodgkin's Disease," *Current Problems in Radiology* 1 (1971): 1–39.

116 Henry S. Kaplan, "Clinical Evaluation and Radiotherapeutic Management of Hodgkin's Disease and the Malignant Lymphomas," *New England Journal of Medicine* 278 (1968): 892–899.

117 Henry S. Kaplan, H. Alan Schwettman, William M. Fairbank,Douglas Boyd, and Malcolm A. Bagshaw, "A Hospital-Based Superconducting Accelerator Facility for Negative Pi-Meson Beam Radiotherapy," *Radiology* 108 (1973): 159–172.

118 Henry S. Kaplan, H. Alan Schwettman, William M. Fairbank, et al., "A Hospital-Based Superconducting Accelerator Facility for Negative Pi-Meson Beam Radiotherapy," *Radiology* 108 (1973): 159–172.

119 Chaim Richman, Henry Aceto, Munduni R. Raju, and Bernard Schwartz, "The Radiotherapeutic Possibilities of Negative Pions," *AJR, American Journal of Roentgenology* 96 (1966): 777–790.

120 M. R. Raju, "Particle Radiotherapy: Historical Development and Current Status," *Radiation Research* 145 (1996): 391–407.

121 C. F. von Essen, M. A. Bagshaw, S. E. Bush, A. R. Smith, and M. M. Kligerman, "Long-term Results of Pion Therapy at Los Alamos," *International Journal of Radiation Oncology Biology Physics* 13 (1987): 1389–1398.

122 Tom Pickles, George B. Goodman, Chris J. Fryer, Julie Bowen, Andrew J. Coldman, Graeme G. Duncan, Peter H. Graham, Michael Mckenzie, William James Morris, Dorianne E. Rheaume, and Isabel Syndikus, "Pion Conformal Radiation of Prostate Cancer: Results of a Randomized Study, *International Journal of Radiation Oncology Biology Physics* 43 (1999): 47–55.

8 Radiation Therapy Politics

Organized radiation therapy actively participated in political activities that supported growth of its devices and departments in the face of its concerns about clinical effectiveness.

Data and Discourse

Clinical Practices and Epidemiological Findings

It was clear by the 1970s that medical care had contributed little to two of the century's three most dramatic cancer mortality trends. Deaths from stomach cancer plummeted, while those from lung cancer skyrocketed (among males first). Incidence changes explained both of these trends. For unknown reasons, fewer people were developing stomach cancer. The cause of the lung cancer epidemic was by then well known. It was tobacco, and nothing medicine did to treat the disease ameliorated its high mortality. Medical care did, however, play a role in the third dramatic trend: reduction in mortality from cancer of the uterine cervix.

Statewide data from California reported a rise in 5-year cervical cancer survival rates from 40 percent in the 1942–46 treatment cohort to 63 percent in 1952–56, as shown in Figure 8.1. The California figures, which included a significant chunk of the US population, were comparable to an ongoing survey initiated by the League of Nations, which found recurrence-free cervical cancer survival rates in selected European, plus a few American, hospitals rising from less than 30 percent in the 1930s to more than 50 percent by the 1960s.[1]

Radiotherapy leaders used temporal correlations between voltage increases and survival gains to claim a causal connection between the two. Canadians T. A. Watson and Harold Johns later asserted that cure rates for cervical cancer rose from 25 to 75 percent "with the introduction of high-energy machines, cobalt units and betatrons."[2] But this was professional hype, and the authors in fact knew better. The 25 percent before figure was spurious, as Watson himself had reported a 45 percent 5-year survival rate for cervical cancer patients treated in Saskatchewan cancer clinics prior to their introduction of megavoltage.[3] Furthermore, Watson had previously attributed much of the postwar gain not to voltage increases but to earlier diagnoses due to the growth of provincial cancer clinics and Pap smear use.[4] Nor did their claim acknowledge the fact that most radiation treatments for cervical cancer at the time entailed radium brachytherapy (not high-voltage teletherapy). The 25–75 percent claim stuck, however, and the radiation therapy industry exploited it.[5]

As Watson appreciated, medicine can take credit for much of the mortality decline in cervical cancer due to recognizing and communicating to women the importance of early diagnosis and treatment before the cancer has had a chance to spread. The proportion of California women diagnosed when their cervical cancers were diagnosed as "localized" rose from 36 percent in the early 1940s to 57 percent in the mid-1950s.[6] Although staging definitions were far from consistent, both the California and the League of Nations–originated studies found increased 5-year survival rates for localized cervical cancer; California's rose from 60 to 85 percent.[7] Yet the rise in survival within the localized category also suggests treatment gain. The major treatment change for cervical cancer in California during this time period was a shift toward surgery and away from radiation. Use of surgery in the first course of treatment for localized tumors rose from 10 percent in 1942–46 to 50 percent in 1952–56.[8] Declining from 79 to 42 percent over the same time period, the use of radiation alone was the sole downward trend in a picture of upward trajectories, as Figure 8.1 so strikingly illustrates.

The shift to surgery—itself advancing in safety—and away from radiation may have been the major treatment contribution to survival of women with localized cervical cancer during the reported decades in California. (Very few women

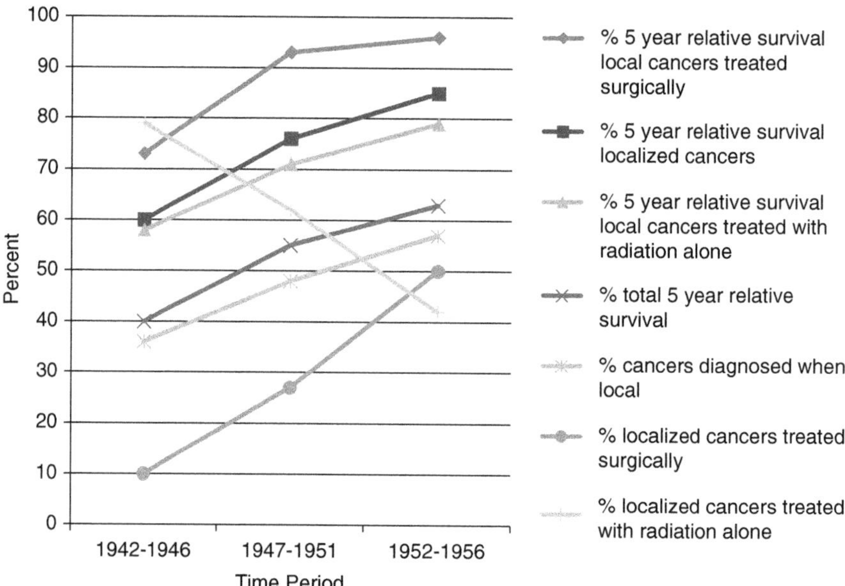

Figure 8.1 Cervical Cancer and Radiation Trends in California, 1942–1956.

Source: California Tumor Registry, *Cancer Registration and Survival in California* (Berkeley: State of California Department of Public Health, 1963).

received both surgery and radiation.) Although both groups gained during the time period, patients treated with surgery alone did better than those treated with radiation alone. Relative 5-year survival rates for California women with localized cervical cancers treated with surgery alone rose from 73 to 96 percent, compared with 58 to 79 percent for those receiving radiation alone.[9] Comparing outcomes of breast cancer treatment with surgery and radiation was more complicated.

While surgeons reigned over breast cancer in the United States with radical mastectomy, radiotherapists in France were treating many women with localized tumors with radiation alone or combined with partial excision (lumpectomy).[10] In Britain also, women physicians and their patients were choosing radiation over the mutilating and dangerous radical mastectomy.[11] The California data may have suggested, however, that radiation alone was not sufficient; of women whose localized breast cancers were surgically removed, 85 percent survived for 5 years compared to 53 percent of women receiving radiation alone.[12]

The fact that cancers of the breast and uterus (cervix and corpus) accounted for more than 40 percent of California's radiation therapy patients meant that significantly more women than men at the time received radiation treatment. In total, 27 percent of females with cancer received radiation in the first course of their treatment, compared to 17 percent of males.[13] Although some radiotherapists may have considered women more expendable (as they seemed to consider poor and minority populations, as touched upon below and further noted in Chapter 10), it seems likely in this case that the predominance of women treated with radiation was largely a matter of supply and demand. As the second and third-highest incidence cancers in California at the time, cancers of the breast and cervix were in good supply and were anatomically accessible to radiation.

Besides sex differences, there were class and race inequities in cancer care, particularly concerning the timing of diagnosis. Compared with patients using county hospitals, nearly twice the proportion of California patients using private hospitals in the 1940s and 1950s had their cancers diagnosed while still localized. The fact that 25 percent of white men in county hospitals had their cancers diagnosed when localized compared to 20 percent of black men also indicated racial inequities; the disparity was even greater within private hospitals, where the figures were 45 and 30 percent. Furthermore, 71 percent of private hospital patients' localized cancers were removed surgically, compared to 57 percent of patients in county hospitals.[14] Since higher proportions of public hospital patients received only radiation for their localized tumors, radiation may have been used as a cheaper alternative to surgery.

In general, cancer treatment trends in California in the 1940s and 1950s moved toward surgery and away from radiation. The total use of surgery in the first course of treatment for all cancers rose from 39 percent in 1942–46 to 55 percent in 1952–56, while the use of radiation declined from 25 to 21 percent.[15] Although improvements in surgical technique and availability of antibiotics to control post-surgical infections would have played a role in the growing preference for surgery, the decline in radiation use in the first treatment course suggests that some doctors were wrestling with their faith in the technology.

Professional Discourse on Relative Effectiveness of Radiation Devices

Despite the warning in a 1950 textbook that strong belief in supervoltage technology would lead to disappointment,[16] leaders continued to hope that the very latest machine would be different. The many descriptive reports on technical features, dosages, and treatment strategies that immediately followed (and even preceded) the installation of each new device advanced the professional positions of their authors and their institutions, as noted in the studies reported in this book. Investigators often acknowledged, however, that observation periods were too short and patient numbers too small to permit scientifically valid conclusions.

Clinicians were chagrined when more time and more patients showed essentially equivalent survival rates for all supervoltage devices—and even, in a number of cases, survival rates equivalent to those of kilovoltage. Disappointingly finding that their new betatron did not increase cancer survival, University of Illinois radiologists nonetheless appreciated that the device's higher energy levels permitted them to complete treatments before patients died of their metastases.[17] They noted that patient referrals grew after they were able to report that their betatron had completely destroyed primary tumors.

Roentgens, Rads, and Riddles, a 1956 symposium report from the Oak Ridge Institute for Nuclear Studies (ORINS), was curiously flippant about the new technologies. Milton Friedman coauthored the comments that radiation therapy had "entered a second childhood and was interested in toys," and that there was no "clinical substantiation of the value of supervoltage irradiation."[18] Baylor University's Vincent Collins wryly observed at the symposium that while many hospitals reported continuous improvement, overall cancer mortality rates did not budge. But medical belief systems, it seems, did not necessarily guide medical practices.

In the same year as the *Riddles* report, radiotherapists resoundingly responded "yes" to the question, "Should We Junk 250 kv?" In fact, their institutions already had junked kilovoltage. New York City's Francis Delafield cancer hospital, which had acquired the first Atomic Energy of Canada, Ltd. (AECL) Theratron B cobalt-60 unit in 1953 and a General Electric (GE) resonance transformer the following year, reported that it was treating two-thirds of its radiation therapy patients with supervoltage.[19] The University of Saskatchewan reported that it was treating 70 percent with supervoltage, despite T. A. Watson's claim that the new technology improved survival rates very little. This was a startling concession coming so soon after his run in the cobalt race. Watson's university, however, would come to appreciate that clinical use of its new betatron and cobalt devices enhanced its national reputation.[20] Despite his disparaging remarks in Oak Ridge, Milton Friedman topped them all: his department used supervoltage—including its new, 2 MeV GE resonance transformer—on 85 percent of its patients. The availability of megavoltage, combined with its use on large numbers of patients in leading institutions, set new *de facto* practice standards that raised the bar in cancer treatment. Questions from the symposium audience reflected community hospital radiologists' anxieties over the competitive consumption. One inquired pointedly, "Should we mortgage ourselves to keep up with the Friedmans?"

Several years later, Friedman privately agreed with San Francisco's Henry Garland that supervoltage provided "no additional benefits to the cancer patient." But, having just moved into a New York University department newly supplied with a cobalt bomb and a linear accelerator, Friedman advised Garland that "the public relations impact of these gadgets is enormous."[21] Friedman was not alone in using the new gadgets for PR purposes.

Radiation therapy leaders at a 1958 National Academy of Sciences meeting, convened to advise the National Institutes of Health and the Donner Foundation on whether they should favor kilovoltage or supervoltage in funding decisions, expressed further doubts about the clinical benefits of the more powerful devices. But, when Robert Stone asked who would be willing to go back to using kilovoltage exclusively, not one hand was raised. Radiotherapists preferred supervoltage for its greater prestige and "convenience."[22] Supervoltage's higher power and higher patient throughput meant higher productivity, more efficient use of staff time, and the achievement of higher revenues by treating more patients. Radiotherapists also perceived supervoltage as more scientific; as their machines got more technologically sophisticated, they tended to assume that clinical treatments using them became more scientifically sophisticated. At the same time, some suggested that basing practice on scientific evidence might be a good idea.

Morton Kligerman reminded his colleagues that the prospective, randomized controlled trial (RCT) was by then the clinical ideal. He proposed at the National Academy meeting that they randomize patients from the beginning of every new technology.[23] But randomization to evaluate new technologies and new procedures was the road not taken. When radiation therapists did design controlled trials, they generally compared different protocols using the latest device rather than compare it with older machines or compare radiation with other treatment modalities. This was partly due to improved beam properties.

It was evident from the beginning that higher-energy rays penetrated the body further than those of lower voltages and delivered larger doses to deep tumors with less superficial tissue burn. Kligerman himself maintained that supervoltage was better than kilovoltage in terms of patient tolerance if not in terms of cure. The ability of supervoltage beams (including those produced by the Van de Graaff, cobalt-60, and linear accelerator) to pass through tender tissues in the cervix and bladder without burning them, he argued, meant considerably less pain for patients.[24] But the improved beam characteristics had a downside: without superficial burn, escalating doses sometimes led to "disastrous" overirradiation of deeper organs.[25] Doctors came to report radiation-induced scarring of patients' kidneys, lungs, hearts, and livers, as well as immunological disruptions and new cancers.

The profession's discourse on complications revealed a fair degree of awareness of radiation therapy's limitations and destructions. It further revealed the extent to which radiotherapists were experimenting on patients as they introduced each new device. Implicitly acknowledging that radiation therapy damaged healthy tissues, the scientific literature promoted each new technology for an improved ability to damage diseased tissues selectively. Henry Kaplan liked to say that supervoltage (particularly his linear accelerator) fired like a rifle instead of a shotgun, a powerful metaphor that still resonates.

Linear Accelerator Versus Cobalt

Many radiation therapy leaders have retrospectively portrayed the linear accelerator as the ultimate in device achievement (or at least until proton beams arrived on the market). The linac's higher energy beam penetrated deeper into the body than cobalt's with less penumbra (fuzzy boundary). Celebrating beam *characteristics*, however, leaders did not necessarily find improved clinical *outcomes*.

British radiation physicist F. T. Farmer declared in 1962 that the betatron, the cobalt-60 irradiator, and the linear accelerator were of "comparable worth" clinically.[26] Like Gilbert Fletcher in Texas, Farmer held that the differences among those devices were primarily of economic, rather than clinical, value (although he acknowledged that cobalt had a beam definition problem). While noting that the price of the linear accelerator was more than double that of the Van de Graaff and cobalt, Farmer advised National Health Service purchasers that the linear accelerator's faster dose rate meant that it was economically more efficient for hospitals because it could treat more patients per day.

Yet the world-wide cobalt boom continued. North America counted 613 installed cobalt-60 devices (compared to 36 linear accelerators) in 1968, Europe 541 cobalts and 26 linacs, and Asia 385 and 10.[27] The global dominance of cobalt at the time meant that few radiation therapy services had the capacity to compare the two. Most major hospitals in New York City and Boston were using cobalt in the mid-1970s, and few of the services with linacs also had cobalt for comparison.[28] Accordingly, most treatment centers were not in a position to test whether linacs produced better clinical results than cobalt on comparable patients with comparable cancers, and the work was not done.

Despite its slow start and evidence dearth, however, linear accelerator growth started to accelerate and came to exceed that of all other devices. The total number of installations in the United States had multiplied to 1000 by the early 1980s (exceeding cobalt's peak), 2000 by the early 1990s, and 3000 by the early 2000s, and it continued growing in the 2010s.[29] Some leaders circularly asserted that the linac's growing dominance over cobalt in itself showed that it was more effective.

Linear accelerator growth was not due to evidence of higher effectiveness, and many nonclinical factors drove it. Blue Cross payments that reimbursed twice as much for linac compared to cobalt treatments generated financial incentives for hospital administrators.[30] Community hospitals staffed by newly trained specialists building new megavoltage departments also wanted the latest device, and the linac was the new new thing. The linear accelerator's higher power conferred greater institutional prestige and permitted faster patient throughput, as Farmer had noted. The greater productivity meant higher hospital revenues per day, as Varian's Edward Ginzton had predicted. The linac's higher purchasing price and operating costs offered a (temporary) means of pricing competing hospitals and private physicians out of the market—including, putatively, the 15 radiotherapy offices in New York City providing cobalt treatment. Finally, no significant competition appeared on the near horizon to challenge the linac's ascendency. The profession continued to engage in political activities that augmented the specialty, its institutions, and its technology development.

Politics and Policy

Two federal programs expanded radiation therapy capacity, while two more tried to organize and control it. The 1965 Regional Medical Programs and the 1971 War on Cancer channeled large doses of money to radiology research, training, and treatment centers. At the same time, the National Health Planning and Certificate of Need programs, intended to control excessive growth of high-cost devices and services, were caught between consolidating services in large medical centers and diffusing high-cost technologies more widely. Radiotherapy leaders worked with all four programs—if not without dissent.

The Great Blue Book Confrontation

While the 1965 Medicare and Medicaid programs paid out substantial sums to medical institutions across the board, Regional Medical Programs (RMP) added to the coffers of three disease categories. The main idea behind President Johnson's blue-ribbon Commission on Heart Disease, Cancer and Stroke (which led to RMP) was to strengthen the elite corps of academic medical centers providing specialty services for those disease categories. RMP established networks that enabled community physicians to refer selected patients to academic centers and designated large geographic regions as their market areas. Not surprisingly, the players behind the regionalization program represented elite academic institutions. Texas Medical Center heart surgeon Michael DeBakey chaired the Texan president's commission, and its members included M. D. Anderson Hospital's R. Lee Clark and other prominent physicians and businessmen.[31]

RMP plunged into the conflict between academic specialists who proposed centralizing high-tech services and community hospital–based specialists who wanted the new technologies for their own departments. Pivotal drivers of diffusion included fee-for-service reimbursements, hospital and specialist ambitions, and manufacturer's marketing. Although RMP law weakened the commission's centralization intent, its operating tactics favored it.

RMP turned to the academically-oriented Committee on Radiation Therapy Studies, chaired by Texas Medical Center's Gilbert Fletcher, to organize the field. The committee's 1968 publication, *A Prospect for Radiation Therapy* (which happened to have a blue cover), identified inadequate systemic coordination as the problem; and competition, mutual distrust, and "Machiavellianism" as the cause. *Prospect* created a three-level service hierarchy—ranked by technological capacity—and advocated centralizing the most powerful devices (and doctors) at the top level.[32] It converted the American College of Radiology's earlier minimum volume standard of 300 patients per radiation therapy service per year to 300 patients per megavoltage machine per year, a major expansion in the number and proportion of patients allotted to the top level. It also advised that major cancer centers needed several megavoltage devices, including cobalt-60 or a linear accelerator. These professional standards became *de facto* national policy as the National Cancer Institute and the American College of Radiology each endorsed the report.

To justify its centralization policy clinically, RMP sought to elicit evidence that highly staffed and equipped hospitals delivered better care. California's RMP sponsored a research project in conjunction with the Department of Radiation Therapy at the University of California, Los Angeles (UCLA) on the *Organization of Radiation Therapy Services Related to Outcome*.[33] Contrary to expectations (and the implications of the title), the study found little relationship between outcomes and organization as defined in terms of availability of full-time radiologist, megavoltage equipment, and a minimum of 300 patients a year. Nevertheless, the study recommended that RMP continue to implement these standards.

In distributing 14,000 free copies of its report, the Committee on Radiation Therapy Studies threw down the gauntlet for what might be called "the great blue book confrontation." Tensions had mounted when a new generation of trained specialists recognized that the new public payment programs could fund their technology dreams. *A Prospect for Radiation Therapy* coincided with the growing numbers of community hospital–affiliated radiotherapists as well as with the introduction of Varian's mass-marketed Clinac® 4, designed particularly for them.

Four years after *Prospect*, a "Subcommittee for Revision of the 'Blue Book' (1968 Report)" issued its own report. Reflecting the ongoing shift in the profession's demographics, the revision committee challenged the policies that granted academic centers a monopoly over the highest-powered equipment. The subcommittee's *Proposal for Integrated Cancer Management* condemned the hierarchical levels system and put forth a free-market rationale that all cancer physicians and hospitals should be allowed to participate in radiation oncology centers.[34] (This publication also signaled the name change of the profession to radiation oncology, in part a response to practitioners' complaints that referring physicians treated them like technicians.) Shortly after *Proposal*'s publication, the American College of Radiology rescinded its earlier preference for designated levels of care—rhetorically conflating regionalization with state medicine—and took the side of the growing segment of its membership seeking to preserve the "private practice of medicine philisophy [sic]."[35] Although they supported opposing distribution strategies, both manifestos (*Prospect* and *Proposal*) were market-oriented proposals that placed specialty development over public need for its services.

Regional Medical Programs might have used the concept of region to match radiation therapy supply with need identified by disease incidence and treatment effectiveness. This is an ideal—if seldom realized—goal of regionalization strategies. Instead, RMP employed a common professional assumption (and *Prospect* reiterated) that at least half of all cancer patients "required" radiation.[36] Although scientific study has not verified it, the 50 percent guideline has remained remarkably consistent over time and technology change—although it is often nudged up to 60 percent and is sometimes applied to newly diagnosed patients alone.

The figure of 50 percent was considerably higher than actual practice in the few geographic areas that actually measured their rates, a fact that might have led to questions about its appropriateness. Instead, it became an ongoing professional goal to expand both supply and demand in order to catch up to the 50 percent assumption. A Utah RMP, for example, was concerned that only 27 percent of its new cancer patients received radiation; at 23 percent, Connecticut's RMP similarly worried that its state's residents were being deprived.[37] The 50 percent standard has served the purpose of supporting international institutional and professional growth, and Varian Associates used it to set linear-accelerator production goals.[38] As the RMP was supporting institutional and technological growth, what's commonly called the *War on Cancer* arrived to throw more money at the same institutions and technologies.

Throw Enough Money ... The Conquest of Cancer Program

Although critics would call the 1971 Conquest of Cancer Program a failure because it did not conquer cancer, the battle successfully endowed the cancer establishment. The war was declared by the American Cancer Society, the American College of Radiology, M. D. Anderson Hospital chief R. Lee Clark, wealthy philanthropist Mary Lasker, and radiation oncologist Henry Kaplan, together with President Richard Nixon. The president undoubtedly hoped that this war would distract public attention from the one in Vietnam. Clark undoubtedly saw funding for M. D. Anderson Hospital when he confidently asserted that medicine could "lick cancer" if Congress would only give it a billion dollars a year for 10 years.[39] Kaplan and other oncology leaders undoubtedly expected to channel cancer-center grants to their own institutions. Megavoltage manufacturers undoubtedly looked forward to the prospect of higher sales.

Even GE considered a comeback; it held managerial meetings on whether the company should reinvest in order to regain its number one position in radiology manufacturing. Because the radiologist was "no longer king," however, the company feared it had lost its hold on hospital purchasing decisions.[40] While projecting a healthy growth rate in radiotherapy, the managers identified "unfavorable" risk factors that might cut into it. Chemotherapy might replace radiation, they suggested, and might even cure cancer in the near future.[41] Although they needn't have worried on that account, GE did not plunge back in.

Unlike GE, Varian Associates was well positioned to benefit from the War on Cancer. Kaplan was a member of its National Panel of Consultants, and Varian exploited the panel's claim that "highly sophisticated" megavoltage technology had produced "remarkable strides" in cancer therapy and that wider use of it could reduce the total cancer death rate by 15–25 percent over the next five years.[42] Although they served to pass the legislation, the panel's figures were not based on evidence.

Kaplan (probably) wrote the radiotherapy section of the panel's report and provided it with figures and an argument that he reproduced in a professional paper a few years later.[43] The report claimed that "representative" 5-year survival rates for several cancers had improved "when treated with megavoltage radiotherapy." The evidence presented in the accompanying table, however, did not measure actual megavoltage treatments against those of lower voltage on comparable patients. Instead, it compared survival rates in the kilovoltage era with survival rates in the megavoltage era. Such an argument—not uncommon in the medical literature—conflates *correlation* with *cause.* The correlation argument neglects other clinical and social variables potentially impacting survival rates. Moreover, some of the figures in the panel's table were spurious. The most misleading figures claimed 50–60 percent 5-year ovarian cancer survival rates in the megavoltage era. It is not clear where the figures came from. California was reporting 24 percent relative 5-year survival for ovarian cancer at the time, Stanford was reporting 42 percent, and M. D. Anderson around 36 percent.[44] Nonetheless, the panel report reinforced professional belief in megavoltage (and Kaplan's linear accelerator in particular). Although one paper held that Kaplan's follow-up publication using panel data "demonstrated decisively the superiority of megavoltage X rays," it was not so decisive.[45] Nonetheless, the Conquest of Cancer successfully funneled many dollars into high-ranking radiation therapy departments.

The National Panel of Consultants advocated centralizing personnel and technologies in major cancer centers. Leaders widely expected that Kaplan's name would be on one of the new centers, but his own colleagues sabotaged him. Perhaps striving to regain power he had lost in the battle over departmental control, Kaplan proposed to build a cancer center with a fully equipped research laboratory, a fully equipped ambulatory care center, and a large number of inpatient beds separate from the main hospital. Fearing that its proposed size and administrative independence would make Kaplan's project a "cancer empire" (and Kaplan its emperor), other Stanford department chairs torpedoed it.[46]

The critics who had initially lambasted the Conquest of Cancer's hype may have felt justified when it turned out that, far from the suggested 15–25 percent reduction, the national cancer mortality rate remained flatlined for two more decades. The war on cancer's hundreds of millions of dollars had boosted oncology professions and institutions, but it had not licked cancer.

As RMPs and the Conquest of Cancer accelerated technological and institutional growth, organized health and hospital planning tried to apply some brakes.

Hospital Planning and Capital Investment in Cobalt

Hospital planning under the Hill–Burton program encouraged technological growth and worked with industry to achieve it. Ten manufacturers contributed sections to the American College of Radiology's *Planning Guide for Radiologic Installations*, which advised hospital administrators to work with the manufacturers to maximize equipment placement in hospital radiology departments.[47] University of Illinois radiologist Roger Harvey advised that all smaller hospitals should have at least one X-ray therapy room and that larger ones should have a second room supplied with the highest voltage available—which, at the time, was the University of Illinois/Allis-Chalmers betatron.[48] Criteria proposed by academic radiologists supported hospital construction plans that built high-tech equipment into hospital architecture and reinforced hospital hierarchy.[49]

Initiated by the hospital industry in 1938 to oversee hospital finances, the Health and Hospital Planning Council of Southern New York established a Cobalt Committee to review hospital investment in that technology in the 1960s. The New York Cobalt Committee adopted the American College of Radiology's levels of care strategy at the time, advising that smaller services should only diagnose and palliate and that they should refer patients to regional centers for "definitive" treatment on the latest equipment.[50]

Struggling against the growing dominance of New York's academic medical centers several years before the first policy blue book, nonacademic radiologists and administrators articulated a range of rationales for why their hospitals required cobalt-60 teletherapy. As an accepted community provider of (kilovoltage) radiation therapy already, one applicant maintained, it required cobalt to keep up with the times.[51] Administrators at another hospital argued that they needed cobalt to attract radiology residents and maintain residency approval.[52] The Planning Council approved most community hospital applications on the condition they establish "meaningful affiliation[s]" with medical schools. *Meaningful*, in one case at least, meant the applicant would purchase equipment the medical school required, allot time for its radiotherapist to teach, send staff for continuing education, and transfer its more complex cases.[53] The Planning Council did not so much contain cobalt teletherapy growth as tie it to the burgeoning medical empires.

Not satisfied with Southern New York's and other hospital councils' voluntary efforts, which were controlling neither rising hospital nor insurance costs, New York political leaders inaugurated the nation's first Certificate of Need program, which required state approval for hospitals' major capital expenditures. Governor Rockefeller's Committee on Hospital Costs, chaired by Eastman Kodak executive (and President Eisenhower's Secretary of Health, Education and Welfare) Marion Folsom, reiterated the idle capital argument of earlier hospital surveys. The hospital costs committee criticized inappropriate capital investment in underused facilities and equipment, naming radiation therapy (and open heart surgery) as "dramatic examples" of excessive service supply in "disproportion to the needs and resources of the community."[54] The needs of the community would remain neglected, however. New York's health commissioner announced that he would assess Certificate of Need applications on the basis of their financial arrangements and whether they could cover project costs and remain economically viable.[55]

With American Hospital Association support, Congress extended Certificate of Need to the nation and linked it to the 1974 National Health Planning program. Preceded by Comprehensive Health Planning, a weaker but more community-minded program, health planning sought in 1974 to restrict unnecessary growth of high-tech, high-cost services by building a set of specialty-based oligopolies. Medical technology, including diagnostic and therapeutic X-ray, *Forbes* magazine diagnosed in 1977, was growing "almost too wildly."[56]

According to an early participant, business interests dominated health planning from the beginning.[57] The National Chamber Foundation encouraged businesses to participate in health-planning activities in order to protect the market-oriented private medical care system.[58] Applying experience from large-scale capitalist enterprise, economists advised health-planning agencies that consolidating hospitals and specialized services would achieve economies of scale, enhance medical productivity, and promote full utilization of costly technologies.[59] A growing army of consultants and think tanks taught health planners how to apply business-management methods to medical care. The Western Center for Health Planning advised public health planners as well as hospital administrators that investment decisions in medical care needed to "follow the rules that guide capital expenditures in the rest of the economy."[60]

Business representatives at a 1976 federally sponsored Capital Investment Conference were concerned about unproductive capital trapped in underutilized medical services. They held that the health care industry was overcapitalized, that it provided insufficient returns on investment, and that hospitals had purchased more high-cost technologies like X-ray than they could use appropriately or efficiently. Goldman Sachs investment bankers at the conference advised Certificate of Need administrators to approve only financially viable hospital projects that would be able to repay their debts.[61]

In turning to specialty and trade associations to formulate health-planning and Certificate of Need standards, the government assigned the foxes to guard the henhouse. The American College of Radiology and the National Electrical Manufacturers Association collaborated in developing guidelines for radiation therapy services.[62] They chose the college's 300-patient minimum-volume criterion, based on an estimated financial break-even point, to ensure that services could support themselves economically. The medical electronics industry also favored minimum volume standards, as larger institutions purchased more equipment.[63] Health planning, as it was implemented under the 1974 law, was primarily a financial strategy.

The financial industry, by then funding over one-third of all short-term hospital capital expenditures, favored large, well-equipped institutions for their healthier financial ratios and bond ratings.[64] Medical leaders held that bigger meant better in terms of quality of care—although radiation oncologists would confess in 2010 that the relationship between volume and outcome had "never been empirically examined for radiation therapy."[65] Nonetheless, the higher financial status of larger hospitals remained a major issue across a wide range of state-based Certificate of Need programs.

Certificate of Need and Radiation Therapy in Washington State

Like New York City hospitals applying to purchase cobalt teletherapy in the 1960s, Washington State hospitals were under competitive pressures in the 1970s to buy the latest devices. Certificate of Need staff generally accepted hospital arguments that increasingly powerful linear accelerators would improve hospital market positions and financial status by attracting more patients.[66] The applicants did not try to make a case that the new devices they were seeking would cure more or harm fewer patients than the cobalt-60 irradiators or the less powerful linacs they already had.

Radiologists based in hospitals contending other hospitals' applications bluntly stated that the newer machines being sought were no more effective than the older ones being replaced. University Hospital's application to replace a lower-powered linear accelerator with a higher-powered Varian Clinac 20 "cannot be justified on the basis of improved results from the increased photon energy as there are no data to suggest an increased efficacy" of 15 MeV photons over 4, 6, 8, or 10 MeV photons, charged one competitor.[67] A contending radiation oncologist from Swedish Hospital further queried University Hospital's administrator, "I presume you are also aware that no documentation exists in medical literature to support definitive improvement in either local tumor control or patient survival with photon energies above the range of 4 MeV?"[68] While conceding that the machine's capacity to produce an electron beam to treat patients with mycosis fungoides was a rationale for it, the Swedish Hospital radiation oncologist maintained that the 10–15 patients in the region expected to present with the disease in any one year could easily be handled by the nearby facility that already had electron beam capacity. He then contended that University Hospital wanted the new machine in order to benefit its faculty practice plan, which, he argued, inappropriately competed with the "private practice of radiation oncology in the community." Affiliated with a powerful tertiary (not community) hospital himself, the oncologist alleged that the state university's practice plan constituted state medicine.

The following year, Swedish Hospital was itself seeking to add a Varian Clinac 20 to its megavoltage collection of one cobalt device and two linear accelerators, and it also claimed it needed electron beam capacity—without mentioning the very small demand for it. "Although we already have three machines," its application whined, "we are limited to photons, whereas Virginia Mason [just a few blocks away] has both photon and electron capability."[69] The very same radiation oncologist who one year earlier refused to endorse the university's purchase of the very same machine on the grounds of no added clinical benefits was now collecting letters of support for his application. In identifying the very latest Clinac as "state of the art," the supporting letters implied that all important hospitals had to have one (and that having one made a hospital important).

Meanwhile, Group Health of Puget Sound, the nearby health maintenance organization with lower status aspirations, claimed that it needed to supplement its cobalt-60 device with a small Varian Clinac 4 just to keep up with the standard of practice in the community.[70] Group Health worried that it was treating only 40 percent of its cancer patients with radiation and argued that a new machine would help it attain what it called the 50 percent standard.

Only three years after getting its Clinac 20 and the same year that Varian's latest upgrade, the Clinac 2500, hit the market, University Hospital was back to get one. The newest machine, its latest application claimed, signified a "major advancement in radiotherapy treatment systems." Writing from company literature (or with the direct aid of company personnel), its application regurgitated verbatim Varian's marketing jargon that the new machine would enable clinicians to simultaneously "individualize, optimize, and simplify treatment delivery techniques."[71]

Hospitals were caught in the escalating power and cost spiral generated by Varian's expanding product line and planned obsolescence just to stay in the radiation-therapy business. Letters supporting and contesting Certificate of Need applications demonstrated how professional and economic competition as well as hospital investment strategies drove the purchase of more and more costly equipment. One relatively small community hospital applied to purchase a 10 MeV Siemens linear accelerator at twice the price of a lower-powered Varian device on the grounds that the more powerful the machine, the better—and the local health planning agency bought the argument.[72] The hospital further threatened that if it did not get the desired machine, its radiology group would buy one for its private office.[73] Hospital administrators hoped that higher-energy machines would catapult them into a higher level in the regional hierarchy and capture larger shares of the radiation therapy market.

Chief executive officers, chief financial officers, and chief operating officers (CEOs, CFOs, and COOs) stressed in Certificate of Need meetings that the new devices would make their hospitals more stable financially. Vindicating Edward Ginzton's advice to Varian executives, hospital administrators claimed that the more powerful devices would generate higher revenues by permitting higher patient throughput and more efficient use of personnel. Hospitals would have to attract significantly more patients to achieve the desired productivity levels, the applicants continued, but they assured that the new machines could do that.

Population *need* held very little place in Certificate of Need application strategies, regulatory analyses, or community deliberations. Need is, of course, notoriously difficult to define. As one Washington State physician wrote, "Whether or not there is a need for [a particular] treatment machine" at a particular hospital "depends on philosophical, as well as political and economic considerations."[74]

Neither the local Health Systems Agencies nor the state Certificate of Need office added up how many additional patients would have to be irradiated in order to amortize the costs of all the new machines, or how much the patients would—or would not—benefit from their treatments. Certificate of Need did not and could not take total system costs into account. Its case-by-case review in place of system-wide prospective planning meant that hospital and regulatory analyses never asked how a new machine in one hospital might reduce efficiency and raise costs in the health care system as a whole. The state Certificate of Need program primarily sought to protect the economic viability of applicant hospitals and their creditors. Because most hospitals financed their purchases with bank loans and/or tax-exempt bonds, Certificate of Need administrators tried to ensure that hospitals could pay the interest on their debts and maintain high bond ratings. When they could feasibly project the 300 patients required by the national guidelines, they got their approval.

Despite its many contradictions, Certificate of Need served (and continues to serve) to bring together disparate interests to appreciate common goals and thrash out differences.

Providers, Payers, Regulators, and Consumers Meet Face-to-Face

Certificate of Need's stab at democratic process may inform future health care policy making. Representatives of the many interests shaping medical delivery assembled in meeting rooms throughout the country to develop Certificate of Need standards and review hospital applications to purchase new technologies. Doctors, nurses, hospital administrators, public health regulators, consumers, insurers, and corporate payers meeting face-to-face acted out the tensions in medical technology development and diffusion described in this chapter. The analysis in this section is based on my personal experiences and observations as health-planning staff, particularly my role in organizing a committee to develop Certificate of Need standards for nuclear magnetic resonance imaging (MRI) in Washington State.[75]

Physicians on Certificate of Need committees generally portrayed themselves as the experts in any particular technology to ensure that their specialty maintained a monopoly over it. Radiologists insisted that every important radiology group required the new technology in order to compete (although radiologists in smaller cities had lower expectations). Aware of having recently lost imaging market share to cardiology and nuclear medicine, the radiologists called MRI "state of the art" even prior to Food and Drug Administration (FDA) and Medicare approval, not to mention research evidence. Radiologists purportedly dropped the word "nuclear" from the previously named *nuclear magnetic resonance* in order to stake their claim on the technology over nuclear medicine.

Reiterating marketing lingo, perhaps from sales staff visiting from General Electric, which had long used the term, radiologists at the committee meetings confidently called the new technology a "turnkey" operation that required no further training before using it on patients. One radiologist wondered why everyone was so concerned about high costs, since, he maintained, "these things pay for themselves." More cognizant of who actually pays for these things, insurance and government representatives argued (successfully, in this case) for setting a limit on the number of MRI devices (three) that the state Certificate of Need program could approve in the first year in the small state. Most hospital administrators supported the limit that restrained their competitors as well as themselves. Nonetheless, one manager whose application was denied accused Certificate of Need of dooming his hospital's radiologists to obsolescence—a compelling concern for a technology-based specialty.

Carrying less authority than doctors but still getting their voices heard, nurses who spent more time with patients tended to be more skeptical about how much patients benefited from the new technologies. Hedging their bets, private insurers as payers sought to reduce company payments by restricting device proliferation, while as investors, they supported device expansion. Consumers variously wanted lower costs, access to everything, and a rational health care system.

The restriction on number of hospital MRIs in Washington State did not last, and the technology subsequently spread throughout hospitals, mobile units, and freestanding facilities. Like many new technologies, it fulfilled some, but not all, of its initial promise and (together with computed tomography [CT] scanning, which had debuted just a few years earlier) duplicated services and considerably raised intervention intensity and medical costs.[76]

In sum, Regional Medical Programs, the Conquest of Cancer, Health Planning, and Certificate of Need each in its own way supported institutional, professional, and technological growth in radiation therapy. At the same time, research findings raised questions about that growth. Although selected outcome improvements and palliative benefits intensified radiation oncologists' political efforts, postwar megavoltage growth owed more to expected professional and economic gain than it did to expected patient gain.

Part II as a whole has demonstrated the competitive adoption of higher and higher powered devices in radiation therapy. Innovative electrical engineers licensed their inventions to manufacturers (some of which they had established), coordinated medical services that applied them, trained specialists in their use, and promoted public policies that supported these activities. Subsidized hospital construction, growing insurance plans, research and training grants, competition among institutions and manufacturers, and a faith that growth itself represented progress coalesced to sustain a radiation-therapy boom. These factors set the stage for the coming financial control of medical care in the name of the market.

Notes

1 J. Heyman, ed., *Annual Report on the Results of Radiotherapy in Carcinoma of the Uterine Cervix* (Geneva: League of Nations, 1937), 148, and subsequent reports in the series.

2 H. E. Johns and T. A. Watson, "The Cobalt-60 Story," *Cancer in Ontario* 1982: 20–24. While their language does not literally claim a causal association, its implication does.

3 T. A. Watson, *Results of Treatment of Cancer in Saskatchewan 1932–44* (Saskatchewan: Saskatchewan Cancer Commission, 1951), 32–44, 51.

4 T. A. Watson, *Results of Treatment of Cancer in Saskatchewan 1945–52* (Saskatchewan: Saskatchewan Cancer Commission, 1958), 10–1.

5 Paul Litt, *Isotopes and Innovation: MDS Nordion's First Fifty Years, 1946–1996* (Montreal: Published for MDS Nordion by McGill-Queen's University Press, 2000), 77.

6 California Tumor Registry, *Cancer Registration and Survival in California* (Berkeley: State of California Department of Public Health, 1963), calculated from data on page 312. Fifty-three hospitals and clinics reported to the registry, covering 1/3 of California's annual new cancer cases.

7 California Tumor Registry, *Cancer Registration and Survival in California* (Berkeley: State of California Department of Public Health, 1963), 101.

8 California Tumor Registry, *Cancer Registration and Survival in California* (Berkeley: State of California Department of Public Health, 1963), 215. Treatment data pertain only to first course of treatment, defined as within 3–4 months of initial diagnosis. Studies in this series following this report did not include treatment data.

9 California Tumor Registry, *Cancer Registration and Survival in California* (Berkeley: State of California Department of Public Health, 1963), 219.

10 Barron H. Lerner, *The Breast Cancer Wars: Hope, Fear, and the Pursuit of a Cure in Twentieth-Century America* (New York: Oxford University Press, 2001), 116, 132–134; Ilana Löwy, "Knife, Rays and Women: Controversies about the Uses of Surgery versus

Radiotherapy in the Treatment of Female Cancers in France and in the US, 1920–1960," In Carsten Timmermann and Elizabeth Toon, eds., *Cancer Patients, Cancer Pathways* (Basingstoke, Hampshire: Palgrave Macmillan, 2012), 103–129.

11 Ornella Moscucci, "The 'Ineffable Freemasonry of Sex': Feminist Surgeons and the Establishment of Radiotherapy in Early Twentieth-Century Britain," *Bulletin of the History of Medicine* 81 (2007): 139–163.

12 California Tumor Registry, *Cancer Registration and Survival in California* (Berkeley: State of California Department of Public Health, 1963), 201. It is possible, of course, that a more favorable subset of women with localized cancer received surgery.

13 California Tumor Registry, *Cancer Registration and Survival in California* (Berkeley: State of California Department of Public Health, 1963), calculated from data on pages 68 and 70.

14 California Tumor Registry, *Cancer Registration and Survival in California* (Berkeley: State of California Department of Public Health, 1963), 121 and calculated from data on page 125. The private-hospital figures are questionable regarding race, as the numbers of black patients admitted to private hospitals were very small.

15 California Tumor Registry, *Cancer Registration and Survival in California* (Berkeley: State of California Department of Public Health, 1963), calculated from data on page 60. The radiation figures include surgery combined with radiation, although only 5–6 percent received both.

16 Franz Buschke, Simeon T. Cantril, and Herbert M. Parker, *Supervoltage Roentgentherapy* (Springfield, IL: Charles C. Thomas, 1950), viii, ix.

17 Lewis L. Haas and Roger A. Harvey, "Clinical Aspects of Betatron Irradiation," *American Journal of Roentgenology, Radium Therapy, and Nuclear Medicine* 76 (1956): 905–918.

18 Milton Friedman, Marshall Brucer, and Elizabeth Anderson, eds., *Roentgens, Rads, and Riddles, A Symposium on Supervoltage Radiation Therapy* (Oak Ridge, TN: Medical Division, Oak Ridge Institute of Nuclear Studies, 1956), ix, x, 269.

19 J. W. J. Carpender, "Supervoltage: Should We Junk 250 kv? A Symposium," Radiology 67 (1956): 481–515.

20 "Events in the History of the University of Saskatchewan; 1948: First Betatron in Canada." http://scaa.usask.ca/gallery/uofs_events/articles/1948.php accessed April 15, 2011.

21 Milton Friedman to Henry L. Garland, July 16, 1963, accompanied by a handwritten note: "Ed: this is interesting Garland is a close friend. Ernie." Edward L. Ginzton Papers, SC 330, Box 4. Special Collections and University Archives, Stanford University Archives.

22 Henry S. Kaplan, ed., *Research in Radiology: Proceedings of an Informal Conference* (Washington: National Research Council, 1958), 203–204.

23 Henry S. Kaplan, ed., *Research in Radiology: Proceedings of an Informal Conference* (Washington: National Research Council, 1958), 157.

24 Morton M. Kligerman, "High Voltage Radiation Therapy," *Annual Review of Medicine* 11 (1960): 303–314.

25 Franz Buschke and George Jack, "Twenty-five Years' Experience with Super-Voltage Therapy in the Treatment of Transitional Cell Carcinoma of the Bladder," *American Journal of Roentgenology, Radium Therapy, and Nuclear Medicine* 99 (1967): 387–392.

26 F. T. Farmer, "Supervoltage Therapy—A Review of Present Day Facilities and Techniques," *Physics in Medicine and Biology* 6 (1962): 505–531.

27 International Atomic Energy Agency, *Directory of High-Energy Radiotherapy Centres* (Vienna: IAEA, 1968), xxv– xxvii, xxxi.

28 International Atomic Energy Agency, *Directory of High-Energy Radiotherapy Centres, 1976 edition* (Vienna: IAEA, 1976), 193–194, 205–214.

29 Jean B. Owen, Lawrence R. Coia, and Gerald E. Hanks, "The Structure of Radiation Oncology in the United States in 1994," *International Journal of Radiation Oncology Biology Physics* 39 (1997): 179–185. The American College of Radiology declined to respond to my e-mail and postal inquiries about these and more recent figures.

30 Paul Litt, *Isotopes and Innovation: MDS Nordion's First Fifty Years, 1946–1996* (Montreal: Published for MDS Nordion by McGill-Queen's University Press, 2000), 158.

31 President's Commission on Heart Disease, Cancer and Stroke, *Report to the President: A National Program to Conquer Heart Disease, Cancer and Stroke, Volume 1* (Washington: 1964).

32 Committee for Radiation Therapy Studies, Subcommittee on Regional Medical Programs, *A Prospect for Radiation Therapy in the United States, Final Report* (Bethesda, MD: National Institutes of Health, 1968), 5–10.

33 Gerald Peter Hanson, "Organization of Radiation Therapy Services Related to Outcome." PhD diss., University of California, Los Angeles, 1971.

34 Committee for Radiation Therapy Studies, Subcommittee for Revision of the "Blue Book" (1968 Report). *A Proposal for Integrated Cancer Management in the United States: The Role of Radiation Oncology* (Bethesda, MD: National Cancer Institute, 1972), 13.

35 Robert G. Parker, ed., *A Planning Guide for Community Radiation Oncology Facilities* ([No publication place]: American College of Radiology, 1974).

36 This proportion compared to a 1950 British estimate of 40 percent. Margaret Tod, *An Inquiry into the Extent to Which Cancer Patients in Great Britain Receive Radiotherapy* (Altrincham: John Sherratt and Son, 1950), 19, 23.

37 Weber Basin Health Planning Council, *Radiation Therapy in Northern Utah* (Ogden UT: Intermountain Regional Medical Program, 1973), 24; L. Todd Berman and G. Pierce Taylor, *Radiation Therapy in Connecticut* (North Haven, CT: Connecticut Hospital Planning Commission, 1972), 16.

38 E. Ginzton to A. Eldredge, March 3, 1978. Edward L. Ginzton Papers, SC 330, Box 16. Special Collections and University Archives, Stanford University Libraries.

39 James S. Olson, *Bathsheba's Breast: Women, Cancer & History* (Baltimore: Johns Hopkins University Press, 2002), 125.

40 "A Technology Review, Medical Systems Business Division," no date; "Medical Economics" notebook, September 29, 1971. GE Archives, NBDO Studies. Schenectady Museum Archives, Schenectady, NY.

41 "Planning Development," September 29, 1971, "Medical Economics" notebook, GE Archives, NBDO Studies. Schenectady Museum Archives, Schenectady, NY.

42 Varian Associates, *Annual Report 1972* 13, 50. Russell and Sigurd Varian Papers, SC 345, Varian Associates Series, Box 1. Special Collections and University Archives, Stanford University Libraries.

43 US Senate, *Report of the National Panel of Consultants on the Conquest of Cancer* (Washington: Committee on Labor and Public Welfare, 1971), 51; Henry S. Kaplan, "Radiotherapeutic Advances in the Treatment of Neoplastic Disease," *Israel Journal of Medical Sciences* 13 (1977): 808–814.

44 California Tumor Registry, *Cancer Registration and Survival in California* (Berkeley: State of California Department of Public Health, 1963), 357; Robert H. Sagerman, Gerald E. Hanks, and Malcolm S. Bagshaw, "Supervoltage Radiation Therapy Use of the Linear Accelerator for Treating Ovarian Adenocarcinoma," *California Medicine* 102 (1965): 118–122; Luis Delclos and Edward J. Quinlan, "Malignant Tumors of the Ovary Managed with Post Operative Megavoltage Irradiation," *Radiology* 93 (1969): 659–663.

45 John S. Laughlin, Radhe Mohan, and Gerald J. Kutcher, "Choice of Optimum Megavoltage for Accelerators for Photon Beam Treatment," *International Journal of Radiation Oncology Biology Physics* 12 (1986): 1551–1557.

46 Charlotte DeCroes Jacobs, *Henry Kaplan and the Story of Hodgkin's Disease* (Stanford: Stanford University Press, 2010), 264–266.
47 Wendell G. Scott, *Planning Guide for Radiologic Installations* (Chicago: Year Book Publishers, 1953), x–xii, 1.
48 Roger A. Harvey, "X-ray Requirements for the Smaller Hospital," In *Transcript of the Institute on Hospital Planning* (Chicago: American Hospital Association, 1948), 169–173.
49 Fred J. Hodges, "X-ray Facilities for the General Hospital," *Architectural Record* 101 (1947): 141–142.
50 American College of Radiology, "Guidelines for Determining Standards of Radiotherapy in Approved Cancer Centers," Chicago, 1964. Archives of the Health and Hospital Planning Council of Southern New York, Box 39, Rare Book Room, New York Academy of Medicine, New York; Health and Hospital Planning Council of Southern New York, "Draft Guidelines for the Establishment of Radiation Therapy Services in Hospitals," March 30, 1966. Archives of the Health and Hospital Planning Council of Southern New York, Box 39, Rare Book Room, New York Academy of Medicine, New York.
51 Russell M. Drum to Jack Haldeman, April 21, 1965. Archives of the Health and Hospital Planning Council of Southern New York, Box 39, Rare Book Room, New York Academy of Medicine, New York.
52 County of Westchester to Jack Haldeman, October 27, 1965. Archives of the Health and Hospital Planning Council of Southern New York, Box 39, Rare Book Room, New York Academy of Medicine, New York.
53 SUNY Downstate to Jack C. Haldeman, January 24, 1968. Archives of the Health and Hospital Planning Council of Southern New York, Box 39, Rare Book Room, New York Academy of Medicine, New York.
54 Governor's Committee on Hospital Costs, *Report of the Governor's Committee on Hospital Costs* (New York: The Committee, 1965), 25–26.
55 Hollis S. Ingraham, "The Article 28 Story; Landmark in Health Facility Planning," no date. Archives of the Health and Hospital Planning Council of Southern New York, Box 143. Rare Book Room, New York Academy of Medicine, New York.
56 "Medical Technology: Too Much of a Good Thing?" *Forbes* June 1, 1977, 67–68.
57 Symond R. Gottlieb, "A Brief History of Health Planning in the United States," In Clark C. Havighurst, ed., *Regulating Health Facilities Construction* (Washington: American Enterprise Institute for Public Policy Research, 1974), 7–25.
58 Paul M. Ellwood, Walter J. McClure, and John C. Rosala, *How Business Interacts with the Health Care System* (Washington: National Chamber Foundation, 1978), x.
59 M. F. Long and P. J. Feldstein, "Economics of Hospital Systems: Peak Loads and Regional Coordination," *The American Economic Review* 57 (1967): 119–129; George P. Schultz. "The Logic of Health Care Facility Planning," *Socio-Economic Planning Sciences* 4 (1970): 383–393; Herbert E. Klarman, "Planning for Facilities" in Eli Ginzburg [*sic* for Ginzberg], ed. *Regionalization and Health Policy* (Washington: US Department of Health, Education, and Welfare, 1977), 25–36.
60 Thomas M. Tierney and Leonard F. Krystynak, *Capital Analysis and Priority Setting: Capital Formation Concerns in the Health Sector* (San Francisco: The Western Center for Health Planning, 1981), 1.
61 Gordon MacLeod and Mark Perlman, *Health Care Capital: Competition and Control* (Cambridge, MA: Ballinger, 1978), xvii–xix, 212, 298–303, 365.
62 Otha W. Linton, *The American College of Radiology: The First 75 Years* (Reston, VA: American College of Radiology, 1997), 147.
63 Alan Kotliar, "A Marketing Study of the Medical Electronics Industry," MBA thesis, University of Pennsylvania, 1959, 60, 87–90.
64 Judith R. Lave and Lester B. Lave, *The Hospital Construction Act: An Evaluation of the Hill-Burton Program, 1948–1973* (Washington: American Enterprise Institute for

Public Policy Research, 1974), 50; Bradford H. Gray, *The Profit Motive and Patient Care* (Cambridge, MA: Harvard University Press, 1991), 71.

65 Benjamin P. Falit, Cary P. Gross, and Kenneth B. Roberts, "Integrated Prostate Cancer Centers and Over-Utilization of IMRT: A Close Look at Fee-for-Service Medicine in Radiation Oncology," *International Journal of Radiation Oncology Biology Physics* 76 (2010): 1285–1288.

66 King County Facilities Review Committee, "Certificate of Need, University Hospital: Lease of a High Energy Linear Accelerator and Necessary Remodeling," April 12, 1978. Puget Sound Health Systems Agency Records, Box 7. Special Collections, University of Washington Libraries. Full disclosure: although this section is based on archival research, I worked in the Washington state health-planning office shortly after this time period.

67 Herbert C. Berry and Arthur J. Gerdes to Carl A. Munding, February 17, 1978. Janet Dana Twight Papers, Box 4, Special Collections, University of Washington Libraries.

68 Donald W. Tesh to James W. Varnum, January 17, 1978. Janet Dana Twight Papers, Box 9. Special Collections, University of Washington Libraries.

69 Swedish Hospital Medical Center, "Certificate of Need Application: Replacement of Radiotherapy Linear Accelerator," May, 1979 and amended August, 1979. Janet Dana Twight Papers, Box 4, Special Collections, University of Washington Libraries.

70 Group Health Cooperative of Puget Sound, "Application for Certificate of Need: To Expand and Update Radiation Therapy Services with the Purchase of a Linear Accelerator," date illegible, but projected date for commencing project April 1, 1977. Janet Dana Twight Papers, Box 4. Special Collections, University of Washington Libraries.

71 Varian Associates, *Annual Report 1979*. Russell and Sigurd Varian Papers, SC 345, Varian Associates Series, Box 1. Special Collections and University Archives, Stanford University Libraries; University Hospital, "Certificate of Need Application, University Hospital for Acquisition of a Varian Clinac 2500 Radiotherapy Linear Accelerator," July 30, 1981. Janet Dana Twight Papers, Box 4. Special Collections, University of Washington Libraries.

72 Puget Sound Health Systems Agency, "Staff Analysis, United General Hospital CoN Application to Replace CO60 Equipment with 10 MEV Linear Accelerator," November 17, 1978. Puget Sound Health Systems Agency Records, Boxes 15 and 59. Special Collections, University of Washington Libraries.

73 United General Hospital, "Certificate of Need Application from United General Hospital," August 10, 1978. Janet Dana Twight Papers, Box 9. Special Collections, University of Washington Libraries.

74 David L. Wishart to David L. Bjornson, February 6, 1978. Janet Dana Twight Papers, Box 9. Special Collections, University of Washington Libraries.

75 I also referred to this experience in my book *The Medical Delivery Business.*

76 Diana Farrell, Eric Jensen, and Bob Kocher, *Accounting for the Cost of Health Care in the United States: A New Look at Why Americans Spend More* (New York: McKinsey Global Institute, 2008), 52.

Part III

Financializing Medicine, 1970s to the 2010s

"Crazy medicine and unsustainable public policy"
— Ezekiel J. Emanuel, M.D. and Steven D. Pearson, M.D.

While entrepreneurship and competition played larger roles in shaping medical care in the first two-thirds of the 20th century, the role of finance grew in the last third. Venture capital and other financial firms enhanced the medical business system as they invested in high-tech specialty services. The radiation oncology specialty continued to engage in political activities to protect its trade, and its research continued to find (only) small clinical gains from radiation treatments of most cancers. Health care development in general continued to express the political and economic environment.

Political and Economic Environment

Postwar economic growth crested around 1970, after which the US economy entered a lengthy decline. For the first time since the Great Depression, unemployment rose substantially, income inequality grew, and the average American saw a reduction in living standards.[1] At the same time, big business got bigger and more powerful, and the rich got richer. University of Chicago economist (not New York University radiologist) Milton Friedman articulated the business-oriented market strategies that provided the basis for the political activities of the time. Business leaders used Friedman's theories to denounce government regulation of commerce, capital investment, and private property. Congress subsequently deregulated the financial industry and reduced taxes on capital gains, large incomes, and inheritance. These activities freed up large amounts of investment capital, much of which flowed into high-tech firms. The creation of capital came to surpass the creation of goods, services, and jobs.[2]

The financial industry intensified its efforts to model medical services according to business and to draw them into the sphere of capital.[3] A large section in the January 1970 issue of *Fortune* magazine advised hospitals to become more competitive and to manage their capital more efficiently.[4] The US Federal Trade Commission (FTC) applied antitrust law to the professions and targeted the American Medical Association's monopoly policies, as noted in Chapter 1.

Upheld by the US Supreme Court in 1975, the FTC rulings explicitly defined medical practice as *trade* and ruled out any alternative economics based on *service*.

Capital investment continued to expand complex medical centers by fueling the horizontal and vertical consolidation of services. Medical centers grew in size and complexity as they bought out competitors and added the latest technologies. Capital infusions prompted for-profit conversions and, where feasible, going "public" by selling stock in the stock markets. Differences between for-profit and not-for-profit narrowed as large nonprofit hospitals restructured for-profit subsidiaries and selected services that would improve margins, market shares, and competitive positions.[5]

Business consultants then advised medical leaders and investors that freestanding specialty units offered cost-efficient competitive alternatives to hospital conglomerates.[6] Management guru Peter Drucker praised freestanding medical units as the essence of innovation, and the American Hospital Association advised radiology departments to develop them.[7] Business school professor Regina Herzlinger similarly recommended "focused factories" that specialized in sets of clinical procedures and processed patients rapidly and efficiently like Jiffy Lube® stations.[8] Consulting companies advocated separate, privately owned specialty procedure unit *carve-outs* that converted medical care into a "portfolio of high-performing products" and integrated physicians into capital-management companies.[9] Cancer centers, the consultants boasted, offered a "means to earn profit as opposed to an end upon itself." Procedure units had already extended the carve-out logic of specialization by designing separate units for different specialty procedures and technologies. Public policy aided and abetted specialty-unit development.

The pharmaceutical industry benefitted first from the 1980 Bayh-Dole Patent and Trademark Act, which handed to universities the patent rights of technologies developed in their federally funded research laboratories. By the end of the century, the medical device industry was catching up.[10] Venture capital companies looked to high-cost, high-return technologies, and device companies came to account for significant portions of their portfolios.[11] Medical device innovation became a global symbol of national scientific progress and economic modernization.[12]

The final decades of the 20th century saw a quantitative leap in market strategies shaping medical care organization and practice. Why, in times of weak economy, was there a race to build treatment centers of uncertain clinical value costing up to $300 million apiece?

Notes

1 Robert L. Heilbroner and Aaron Singer, *The Economic Transformation of America: 1600 to the Present* (Fort Worth: Harcourt Brace, 1994), 341–357.

2 Greta R. Krippner, *Capitalizing on Crisis: The Political Origins of the Rise of Finance* (Cambridge: Harvard University Press, 2011), 29; Thomas Piketty, trans. Arthur Goldhammer, *Capital in the Twenty-First Century* (Cambridge: Harvard University Press, 2014), 195–212, 291–296.

3 Bob Jessop, "From Hegemony to Crisis? The Continuing Ecological Dominance of Neoliberalism," In Kean Birch and Vlad Mykhnenko, eds., *The Rise and Fall of*

Neoliberalism: The Collapse of an Economic Order? (London: Zed Books, 2010), 171–187.

4 "Our Ailing Medical System," *Fortune* January 1970, 80–81, 96,128,130. Yet, illustrating the political shift since that time, some of the articles accepted goals of equitable access to health care, paying fair wages to health care workers, and union-sponsored national health insurance.

5 Patricia J. Arnold, "The Invisible Hand in Health Care: The Rise of Financial Markets in the U.S. Hospital Industry," In John L. Campbell, J. Rogers Hollingsworth, and Leon N. Lindberg, eds., *Governance in the American Economy* (Cambridge: Cambridge University Press, 1991), 293–316.

6 Jeff Goldsmith, "Death of a Paradigm: The Challenge of Competition," *Health Affairs* 3 (1984): 5–19.

7 Peter F. Drucker, *Innovation and Entrepreneurship: Practices and Principles* (New York: Harper and Row, 1985), 24, 61; Suzanna Hoppszallern and Christine M. Hughes, *Outpatient Radiology Service: Successful Business Strategies* (Chicago: American Hospital Association, 1988).

8 Regina E. Herzlinger, *Market-Driven Health Care: Who Wins, Who Loses in the Transformation of America's Largest Service Industry* (Reading, MA: Addison-Wesley, 1997), 163, 166.

9 Tiber Group, *The "Carve-Out" Guide* (Chicago: Tiber Group, 1997), 1, 5; Tiber Group, *Can Local Products Compete in a National Marketplace? The Carve-Out Guide II* (Chicago: Tiber Group, 2000), 8.

10 Hamilton Moses, E. Ray Dorsey, David H. M. Matheson, and Samuel O. Their, "Financial Anatomy of Biomedical Research," *JAMA* 294 (2005): 1333–1342.

11 D. Clay Ackerly, Ana M. Valverde, Lawrence W. Diener, K. L. Dossary, and K. A. Schulman, "Fueling Innovation in Medical Devices (and Beyond): Venture Capital in Health Care" *Health Affairs* 28 (2009): w68–w75.

12 Jing Wang, Xiaodong Wu, Yuguo Tang, et al., "A Comprehensive Evaluation System for the Application and Promotion of Chinese Medical Devices," advertisement in *Science* 344 (2014): unpaginated.

9 Speculating on Proton Therapy

Radiation physics investigators counseled in the mid-1980s that photon energies had reached peak clinical performance and that further photon energy rise would not further clinical gain.[1] An implication of this advice was that the future lay in particles. But several US and European institutions had used neutrons after the war and had not found noteworthy clinical gain. University of Washington researchers found that neutrons seemed to offer better results (only) for local control of cancers of the salivary gland. They explained, however, that the capital intensity of neutron facilities meant that they "must operate over decades to recoup the original investment."[2] By 2008, not one of 25 randomized controlled trials had demonstrated neutrons to be more effective than X-ray or cobalt-60 photons in treating cancer, and many studies reported delayed morbidity to be a serious problem.[3]

At the same time that some universities were treating patients with neutrons from their physics departments' cyclotrons, others were using the physics machines to treat patients with beams of protons. After 40 years of such use, an innovation in medical delivery escalated the capitalization of radiation therapy to stratospheric heights. Proton treatment centers costing $100–300 million each more than complied with a 1984 business guide's advice to radiology administrators to maximize their capital expenditures.[4] Proton centers are specialty procedure units on steroids.

Raising the Stakes

Harvard University physicist Robert R. Wilson later recalled that he had suggested using proton beams to treat cancer in 1946 as "atonement for involvement in the development of the bomb at Los Alamos."[5] John Lawrence and his colleagues initiated proton-beam treatments at their Berkeley laboratory in 1954 and switched to heavier particles when the physicists reset the cyclotron to hurl them. They were primarily aiming to destroy the pituitary glands of patients with acromegaly, diabetic retinopathy, and metastatic breast cancer.[6] Sweden's University of Uppsala initiated clinical use of protons in 1957, and the Massachusetts General Hospital did so in 1961, using the synchrocyclotron in the Harvard physics department.

Massachusetts General Hospital/Harvard University

William Sweet, the Massachusetts General Hospital neurosurgery chief who was rendering patients' pituitary glands dysfunctional in a variety of ways, hoped that protons might avoid the serious brain damage generated by X-rays. Sweet sent junior colleague Raymond Kjellberg to Sweden for training, and Kjellberg subsequently sent patients across the river for treatment on the Harvard machine. The National Aeronautics and Space Administration (NASA) funded the medical annex to the cyclotron in order to learn more about radiation risks to astronauts.[7] The clinical program came to support itself entirely—and the cyclotron to boot—with income from patient treatments. The Harvard unit was the country's only active proton-beam treatment facility for more than three decades without inspiring other proton facilities—until a new entrepreneurial idea came along.

The Proton [later Particle] Therapy Cooperative Group (PTCOG) started up in 1983 with the goal of initiating a hospital-based proton facility. Harvard researchers announced the following year at the first annual meeting of the American Society for Therapeutic Radiology and Oncology (ASTRO, which subsequently changed its name to American Society for Radiation Oncology but retained the acronym) that they were designing a proton treatment machine that might sell for around $2 million.[8] But Harvard did not develop a commercial device or open the first hospital-based proton unit.

Loma Linda University/Fermilab

Some PTCOG members were chagrined when it was California's Loma Linda University that announced it was building the first hospital-based proton treatment center. James Slater, Loma Linda's radiation medicine chief, was the first to come up with the money when PTCOG [under]estimated that a hospital-based proton center would cost around $20 million.[9] Loma Linda sent some of its engineers to work with physicists at the Fermi National Accelerator Laboratory (Fermilab) on building a clinical proton-accelerating synchrotron.

Jointly funded by government and private donors, Loma Linda's proton center benefitted from a US Department of Energy grant initiated by Congresswoman Lindy Boggs, whose daughter had died of choroidal melanoma. Haughtily distinguishing Congressionally-directed grants from National Institutes of Health (NIH) largesse, Harvard later declared that it, too, could have gotten a leg up from the special appropriation, but that it rejected "pork barrel" monies.[10] Loma Linda widely publicized the 1990 opening of its new proton center. The *Wall Street Journal* greeted the proton device as "unquestionably the most expensive piece of medical equipment ever built."[11] Annual payments for radiation treatments in the United States exceeded the $1 billion mark around that time,[12] and proton therapy portended a massive leap above that.

Loma Linda engineers who had worked on the synchrotron at Fermilab launched the Optivus Proton Therapy company in 1993. While one Slater son succeeded his father as chief of radiation medicine at Loma Linda, another became president of Optivus. The company licensed the Fermilab technology and linked with defense contractor Scientific Applications International to set a goal (which would not be met) of supplying the US medical market with 20 proton devices in its first decade. Optivus was not among the bidders to build a device for the Massachusetts General Hospital.

Massachusetts General Hospital/IBA

Massachusetts General Hospital surgeons and radiation oncologists, as well as ophthalmologists from the contiguous Massachusetts Eye and Ear Infirmary, had been sending patients to Harvard's cyclotron for 30 years. But, after Loma Linda opened its proton center, the Harvard teaching hospital had to have one, too. Three companies responded when the hospital issued a request for bids: Ion Beam Applications (IBA), Maxwell-Brobeck in association with Varian, and Siemens. IBA won.

IBA was a spin-off of the Cyclotron Research Center of Belgium's Catholic University of Louvain-la-Neuve. Louvain had long played a major radiotherapy role in the country that had extracted radium from its colony in the Congo. Belgium had boasted the "largest radium beam therapy apparatus in the world" at the 1950 International Congress of Radiology.[13] Yves Jongen, who had been a member of Louvain's neutron-beam treatment team, left the university in 1986 to found Ion Beam Applications.[14] Presenting its cyclotron to the Proton Therapy Cooperative Group in 1990, the company rapidly became the world's leading commercial source of clinical proton accelerators. By 2014, IBA had placed its devices in half of the world's proton-therapy centers, and the company projected "tremendous growth potential" if radiation oncologists would only treat 20 percent of their patients with protons.[15]

With the National Cancer Institute covering half its costs, Massachusetts General Hospital (Mass General) built its proton-treatment center across an alley from the hospital on the property of the former Charles Street Jail.[16] The hospital devoted the rest of its newly acquired property to a luxury hotel that would accommodate wealthier patients using hospital facilities. The new proton center treated its first patient in 2001, four decades after the hospital initiated clinical use of protons and one decade after Loma Linda opened its proton center. The Loma Linda and Mass General centers together cracked the US proton-center market wide open. The next in line was the Texas Medical Center.

Texas Medical Center

Reflecting contemporary economic (and social) thought, Texas's president and CEO called the world's largest medical center, which looks like a mid-sized city, a "testament to what free men can achieve in a free society."[17] Texas characteristically held that if not first, its proton center was the "largest and most sophisticated facility of its kind in the world."[18] M. D. Anderson Hospital director John Mendelsohn credited the economics text *Competitive Advantage* when he included a proton center as an important element in the hospital's growth strategy.[19] Responding to the hospital's request for a joint venture in proton therapy, private investors and companies proposed to build a new facility on state-owned medical center land and lease it to a new proton center company. M. D. Anderson would staff the center, organize its publicity, and confer its brand upon it. The proposal projected annual gross revenues of $100 million when the proton center was fully operational.[20] Seeking to challenge IBA's incipient domination of the world proton-therapy market, Hitachi supplied, installed, and maintained M. D. Anderson's synchrotron.[21]

In addition to Hitachi, other key partners in the Texas venture included Sanders Morris Harris, the largest investment bank in the state; and the Styles Company, a property developer. The nominally not-for-profit M. D. Anderson Hospital held 15 percent of the equity of the for-profit proton center and expected to reap a minimum of 15 percent of its profits after the partners recouped their investment plus interest.[22] The new center had to set its charges high and treat large numbers of paying patients in order to cover its overhead, debt costs, and profit allocations. Charged with raising the required capital, John Styles allotted 1 percent of the proton center's future profits to a company that connected him with important investors.[23] The company did not have far to look. Although warned of financial risk, the Houston Police Officers' Pension System and the Houston Firefighters' Relief & Retirement Fund became heavily invested in the financial success of proton treatment in Houston.

Early proton adopters thought they were securing a comfortable lead due to the technology's extremely high entry costs, but they did not take into account the massive amount of investment capital seeking profitable outlets. A wide variety of property development, finance, and physician management companies started up to partner with medical providers and manufacturers to build new proton centers.

Management Company/Manufacturing Alliances

ProCure/IBA

John Cameron, a particle physicist who had helped build the Indiana University Health Proton Therapy Center (which would close in 2014), founded ProCure Treatment Centers in 2005 in conjunction with Wall Street banker Hadley Ford. Offering a "complete turnkey outsourcing solution," ProCure initially noted on its web site that it would own, design, finance, construct, staff, and manage the day-to-day operations of its treatment centers. The founding banker drew up the business plan arranging for ProCure to own 70–80 percent of the equity of each for-profit proton center, with participating oncology groups and hospitals holding minority stakes. The plan projected that each proton center would be 80 percent bank-financed and yield 15–20 percent annual returns on investment when running at full capacity.[24]

ProCure partnered with two local radiation oncology groups and announced that the Belgian financial institutions Fortis and KBC were financing its IBA-equipped center in Oklahoma City.[25] After Oklahoma, ProCure outcompeted a project in the affluent Chicago suburbs. Northern Illinois University had linked with the Northwestern Medical Faculty Foundation to plan the Northern Illinois Proton Treatment and Research Center (NIPTRC). NIPTRC contracted with Varian Medical Systems to purchase the cyclotron the company was building in Germany, having purchased Siemens's offspring Accel Instruments in 2007. But in 2010, the Illinois project ran into "tough economic conditions" (its bonds were not selling) and a tough economic competitor.[26]

ProCure had entered a joint venture with Central DuPage Hospital and the Chicago area's largest private-practice radiation oncology group to develop a proton-treatment center of its own in the Chicago suburbs. Aggressively pursuing its project, ProCure sued when NIPTRC received state Certificate of Need (CoN) approval, accusing NIPTRC of violating antitrust law.[27] Illinois regulators initially rejected ProCure's own CoN application, but the company won on appeal and withdrew its lawsuit. Calling the ProCure project a "cash register for greedy investors," NIPTRC leaders insinuated that campaign donations to the then governor Rod Blagojevich might have lubricated the CoN reversal. Any allegations of wrongdoing, ProCure CEO Hadley Ford retorted, were "baloney."[28] Central DuPage Hospital loaned ProCure $40 million to build its Illinois proton center and invested a further $18 million in the project. The new proton center installed an IBA cyclotron, and the 2009 IBA–ProCure press release announced that it had set a world record in taking just over 2 years from breaking ground to irradiating patients. Other ventures in the making undoubtedly took note of the corporate proton-therapy model.

In 2013, however, with two more ProCure centers in progress, the company was headed toward default on a $3.6 million interest payment due on its loan from Central DuPage Hospital. Proton therapy was not itself in doubt, managers hastened to assure the public, claiming [inaccurately] that "a growing body of research confirms the efficacy of proton therapy."[29] A few months later, Cadence Health filed papers to purchase ProCure's 70 percent ownership interest in the DuPage proton center. Cadence was the recent product of a "blockbuster merger" that had incorporated Central DuPage Hospital into a vertically-integrated health care network.[30] When Cadence merged with Northwestern Medicine in 2014, the university health plan got the proton center it failed to get with NIPTRC.

Having announced its proton device at the 2010 meeting of the Particle Therapy Cooperative Group and losing out at NIPTRC, Varian still urgently needed to get in the game. A San Diego company gearing up to challenge ProCure's lead in corporate proton therapy provided the opportunity.

Advanced Particle Therapy/Varian

Advanced Particle Therapy targeted academic medical centers and other major medical systems as partners in its investor-owned proton-therapy centers.[31] Their money would be safer, Advanced Particle's president and CEO assured potential investors, when connected to prestigious institutions unlikely to go bankrupt. As developer, owner and manager of its proton-therapy centers, the company would analyze their markets, design layout for rapid patient throughput, supervise construction, select vendors, and manage debt and equity financing.

Advanced Particle partnered with Varian to place the manufacturer's previously NIPTRC-bound cyclotron in the Scripps Health system. The $220 million Scripps proton center was expected to be 35 percent equity and 65 percent debt financed. Varian reportedly agreed to loan up to $115 million to the San Diego center in exchange for 4 percent of its gross revenues for 35 years.[32] Varian brought in JP Morgan Chase Bank to finance part of its debt as well as Orix Capital Markets, which chipped in $50 million for another share of the proton center's future revenues.[33] Each partner brought in along the way held an interest in the clinic's financial success.

Varian had finally entered the business it had eschewed in the early 1970s.[34] The Stanford–Varian team had instead continued to develop its linear electron accelerator line as well as technological upgrades and software systems for it. Varian had done very well with its intensity-modulated radiation therapy (IMRT) system. Comprising filters or collimators to shape radiation beams and computer software to guide them, the innovation was the package rather than the separate components in it.[35] IMRT became a huge success for Varian, and the company credited the technology with contributing to its business strategy of increasing transaction prices while shortening product replacement cycles.[36] Some radiation oncologists would criticize IMRT's rapid adoption without sufficient testing, pointing out that IMRT exposed patients to more total radiation than conventional radiotherapy did.[37] But hospital administrators and specialists convinced insurers to pay substantially higher rates for it, and IMRT rapidly became the standard of care against which researchers and clinicians measured alternative techniques, including protons.

Varian's product line enabled the company to dominate the domestic external beam radiotherapy market and to claim half of the global market by 2014. Varian marketed its products in professional symposia, investment bank–sponsored health care conferences, consumer-oriented educational programs, and investor meetings held at professional conventions.[38] The company further promoted itself by advertising on street corners, as shown in Figure 9.1. Presumably not marketing to the large homeless population in the area, the San Francisco poster seemed to be selling the company brand to the nearby City Hall. It displayed another poster in the financial district.

Despite Advanced Particle Therapy's tactic of partnering with academic medical centers that were unlikely to go bankrupt, its planned Dallas Proton Treatment Center affiliated with the University of Texas Southwestern filed for bankruptcy protection in 2015, and the following year, investors in the company's Emory Proton Therapy Center in Atlanta tried to force the same route.[39] Billionaire investors in both cases wanted to pull their money out of financially struggling, partially built facilities.

While ProCure/IBA and Advanced Particle Therapy/Varian and their allied property development and finance firms were positioning themselves in (and crashing out of) the proton-therapy market, second-generation technologies were

OUR
CANCER-
FIGHTING
TECHNOLOGY
HAS BEEN
MAKING
THE NEWS
SINCE 1948.
VARIAN
A partner for life

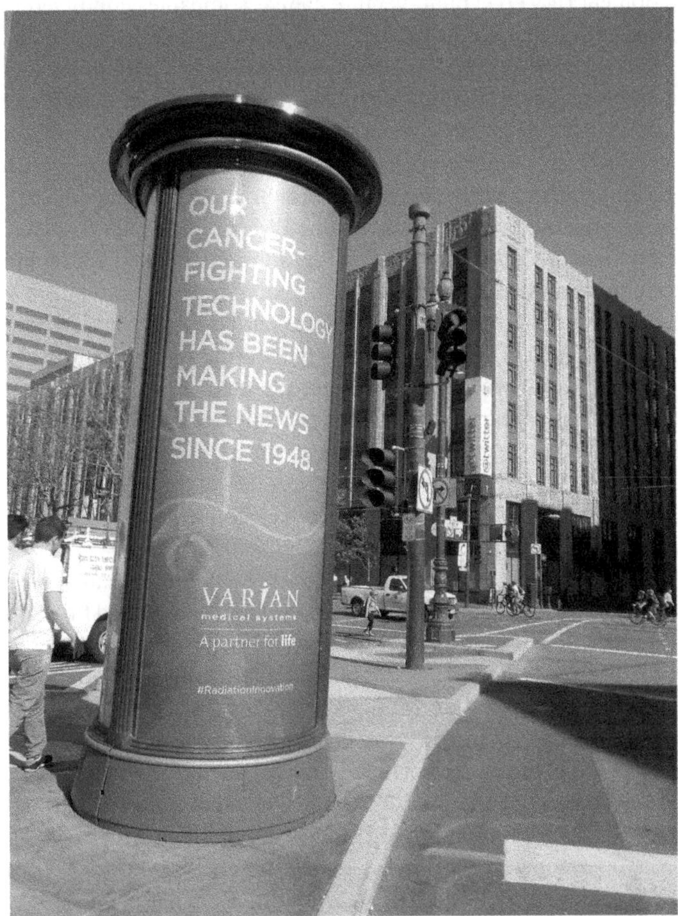

Figure 9.1 Varian Medical Systems Advertises on Street Corners. Intersection of Market and Fell, San Francisco, September 23, 2014.

Photograph: Barbara Bridgman Perkins.

coming along faster than expected. Spurred by the booming market, a variety of manufacturers acquired patents or exclusive licenses for cheaper ways to accelerate protons. One of them beat Varian to the ribbon-cutting ceremony.

Proton Manufacturing Accelerates

Located in Boston's high-tech corridor, Still River Systems licensed an accelerator developed in a federally funded laboratory at the Massachusetts Institute of Technology (MIT).[40] The company expected to achieve competitive advantage in the proton-therapy market with a device that was significantly smaller and cheaper than those of its competitors. Although the 2008 economic implosion reduced research and development (R&D) capital, venture capital companies continued to pump tens of millions of dollars into Still River.[41] The venture capitalists expected that a price tag of $20–35 million could out-compete the IBA and Varian devices that were coming in closer to $100 million for the machines alone. Still River attracted the attention of radiology service company American Shared Hospital Services, which acquired an equity interest in it.[42] St. Louis's Barnes-Jewish Hospital opened the first American Shared Services proton treatment center in 2013 with a device from the manufacturer by then renamed Mevion Medical Systems. When the Ackerman Cancer Center in Jacksonville, Florida installed a Mevion device, it became the first private medical practice to claim proton treatment.

After accumulating over $140 million from venture capital firms, Mevion filed an Initial Public Offering (IPO) in 2014. Customers purchasing its device, Mevion suggested in its IPO prospectus, would be able to recoup their capital outlays and installation costs within 3 or 4 years—provided they attained a minimum of 275 patients per treatment room per year. To ensure this number, the company advised radiation oncologists, they needed to treat at least 15 percent of their patients with protons.[43] Both Mevion and American Shared Hospital Services ran into trouble on Wall Street in 2015, however, and Mevion cancelled its IPO.

Other manufacturers acquired patent rights to other (relatively) small proton accelerators and were rushing to get them on the market. The Texas-based ProTom International acquired exclusive US rights to a Russian synchrotron and offered partnerships with medical providers in developing, constructing, and operating proton centers. ProTom contracted with McLaren Health Care to locate its first proton facility in Flint, Michigan.[44] In 2014, ProTom announced that US Food and Drug Administration (FDA) "clearance" officially put its device on the market.[45] The FDA's 510(k) process, ProTom's CEO asserted, entailed a "thorough and rigorous FDA review of the safety and effectiveness" of the device. Chapter 10 describes how the 510(k) notification process entails no such review. ProTom filed for bankruptcy protection the following year, but McLaren announced that it was proceeding with its proton center.[46] After finding lead in the city's water supply a few months later, Flint residents might be justified in thinking that safe drinking water would do more for their health than a new proton center.

Like radiology manufacturers before them, proton device companies did not just put their machines on the market and wait for buyers to appear, they built up the market also. The companies expanded the platoon of sales representatives appearing in radiation oncology offices on a weekly basis.[47] Vendor ability to provide financing played a key role in device marketing, and European banks frequently invested in American proton centers. IBA arranged financing of its proton centers with Belgian banks, and Varian turned to Deutsche Bank.[48] Each leap in medical care capitalization called for more connections, and each of them raised the number of interests holding stakes in the commercial success of proton therapy. Although smaller machines were cheaper and less likely to require management company involvement, some medical providers continued to choose the high productivity, prestige, and potential profits of the larger machines.

Specializing in a single technology, gleaming proton centers—many of which look like whole hospitals—exemplify a Jiffy Lubrication of medicine, whether they are strategic business units in medical complexes or whether they follow the independent boutique model. Since many separately owned carve-outs were located on or near hospital campuses and took advantage of the hospital brand, the shift in corporate status was not always perceptible to patients moving from one to another. Although each freestanding unit may individually achieve an efficient and high-quality delivery of specialty interventions, their proliferation leads to an inefficient and uncoordinated health care system. Specialists turning their private offices into procedure units by installing costly technologies like CT scanning or radiation therapy also extended the logic of specialism as well as that of capitalism. Perhaps, not unlike the drive-in doc-in-a-box cartoon in Chapter 1, we will drive to the nearest Zippy Zap station for accelerated radiation treatments.

Reading company prospectuses, hospital brochures, newspaper headlines, and media stories, investors and consumers alike may have felt justified in thinking that proton-therapy growth was based on scientific evidence of effectiveness. Radiation oncologists rationalized proton centers' high costs by maintaining that the dose distribution properties of protons would "almost certainly" improve outcomes.[49] Was their near certainty justified?

Practice versus Science

In 1966, *Time* magazine celebrated new medical technologies that included Massachusetts General Hospital's use of the Harvard cyclotron for proton beam treatment. The magazine also quoted hospital director John Knowles as saying that while many of the new technologies increased medical costs "astronomically," they were "relatively useless" clinically.[50] Some of his hospital's staff obviously did not agree with Knowles in the case of proton therapy, but they were not in fact producing clear evidence of its utility. Instead, they maintained that the dose distribution properties of proton beams "should translate into improved local control and reduced morbidity."[51] The argument is reasonable. Proton beams unloose most of their energy at a predictable depth in the body and, unlike X-rays, they do not continue a destructive path through the body after that point.

The media popularized the dose distribution argument. The *Wall Street Journal* declared that protons act like "crack combat troops" that target precisely the right area. Yet when the *Journal* asked radiation oncologist Joseph Imperato about Loma Linda's new proton center, Imperato grumbled, "I can't understand why the hell they built this ridiculous unit" ... "it's a great physics project, but some of the medical claims are lunatic."[52] As a hypothesis, the argument that the dose distribution should translate into improved outcomes is not lunatic, and a scientific approach would test it.

But assuming *a priori* that the dose distribution translated into improved cancer outcomes meant that advocates were not eager to test the validity of that assumption. Three 2007 worldwide literature reviews revealed a huge evidence gap. One review suggested that proton (and other particle) treatments might lead to better outcomes only for some patients with ocular tumors and chordomas of the base of the skull.[53] The second recognized local control of pediatric intracranial tumors, but noted that some children subsequently suffered neuropsychological impairment, hypopituitarism, and cataracts.[54] The third found insufficient evidence of increased effectiveness or reduced damage for recommending proton-beam treatment for any disease site.[55]

Some critics within radiation oncology accused that economic, political, and professional considerations had overridden scientific ones in the growth of proton treatment.[56] Anthony Zietman, ASTRO's 2007 president, criticized billboard advertising and called proton centers "prestige projects for marketing purposes without proof of real benefit."[57] Another radiation oncology professor charged that growth in proton therapy was "driven by the business model, not by any evidence of clinical need."[58] Some leaders, however, maintained that proton therapy did not require evidence of improved outcomes.

Face-to-face with a cancer patient, some clinicians reject randomized controlled trials (RCTs) in favor of their own clinical judgments.[59] And some of their patients do well. Although one had praised his field for early adoption of RCTs and the other had proclaimed a "clear need" for them 20 years earlier, M. D. Anderson Hospital radiation oncologist James Cox and Massachusetts General Hospital radiation physicist Michael Goitein controversially declared in 2008 that RCTs were not necessary for proton therapy.[60] They argued that it was unethical for clinicians who believed in the effectiveness of a particular treatment to conduct trials (to test that belief). They invoked the principle of *equipoise*—or balance of interests—which holds that there must be a level of uncertainty regarding the benefit of a particular treatment in order to ethically withhold it from any patient. The implication of this interpretation of equipoise is that individual provider certainty trumps scientific evidence.

Challenging Cox and Goitein's argument, a paper in the *Journal of Medical Ethics* made the case that equipoise required uncertainty at the level of the relevant expert community rather than that of the individual practitioner, and that the radiation oncology community was indeed uncertain about the effectiveness of proton treatment.[61] Supporters of this argument suggested that practitioners rejecting trials had professional interests to protect and feared that the "emperor may in fact be naked."[62]

The emperor's state of dress remained unexposed. The US Agency for Healthcare Research and Quality (AHRQ) reported in 2009 that research studies still did not support assumptions of better outcomes with proton beams.[63] It further revealed that debilitating, irreversible, and even life-threatening treatment complications were inconsistently reported. The American Society for Radiation Oncology (ASTRO) was more optimistic, announcing in 2012 that proton beams appeared to be superior in treating large ocular melanomas, chordomas, and perhaps central nervous system (CNS) cancers in children.[64] ASTRO further deemed protons effective but not superior to X-rays in treating prostate cancer, and it found insufficient evidence to recommend proton therapy for cancers of the lung, head and neck, gastrointestinal tract, and pediatric non-CNS malignancies. In the same year, AHRQ again criticized the escalating use of proton therapy despite the ongoing dearth of outcomes evidence.[65]

In a 2012 reprise of the debate on trials, a radiation oncologist holding for the proposition (circularly) argued that clinical "trials are not necessary because it is obvious that protons are better" on the grounds that they deliver lower radiation doses to nontarget tissues. Furthermore, he maintained that it would be inefficient to conduct randomized controlled trials because they were "likely to demonstrate no major differences in cure rates."[66] The radiation oncologist arguing against the proposition charged that refusing to conduct trials was unscientific. He called belief in proton superiority in the absence of adequate evidence "faith-based medicine."

The evidence drought persisted. American College of Radiology/American Society for Radiation Oncology joint-practice parameters advised in 2014 that there was still insufficient evidence to conclude that protons were superior to conventional radiotherapy.[67] Even if protons did not improve immediate outcomes, users continued to hope they would induce less coronary artery disease, lung fibrosis, and malignancy.[68] The proton boom continued, and many centers bet their futures on prostate cancer.

The Case of the Prostate Gland

Projections of profitably treating patients with prostate cancer spurred proton-center growth. Most American men with prostate cancer are over 65 and are covered by Medicare. Furthermore, the gland's radiation treatment is considered a relatively simple procedure that permits rapid processing of large numbers of patients.[69] One study estimated that a proton center costing $125 million would have to treat at least 2000 patients a year in order to generate the $50 million in annual revenues required just to cover its costs.[70] Many proton-center business plans projected prostate cancer as comprising 50–80 percent of their patient loads in order to succeed financially. Without prostate cancer, their accountants advised, it was nearly impossible.

As the most common cancer among US males, prostate cancer offers a huge patient population. "The easiest group to market to," one hospital administrator observed, was "men worrying about the functioning of their penis."[71] Many older men, possibly two-thirds of them in their 70s, have lurking in their prostate glands cells that can be diagnosed microscopically as cancerous but that do not metastasize. Many of these cells remain this way and are not life threatening so long as they do—although it is often not predictable which ones will become dangerous. The paradox is that trouble usually starts when the cancerous cells come to medical attention. A simple blood test drove the politics of prostate cancer by expediting discovery of these cells.[72]

The number of prostate-cancer diagnoses spiked in the early 1990s after scientists at Roswell Park Cancer Institute patented a test measuring blood levels of a protein they called prostate-specific antigen (PSA). Biotech companies commercialized the test, the FDA approved it, and doctors and device manufacturers added it to their panels of routine metabolic measurements. Fear of cancer, fear of lawsuits, and product advertising rapidly made the PSA test standard practice in many medical venues.

A PSA number on the upper side of the normal bell curve came to define a disease that called for medical attention.[73] Yet the protein is a normal product of the prostate gland and it is not cancer specific, and many factors besides cancer (including aging, exercise, and sexual activity) can affect its circulating levels. Consequently, using PSA measurement as a screening tool for cancer can incur false positive rates approaching 75 percent. False positives were leading to unnecessary biopsies on more than a million American men a year, the independent US Preventive Services Task Force cautioned in 2011.[74] Although PSA screening does detect more prostate cancers, the Task Force concluded that screening did not reduce 10-year prostate cancer-specific mortality rates. The Task Force explicitly recommended against PSA screening in 2012.[75] The Cochrane Collaboration's 2013 analysis of five randomized controlled trials concluded that PSA screening did not decrease mortality but that it did increase treatment-related harms.[76] When cancerous cells appear in the microscope, clinical protocols typically dictate treatment.

Many patients—and their doctors—believe that survival after cancer treatment means that the treatment worked, and high prostate-cancer survival rates seem to support that belief. But it is easy to misinterpret the higher survival rates that followed widespread use of the PSA test. Adding men with microscopic prostate-cancer cells to the calculation dilutes the total number of diagnosed cases with nonthreatening cancers and in itself raises the measured proportion of survivors. Many men live healthy lives without any treatment of their prostate cancer cells. Although 26,000 US men do die each year of prostate cancer, it is a small proportion of all prostate cancer cases, and 70 percent of those men are over 75 years of age.[77] More treatment may or may not have extended the lives of some of them by a few years (or months). The goal of cancer treatment is not to prevent death (which medicine never does, of course) but to prevent disability, discomfort, and premature death.

Many radiation oncologists hoped that proton beams would treat prostate cancer more effectively than X-rays, but, as noted earlier in this chapter, this did not seem to be the case. A 2008 textbook advised that proton beam irradiation did not increase the already high prostate-cancer survival rates or decrease complication rates from radiation therapy.[78] Doctors and their patients also hoped that radiation would do less damage than prostate surgery, long known to lead to impotence and incontinence in many men. The evidence on this was mixed; some studies have suggested that radiation leads to less erectile dysfunction and less urinary incontinence but more bowel damage than surgery. Somewhere between the not-very-helpful range of 2–58 percent of patients reported short- and/or long-term fecal incontinence following radiotherapy for prostate cancer.[79] The greatest prostate-cancer risk, one oncologist concluded, stems "from the active treatments triggered by a cancer diagnosis."[80]

Ironically, perhaps, US practice patterns seemed to be shifting away from irradiating prostate-cancer patients even as proton centers were recruiting them. The shift was due in part to an ongoing competition between radiation oncologists and urologists for prostate-cancer patients. Trained in surgery and already treating prostate cancer with brachytherapy, urologists eagerly purchased the new robotic surgery devices. Although the data do not indicate the proportion using robots, surgery as the sole initial treatment of prostate cancer rose from 35 percent in 2000 to 54 percent in 2013, and the use of radiation (alone or with other treatments) declined from 47 to 31 percent.[81]

In the midst of the interspecialty tug-of-war over prostate-cancer patients, The American Society for Radiation Oncology advised against routine proton beam treatment of prostate cancer outside of clinical trials and counseled that physicians discuss with their low-risk patients "active surveillance" versus immediate active intervention.[82] Concerned about overtreatment of cancer at high cost to patients as well as to society, some medical experts called for professional and/or public policy to control proton-therapy growth.

Public and Private Health Policy

Proton therapy was "crazy medicine and unsustainable public policy," medical advisors Ezekiel Emanuel and Steven Pearson contended.[83] Not quite so outspoken, the Center for American Progress identified the proton-therapy boom as a "prime example of our health system rushing headlong into an unproven, costly treatment."[84] But there were few regulatory mechanisms to address the problem, and those that did exist were indifferently applied or overwhelmed by market strategies.

Announcement of one proton center in a city frequently triggered a competing announcement in the same city—the very duplication of services that Certificate of Need (CoN) was designed to mitigate. Yet when Johns Hopkins Medicine and MedStar Health each submitted CoN applications to build proton centers just a few miles apart, the District of Columbia's CoN approved both.[85] MedStar proposed a center at MedStar Georgetown University Hospital, the centerpiece of its hospital–physician–pharmaceutical system. Johns Hopkins proposed to build its proton center at a former community hospital that Hopkins was in the process of transforming into an expansion of its Baltimore-based tertiary level system.

In contrast to DC, New York State's planning agency took a route advocated by health-policy professor Howard Berliner: solicit collaborative proposals for a proton center and select one.[86] The agency chose the application of a consortium of New York City hospitals led by Memorial Sloan-Kettering Hospital. The consortium's proposed $300 million proton center would be an attraction in the upcoming East Harlem Media, Entertainment and Cultural Center.[87] Tax exemptions as well as JP Morgan Chase and Goldman Sachs financial firms facilitated the proposed conversion of a low-income neighborhood into a high-priced playground.[88] Despite New York's (first round) CoN example, public policy generally had a small impact on the competitive multiplication of proton centers.

Capital investment powered proton-center growth. Projections of a $15 billion domestic proton-therapy industry and annual growth rates upwards of 17 percent continued to draw investors in the face of concerns of a proton bubble.[89] Low interest rates and a stagnant economy in other sectors encouraged speculation in medical care. Proton centers were a comparatively low-risk investment, since cancer is a disease of older people and the American taxpayer paid for their high-cost treatments under the Medicare program. The private sector chose what to build and the public sector paid for it. Multiplying medical price, cost, and debt by an order of magnitude, proton centers integrated the financial industry into medical delivery more than ever before.

By mid-2016, 23 proton centers were in operation in the United States, and 13 more were officially under development. One center had closed, and several of those under construction were in bankruptcy disputes. A dozen or two other previously announced centers had dropped out of the race—at least temporarily. A growing dilemma was not professional or government policy; it was the insurance industry.

The Insurance Industry Challenges Proton Therapy

Payment structures are the conventional means of reinforcing or restricting US medical care supply, and generous reimbursements paid for proton-center growth. Medicare and private insurance companies rapidly approved proton beam therapy as standard rather than experimental treatment and permitted providers to factor overhead costs into their rates. Basing its reimbursements on hospital expenditure reports, Medicare paid nearly twice as much for proton treatments of prostate cancer as it did for intensity-modulated radiation therapy (IMRT)—which had itself nearly doubled the price of radiation treatment.[90]

Paying attention to the scanty scientific literature on effectiveness as well as to their costs, insurers started to deny or reduce payments for proton therapy. (It could not have hurt that the denials coincided with their own financial interests.) Regence, a Blue Cross/ Blue Shield insurer operating in the Pacific Northwest, started to refuse coverage for proton treatments of localized prostate cancer in 2010; Blue Shield of California and Aetna did so in 2013, and Cigna followed suit.[91] With the exception of maintaining full coverage for children with cancer—who understandably elicit emotional responses and who are particularly vulnerable to X-rays—insurers started to restrict proton-therapy coverage to intracranial arteriovenous malformations, melanomas of the uveal tract (iris, choroid, and ciliary body of the eye), and skull-based tumors such as chordomas and chondrosarcomas. One insurer explicitly asserted that proton therapy was "unproven and not medically necessary for treating ALL other indications."[92]

Providers and professional associations fought back against the payment restrictions. The Proton Therapy Consortium and the Particle Therapy Cooperative Group—North America formulated an alternative reimbursement policy. In addition to the conditions named above by the insurance companies, they asserted that medical experts considered proton-beam therapy to be "reasonable and necessary" for the numerous cancers of the head and neck, urinary and gastrointestinal tracts, prostate, female pelvis, and lung.[93] Nashville's Provision Center for

Proton Therapy took a not unusual step of instigating a bill in the state legislature mandating insurance coverage of proton treatment for most cancers. Despite the seven lobbyists promoting the bill, it died in committee (the first time around, anyway).[94] US payment restrictions did not seem to impede international investment, and the proton-center model rapidly spread.

Globalizing Particle Centers

The proliferation of staggeringly high-cost proton treatment centers of uncertain clinical value may serve as a warning to global authorities seeking to import market reforms into their health care systems. Some American proton treatment centers saw the world as their market. The Mayo Clinic, for example, made proton therapy the centerpiece of a $6 billion initiative to secure the clinic's status as a "global medical destination center."[95] At the same time, European and Asian initiatives grew as enterprising radio-oncologists, hospitals, and management companies built their own proton-treatment centers.

European proton treatment had located initially in research institutions in Sweden, Switzerland, and Russia. In 2011, a consortium of Swedish counties with university hospitals announced that it would build a €100 million IBA-equipped proton center adjacent to Uppsala University Hospital.[96] Opening in 2015, the centralized facility included a hotel to accommodate patients and families travelling long distances. Sweden's collaboration was not the general rule, however; many planned European proton centers were individual initiatives.

Physician-entrepreneur Hans Rinecker opened the €150 million Varian-equipped Rinecker Proton Therapy Center in Munich in 2009. He also directed the company established to operate the proton center and provided hospital backup at The Dr. Rinecker Surgical Hospital.[97] Calling it the first "fully certified proton radiation centre" in Europe, Rinecker wrote in *Medical Tourism Magazine* that the center offered a premium package for international patients that included travel arrangements, hotel accommodations, limousine service, personal trainers, and other assistance that would help them enjoy their stay in Munich.[98]

Germany led the European particle center initiative. A construction company initially partnered with IBA to build one of its centers, the West German Proton Therapy Centre, after which a banking syndicate loaned money to the University Hospital of Essen to purchase the center as a hospital subsidiary.[99] Essen Hospital administrators projected that treatment payments would make the center self-supporting and paying back on its debts within a few years.

IBA came home to Belgium in 2016 when several university hospitals partnered with industry to propose a proton research and treatment center in Leuven equipped with the company's compact *Proteus®ONE* system.[100] Along with other big machine manufacturers, IBA had developed a cheaper, more compact device to compete with manufacturers like Mevion Medical Systems.

Mevion also had international aspirations. After withdrawing its Initial Public Offer, the company used a new round of venture capital financing to market its wares in Europe and China. Mevion teamed up with an oncology development company and a university hospital to build a joint venture in Lausanne, Switzerland.[101] The oncology company cited the Mevion device's relatively low cost and high patient throughput as deciding factors in its choice of devices. Mevion also entered a $200 million venture with Chinese and US investors to provide proton treatments to the growing middle class in China.[102] Other companies were also looking to China's huge market. Tennessee's Provision Healthcare, which had been the first facility in the world to have two proton devices when its ProNova partner's device became available,[103] joined with a Chinese pharmaceutical conglomerate to bring ProNova proton therapy to newly built cancer-treatment centers in China.[104]

As a public organization responsible for both health care delivery and its funding, Britain's National Health Service (NHS) had held back from committing its limited resources to proton therapy. Professional pressures, however, pushed the country to keep up with global leadership. Seeking what it called "world class" service, the specialty consultant-based National Radiotherapy Advisory Group proposed in 2007 that the public NHS build a proton center in partnership with industry.[105] Public and media pressure also responded to the emotional issue of a child with a brain tumor by promoting proton treatment. In 2012, the NHS announced two forthcoming proton centers at University College London Hospitals and the Christie Hospital in Manchester, and Varian Medical Systems announced 3 years later that it would be the vendor.[106] By then, private medicine had made major plans for proton therapy in the United Kingdom.

Due in part to a growth in private health insurance, which international corporations often offered their British employees, private medical delivery companies saw Britain as fertile ground for the high-cost technology. Advanced Proton Solutions proposed a center for London's financial district. Advanced Oncotherapy sought to develop three centers in collaboration with BMI Healthcare, a private-hospital operator owned by Apax Partners, a French private equity firm; and Netcare, a holding company whose subsidiaries operated private hospitals in South Africa and the United Kingdom.[107] Proton Partners International also announced that it would build three UK proton centers with £100 million in financial backing from institutional and private investors.[108] The private centers would be accessible to NHS patients if the government chose to cooperate with them.

Alongside of proton accelerators, research institutes in Germany and Japan were collaborating with manufacturers to build even more costly cancer guns shooting beams of heavier particles or ions (atomic nuclei stripped of electrons)—particularly those of carbon. Some US companies geared up to manufacture carbon ion accelerators if the market looked favorable, and others were building carbon-beam capability into their proton devices.[109] By the mid-2010s, Europe was equipped with roughly the same number of proton and other particle treatment centers as the United States, and Asia closely followed.[110] The proliferation of particle centers and their partnerships with industry demonstrated not only the globalization of particle therapy but also the role of particle centers in propagating corporate medical care.

Ironically condoning corporate medicine, an article on the World Socialist web site criticized the Siemens company for "putting profits before health" when it dismantled a particle-treatment center it had been building in Germany after its accountants projected that the center would not turn a profit. Siemens was closing the door on a technology that was "often the last hope for very sick people," the article accused, rhetorically advising that particle-treatment facilities "must not be subordinated to the profit interests of capitalist corporations."[111] What the article did not take into account was that the particle-center movement was itself a finance-driven project, that proton-center expansion also put profits before health, and that widespread belief that proton centers were what the author called a "social necessity" was based more on product promotion than on scientific evidence.

Despite meager evidence showing that particle beams improved clinical outcomes,[112] proponents supported international particle-center growth on the grounds that radiotherapy was naturally evolving from X-rays to particles and that particle treatment had "reached a mature state that allows a wide-spread clinical application."[113] As with earlier radiation therapy development, new technologies and delivery innovations drove a momentum that defined the latest development as synonymous with progress despite insufficient evidence of clinical benefit—and few hospitals or specialists wanted to be left behind.

At the same time—and perhaps surprisingly—the use of cobalt teletherapy persisted. Economic recessions, it seemed, led to a "renewed appreciation of the virtues of the cobalt-60 units."[114] Theratronics International, AECL's successor, had continued to sell cobalt devices to less wealthy hospitals and countries. Comprising 11 percent of teletherapy installations in the United States in the 1990s, cobalt accounted for 24 percent of those in France around that time, 31 percent of China's, 43 percent of Thailand's, and 82 percent of Bangladesh's.[115] Its users cited lower costs, lower electricity consumption, and less down time as the reasons they chose cobalt over linear accelerators.[116] With a few design improvements, Theratronics hinted, cobalt devices might recapture up to a third of the Western market and, in so doing, reduce overall radiation therapy costs.[117] But the global gold rush for particles was on.

Capital investment was a powerful force in proton-center growth. Astronomical investment levels upped the capital ante to practice medicine, required business rules of operation, and further opened the door to corporate medicine. Whether intentional or not, developing high-cost, highly indebted treatment centers reinforces the broader neoliberal market agenda to privatize health care systems worldwide and open them up to financial industry penetration. Spread of the American proton-center innovation meant that the most market-driven health care system in the developed world was imposing its private, high-debt mode of operation on the rest of the globe.

As a report on contemporary activities, the description of proton-center development in this chapter cannot benefit from the perspective of time, nor can it wrap up the episode. It has necessarily relied on (perhaps inaccurate) media sources and corporate press releases and has left some proton centers and companies on the brink of financial insolvency. With so many bankruptcies, failed IPOs, and loan defaults, it remained an open question whether proton therapy was a boon or a boondoggle. Would there be a scientific breakthrough that justified the venture? Would many more providers and investors have to write off sunk costs? Would a (large or small) number of proton centers survive to blend in with the radiation therapy repertoire?

While some investigators advocated a moratorium on further particle-center growth pending scientific evidence of effectiveness, public policy efforts did not suit the hegemony of the market economy.

Notes

1 John S. Laughlin, Radhe Mohan, and Gerald J. Kutcher, "Choice of Optimum Megavoltage for Accelerators for Photon Beam Treatment," *International Journal of Radiation Oncology Biology Physics* 12 (1986): 1551–1557. I follow the simplified convention that calls hydrogen, helium, carbon, and other nuclei stripped of electrons, in addition to electrons and neutrons, *particles.*

2 George E. Laramore, "The Use of Neutrons in Cancer Therapy: A Historical Perspective through the Modern Era," *Seminars in Oncology* 24 (1997): 672–685; George E. Laramore, Robert Emery, David Reid, Stefani Banerian, Ira Kalet, Jonathan Jacky, and Ruedi Risler, "University of Washington Clinical Neutron Facility: Report on 26 Years of Operation," *AIP Conference Proceedings* 1412 (2011): 311–318.

3 Thomas F. Delaney and Hanne M. Kooy, eds., *Proton and Charged Particle Radiotherapy* (Philadelphia: Wolters Kluwer, 2008), 110.

4 Wayne T. Stockburger, *Radiology Administration: A Business Guide* (Philadelphia: J.B. Lippincott, 1989), 123–125.

5 Richard Wilson, *A Brief History of the Harvard University Cyclotrons* (Cambridge: Harvard University Department of Physics, 2004), 9. Robert R. Wilson and Richard Wilson were two different physicists.

6 Max L. M. Boone, John H. Lawrence, William G. Connor, Richard Morgado, John A. Hicks, and Richard C. Brown, "Introduction to the Use of Protons and Heavy Ions in Radiation Therapy: Historical Perspective," *International Journal of Radiation Oncology Biology Physics* 3 (1977): 65–69.

7 Richard Wilson, *A Brief History of the Harvard University Cyclotrons* (Cambridge: Harvard University Department of Physics, 2004), 2, 27.

8 J. M. Sisterson and B. Gottschalk, "Hospital-Based Acceleration for Proton Radiotherapy," *International Journal of Radiation Oncology Biology Physics* 10, supplement 2 (1984): 165.

9 Yves Jongen, "Review on Cyclotrons for Cancer Therapy," *Proceedings of Cyclotrons 2010,* Lanzhou, China, 398–403.http://cyclotrons10.impcas.ac.cn/JACoWPub/papers/frm1cio01.pdf accessed August 10, 2011.

10 Richard Wilson, *A Brief History of the Harvard University Cyclotrons* (Cambridge: Harvard University Department of Physics, 2004), 44.

11 Frank E. James, "Proton Device to Fight Cancer is a Boondoggle—Or a Breakthrough?" *Wall Street Journal* March 17, 1989, A1.

12 James Hayman, Jane Weeks, and Peter Mauch, "Economic Analyses in Health Care: An Introduction to the Methodology with an Emphasis on Radiation Therapy," *International Journal of Radiation Oncology Biology Physics* 35 (1996): 827–841.

13 Sixth International Congress of Radiology, *Handbook and Guide to the Technical Exhibition* (London: The Congress, 1950), 85.

14 Yves Jongen, "Review on Cyclotrons for Cancer Therapy," *Proceedings of Cyclotrons 2010,* Lanzhou, China, 398–403.http://cyclotrons10.impcas.ac.cn/JACoWPub/papers/frm1cio01.pdf accessed August 10, 2011.

15 Andrew Clapham, "Ion Beam Sees Strong Year with 50 Potential Proton Deals," *Bloomberg* January 22, 2015. http://www.bloomberg.com/news/2015-01-22/ion-beam-sees-strong-year-with-50-potential-proton-deals.html accessed January 25, 2015.

16 Personal note: as an electron microscopy research technician at the Massachusetts Eye and Ear Infirmary (MEEI), I used to look out the window and see the prisoners milling around the yard. MEEI wanted the property for its own hospital expansion but didn't get it.
17 Richard E. Wainerdi, *Texas Medical Center* (New York: Newcomen Society of the United States, 1993), 19, 24.
18 M. D. Anderson Hospital, "Proton Pencil Beam Therapy," *Cancer Newsline* March 30, 2009. http://www.mdanderson.org/newsroom/cancer-newsline/cancer-newsline-topics/2009/cancer-newsline-03-30-09-proton-pencil-beam-therapy.html accessed February 9, 2015.
19 James S. Olson, *Making Cancer History: Disease and Discovery at the University of Texas M.D. Anderson Cancer Center* (Baltimore: Johns Hopkins University Press, 2009), 248–249, 277–280.
20 Dan Feldstein, "Proton-Therapy Costs vs. Benefits Debated," *Houston Chronicle* October 23, 2005. http://www.chron.com/news/houston-texas/article/Proton-therapy-costs-vs-benefits-debated-1920064.php accessed March 4, 2015.
21 Hitachi, "Hitachi to Supply Proton Beam Therapy System to the University of Texas M.D. Anderson Cancer Center," News release, May 7, 2003. http://www.hitachi.us/press/05072003 accessed August 7, 2016.
22 "M. D. Anderson, Partners Break Ground on Proton Therapy Center," M. D. Anderson News Release, May 7, 2003.http://www.mdanderson.org/newsroom/news-releases/2003/05-07-03-m-d-anderson-partners-break-ground-on-proton-therapy-center.html accessed February 9, 2015.
23 Dan Feldstein, "Police, Fire Pensions Warned About Deal," *Houston Chronicle* October 23, 2005. http://www.chron.com/news/houston-texas/article/Police-fire-pensions-warned-about-deal-1487556.php accessed March 4, 2015.
24 David Whelan and Robert Langreth, "The $150 Million Zapper," *Forbes* February 26, 2009. http://www.forbes.com/forbes/2009/0316/062_150mil_zapper.html accessed February 11, 2015.
25 ProCure, "ProCure Secures Financing for Proton Therapy Cancer Treatment Center in Oklahoma City," press release, April 19, 2007. http://www.procure.com/Financing-Secured-for-ProCure-Center-in-OK accessed February 11, 2015.
26 Northern Illinois University, "Northern Illinois Proton Center Delayed by Tough Economic Conditions," press release, March 1, 2010. http://www.niu.edu/northerntoday/2010/march1/proton1.shtml accessed February 11, 2015.
27 James Kimberly, "Procure Treatment Centers Inc. Sues NIU Over Plans to Build Proton Therapy Facility," *Chicago Tribune* July 23, 2008. http://articles.chicagotribune.com/2008-07-23/news/0807220600_1_proton-therapy-niu-facility accessed February 11, 2015.
28 David Whelan and Robert Langreth, "The $150 Million Zapper," *Forbes* February 26, 2009. http://www.forbes.com/forbes/2009/0316/062_150mil_zapper.html accessed February 11, 2015. Blagojevich was subsequently imprisoned for corruption.
29 Kristen Schorsch, "Partner in CDH Proton Center Hits Financial Snag," *Crain's Chicago Business* May 30, 2013.http://www.chicagobusiness.com/article/20130530/NEWS03/130539993/partner-in-cdh-proton-center-hits-financial-snag accessed September 30, 2013.
30 Claire Bushey, "Cadence Health Revenue Tops $1 Billion," *Crain's Chicago Business* October 16, 2012. http://www.chicagobusiness.com/article/20121016/NEWS03/121019854/cadence-health-revenue-tops-1-billion accessed February 11, 2015.
31 Nancy Ryerson, "Q&A with Jeff Bordock of Advanced Particle Therapy," *DOTmed Daily News* September 26, 2013. http://www.dotmed.com/news/story/21694&ct=ga&cd=NDY0NDQzNjc1NDY0OTgyMzU2NA&cad=CAEYAA&usg=AFQjCNFrB6vDzcx-wFhRN6Y_G-vR4_jWGQ accessed December 1, 2014.

32 Jaimy Lee, "Proton-beam Centers Sprout Despite Evidence Drought," *Modern Healthcare* April 12, 2014. http://www.modernhealthcare.com/article/20140412/MAGAZINE/304129979 accessed February 24, 2015.

33 Jessica Griffith, "Proton Beam Centers Taking Off Despite High Costs," *Healthcare Real Estate Insights* September 2010, 12–15. http://www.proton-therapy.org/documents/hre_insights.pdf accessed January 31, 2014; Varian Medical Systems, "Varian Medical Systems Books $88 Million Order to Equip Proton Treatment Center," press release, October 3, 2011. http://newsroom.varian.com/pressreleases?item=103375 accessed August 8, 2016; Varian Medical Systems, "JPMorgan Chase Bank, NA to Assume $45 Million of Varian Medical Systems Loan Commitment for the Scripps Proton Therapy Center," press release, June 16, 2014. http://newsroom.varian.com/2014-06-16-JPMorgan-Chase-Bank-N-A-to-assume-45-million-of-Varian-Medical-Systems-loan-commitment-for-the-Scripps-Proton-Therapy-Center accessed November 19, 2014.

34 M. R. Raju, "Particle Radiotherapy: Historical Development and Current Status," *Radiation Research* 145 (1996): 391–407.

35 David I. Thwaites and John B. Tuohy, "Back to the Future: The History and Development of the Clinical Linear Accelerator," *Physics in Medicine and Biology* 51 (2006): R343–R362.

36 Wendy Diller, "How Varian Medical Stays on Top," *Windhover's In Vivo: The Business & Medicine Report* 21 (2003): 1–8.

37 Eli Glatstein, "Intensity-modulated Radiation Therapy: The Inverse, the Converse, and the Perverse," *Seminars in Radiation Oncology* 12 (2002): 272–281.

38 Wendy Diller, "How Varian Medical Stays on Top," *Windhover's In Vivo: The Business & Medicine Report* 21 (2003), 1–8.

39 Bill Hethcock, "Dallas Proton Treatment Center Files Chapter 11, Billionaire Kelcy Warren Wants His $20M back," *Dallas Business Journal* September 28, 2015. http://www.bizjournals.com/dallas/news/2015/09/25/dallas-proton-treatment-center-files-chapter-11.html accessed December 5, 2015; Katy Stech, "Investors Try to Push Half-Built Cancer Center into Bankruptcy," *Wall Street Journal* March 7, 2016.

40 Massachusetts Institute of Technology, "MIT Proton Treatment Could Replace X-ray Use in Radiation Therapy," *MIT News* August 28, 2006. http://web.mit.edu/newsoffice/2006/proton.html accessed July 20, 2011.

41 Mass Device staff, "Still River Systems Lands $33 Million Investment Round," *Mass Device*, March 17, 2009. http://www.massdevice.com/still-river-systems-lands-33-million-investment-round/ accessed August 6, 2016.

42 American Shared Hospital Services, "American Shared Hospital Services Increases its Equity Investment in Still River Systems, Developer Of The Clinatron 250 Proton Beam Radiation Therapy Device," press release, September 10, 2007. http://www.ashs.com/pr09-10-07.html accessed September 26, 2011.

43 United States Securities and Exchange Commission, "Form S-1. Mevion Medical Systems, Inc.," September 11, 2014, 3. http://www.sec.gov/Archives/edgar/data/1326730/000119312514339250/d730478ds1.htm accessed December 7, 2014.

44 McLaren Health Care, "McLaren Bringing First Proton Therapy Center to Michigan," press release, January 10, 2012. http://www.mclaren.org/Main/News/279.aspx accessed February 13, 2015.

45 Charles Moore, "ProTom International Inc.'s Proton Cancer Therapy Technology A Texas Biotech Success Story," *Bionews Texas* May 14, 2014. http://bionews-tx.com/news/2014/05/14/protom-international-inc-s-proton-cancer-therapy-technology-a-texas-biotech-success-story/ accessed November 6, 2016.

46 Jay Greene, "McLaren's Proton Beam Center Delayed until Next Spring," *Crain's Detroit Business*, November 1, 2015. http://www.crainsdetroit.com/article/20151101/NEWS/311019985/mclarens-proton-beam-center-delayed-until-next-spring accessed August 6, 2016.

47 Thomas E. Goffman and Eli Glatstein, "The Vulnerability of Radiation Oncology within the Medical Industrial Complex," *International Journal of Radiation Oncology Biology Physics* 59 (2004): 1–3.
48 Varian Medical Systems, "Maryland Proton Therapy Center Financing Completed," press release, May 13, 2015. http://newsroom.varian.com/2015-05-13-Maryland-Proton-Therapy-Center-Financing-Completed accessed July 9, 2016.
49 Herman D. Suit, James Becht, Joseph Leong, Michael Stracher, William C. Wood, Lynn Verhey, and Michael Goitein, "Potential for Improvement in Radiation Therapy," *International Journal of Radiation Oncology Biology Physics* 14 (1988): 777–786.
50 *Time*, "The Machines of Progress," October 7, 1966, 72–77.
51 A. P. Brown, M. M. Urie, R. Chisin, and H. D. Suit, "Proton Therapy for Carcinoma of the Nasopharynx: A Study in Comparative Treatment Planning," *International Journal of Radiation Oncology Biology Physics* 16 (1989):1607–1614.
52 Frank E. James, "Proton Device to Fight Cancer is a Boondoggle—Or a Breakthrough?" *Wall Street Journal* March 17, 1989, A1.
53 Mark Lodge, Madelon Pijls-Joannesma, Lisa Stirk, Alastair J. Munro, Dirk De Ruysscher, and Tom Jefferson, "A Systematic Literature Review of the Clinical and Cost-effectiveness of Hadron Therapy in Cancer," *Radiotherapy and Oncology* 83 (2007): 110–122.
54 Dag Rune Olsen, Øyvind S Bruland, Gunilla Frykholm, and Inger Natvig Norderhaug, "Proton Therapy—a Systematic Review of Clinical Effectiveness," *Radiotherapy and Oncology* 83 (2007): 123–132.
55 Michael Brada, Madelon Pijls-Johannesma, and Dirk De Ruysscher, "Proton Therapy in Clinical Practice: Current Clinical Evidence," *Journal of Clinical Oncology* 25 (2007): 965–970.
56 Michael L. Steinberg and Andre Konski, "Proton Beam Therapy and the Convoluted Pathway to Incorporating Engineering Technology into Routine Medical Care in the United States," *The Cancer Journal* 15 (2009): 333–338.
57 Eric T. Rosenthal, "How and Why are Patients Referred for Proton Beam Therapy in the US and What Proven Benefits Does it Really Have?" *Oncology Times UK* 9 (2010): 19, 21.
58 Sara Solovitch, "Vying for Big New Cancer Centers," *Silicon Valley Business Journal* February 4, 2008. http://www.bizjournals.com/search?q=%22Procure+Treatment+Centers%22&s=3&pl=2 accessed February 10, 2014.
59 Charles Bosk, *Forgive and Remember: Managing Clinical Failure* (Chicago: University of Chicago Press, 1979), 33; Jeanne Daly, *Evidence-Based Medicine and the Search for a Science of Clinical Care* (Berkeley: University of California Press, 2005), 107–108.
60 James D. Cox and Simon Kramer, "Strategic Plan for Radiologic Sciences: Outcome Analysis," *Cancer Treatment Symposia* 1 (1984): 169–175; Michael Goitein and John Munzenrider, "Proton Therapy: Good News and Big Challenges," *International Journal of Radiation Oncology Biology Physics* 10 1984): 319–320; Michael Goitein and James D. Cox, "Should Randomized Clinical Trials Be Required for Proton Radiotherapy?" *Journal of Clinical Oncology* 26 (2008): 175–176.
61 Mark Sheehan, Claire Timlin, Ken Peach, et al., "Position Statement on Ethics, Equipoise and Research on Charged Particle Radiation Therapy," *Journal of Medical Ethics* 40 (2014): 572–575. Benjamin Freedman had made a similar argument in "Equipoise and the Ethics of Clinical Research," *The New England Journal of Medicine* 317 (1987): 141–145.
62 Fergus R. Macbeth and Michael V. Williams, *Journal of Clinical Oncology* 26 (2008): 2590–2591.
63 Thomas A. Trikalinos, Teruhiko Terasawa, Stanley Ip, Gowri Raman, and Joseph Lau, *Particle Beam Radiation Therapies for Cancer. Technical Brief No. 1* (Rockville, MD: Agency for Healthcare Research and Quality, 2009).

64 Aaron M. Allen, Todd Pawlicki, Lei Dong, et al., "An Evidence Based Review of Proton Beam Therapy: The Report of ASTRO's Emerging Technology Committee," *Radiotherapy and Oncology* 103 (2012): 8–11.

65 Stephanie Jarosek, Sean Elliott, and Beth A. Virnig, *Proton Beam Therapy in the U.S. Medicare Population: Growth in Use between 2006 and 2009* (Rockville, MD: Agency for Healthcare Research and Quality, 2012).

66 Hideyuki Sakurai, W. Robert Lee, and Colin G. Orton, "'We Do Not Need Randomized Clinical Trials to Demonstrate the Superiority of Proton Therapy,'" *Medical Physics* 39, (2012): 1685–1687.

67 American College of Radiology and American Society for Radiation Oncology, "ACR-ASTRO Practice Parameter for the Performance of Proton Beam Radiation," 2014. http://www.acr.org/~/media/7BEBF7E77E1141578CB8722F997BDE9B.pdf accessed December 2, 2014.

68 "SCCA Proton Therapy Center to Participate in PCORI Trial," Seattle Proton Center, October 1, 2015. http://www.newswise.com/articles/proton-therapy-offers-hope-for-patients-with-locally-advanced-stage-iii-breast-cancer accessed December 5, 2015.

69 P. Johnstone, J. Kerstiens, M. Williams, and R. Helsper, "Proton Facility Economics: The Essential Role of Prostate Cancer (CaP)," *International Journal of Radiation Oncology Biology Physics* 78 (2010): S564.

70 Topher Spiro, Thomas Huelskoetter, and Gina Phillipi, "Prostate Cancer Treatment: Unproven Proton Radiation Therapy Wastes Millions of Dollars," Washington: Center for American Progress, July 17, 2014.

71 Robert Langreth Bloomberg, "Proton Therapy for Prostate Cancer Comes at a Cost," *Daily Herald* Arlington Heights, IL: April 2, 2012, 5. https://www.questia.com/read/1G1-284991664/proton-therapy-for-prostate-cancer-comes-at-a-cost accessed February 24, 2015.

72 Keith Wailoo, *How Cancer Crossed the Color Line* (New York: Oxford University Press, 2011), 151–153; Helen Valier, "Uncertain Enthusiasm: PSA Screening, Proton Therapy and Prostate Cancer," In Carsten Timmermann and Elizabeth Toon, eds., *Cancer Patients, Cancer Pathways* (Basingstoke: Palgrave Macmillan, 2012), 186–203.

73 Lowered PSA levels also became a surrogate of treatment success. Medical historians have pointed out a number of cases in which biochemical or biophysical measurement became the disease definition, such as high blood pressure and high cholesterol. Jeremy Greene, *Prescribing by Numbers: Drugs and the Definition of Disease* (Baltimore: Johns Hopkins University Press, 2007).

74 Roger Chou, Jennifer M. Croswell, Tracy Dana, et al., "Screening for Prostate Cancer: A Review of the Evidence for the U.S. Preventive Services Task Force," *Annals of Internal Medicine* 155 (2011): 762–771; Richard J. Ablin with Ronald Piana, *The Great Prostate Hoax: How Big Medicine Hijacked the PSA Test and Caused a Public Health Disaster* (New York: Palgrave Macmillan, 2014), 6, 15, 88.

75 Virginia A. Moyer, "Screening for Prostate Cancer: U.S. Preventive Services Task Force Recommendation Statement," *Annals of Internal Medicine* 157 (2012): 120–134.

76 Dragan Ilic, Molly M. Neuberger, Mia Djulbegovic, and Philipp Dahm, "Screening for Prostate Cancer," *Cochrane Library* January 31, 2013. http://onlinelibrary.wiley.com/doi/10.1002/14651858.CD004720.pub3/abstract accessed January 8, 2015

77 US National Cancer Institute, "SEER Stat Fact Sheets: Prostate Cancer," http://seer.cancer.gov/statfacts/html/prost.html accessed April 9, 2015.

78 Thomas F. Delaney and Hanne M. Kooy, eds., *Proton and Charged Particle Radiotherapy* (Philadelphia: Wolters Kluwer, 2008), 219.

79 Yasuko Maeda, Morten Høyer, Lilli Lundby, and Christine Norton, "Faecal Incontinence Following Radiotherapy for Prostate Cancer: A Systematic Review," *Radiotherapy and Oncology* 98 (2011): 145–153.

80 Robert Aronowitz, "'Screening' for Prostate Cancer in New York's Skid Row: History and Implications," *American Journal of Public Health* 104 (2014): 70–76.

81 American College of Surgeons, National Cancer Data Base, *NCDB Public Benchmark Reports*. https://www.facs.org accessed February 24, 2015 and July 12, 2016. This data base may overenumerate surgery. Most of the radiation treatments in 2013 were external beam.

82 American Society for Radiation Oncology, "ASTRO Releases List of Five Radiation Oncology Treatments to Question as Part of National Choosing Wisely® Campaign," September 23, 2013. http://www.choosingwisely.org/astro-releases-list-of-five-radiation-oncology-treatments-to-question-as-part-of-national-choosing-wisely-campaign/ accessed August 9, 2016.

83 Ezekiel J. Emanuel and Steven D. Pearson, "It Costs More, but Is It Worth More?" *New York Times* January 2, 2012.

84 Topher Spiro, Thomas Huelskoetter, and Gina Phillipi, "Prostate Cancer Treatment: Unproven Proton Radiation Therapy Wastes Millions of Dollars," Washington: Center for American Progress, July 17, 2014.

85 Jenny Gold, "Proton Beam Therapy Heats Up Hospital Arms Race," *Kaiser Health News* May 31, 2013. http://www.kaiserhealthnews.org/stories/2013/may/31/proton-beam-therapy-washington-dc-health-costs.aspx accessed February 13, 2014.

86 Jenny Gold, "NYC's Answer to Proton Therapy Controversy: One For All," *Kaiser Health News* June 12, 2013. http://www.kaiserhealthnews.org/stories/2013/june/11/proton-therapy-new-york-city.aspx accessed February 13, 2014; Howard Berliner, personal communication, May 15, 2015.

87 Jan Ransom, "Rare Cancer Treatment Center May Call East Harlem Home in New City Development Project," *New York Daily News* September 16, 2014. http://www.nydailynews.com/new-york/uptown/beams-true-new-east-harlem-cancer-treatment-center-article-1.1942243 accessed February 11, 2015. Has high-tech medicine become high-tech entertainment?

88 Gus Iversen, "NYC's First Proton Facility to Open in 2018 with Varian's ProBeam," *Daily News* July 22, 2015. http://www.dotmed.com/news/story/26427 accessed July 29, 2015.

89 RNCOS Business Consultancy Services, "US Proton Therapy Potential Market Stands Tall at US $15 Billion," press release, January 21, 2013. http://www.rncos.com/Press_Releases/US-Proton-Therapy-Potential-Market-Stands-Tall-at-US-15-Billion.htm accessed August 9, 2016.

90 James B. Yu, Pamela R. Soulos, Jeph Herrin, Laura D. Cramer, Arnold L. Potosky, Kenneth B. Roberts, and Cary P. Gross, "Proton Versus Intensity-Modulated Radiotherapy for Prostate Cancer: Patterns of Care and Early Toxicity," *Journal of the National Cancer Institute* 105 (2013): 25–32. In defense of high proton-therapy costs, James Cox claimed that the M. D. Anderson Cancer Center spent $92 million in 2008 on the top four cancer chemotherapy drugs alone. Gustavo Montana and Herman Suit, "An Interview with James Cox, MD, FASTRO," June 17, 2011. https://www.astro.org/About-ASTRO/History/James-Cox/ accessed May 18, 2016.

91 Ron Winslow and Timothy W. Martin, "Prostate-Cancer Therapy Comes Under Attack," *Wall Street Journal* August 28, 2013.

92 UnitedHealthCare, "Proton Beam Radiation Therapy: Medical Policy," November 1, 2016, emphasis original. https://www.unitedhealthcareonline.com/ccmcontent/ProviderII/UHC/en-US/Assets/ProviderStaticFiles/ProviderStaticFilesPdf/Tools%20and%20Resources/Policies%20and%20Protocols/Medical%20Policies/Medical%20Policies/Proton_Beam_Radiation_Therapy.pdf accessed November 6, 2016.

93 Proton Therapy Consortium and Particle Therapy Cooperative Group—North America, "Model Policy: Coverage of Proton Beam Therapy," March 31, 2014. http://npc2014.

com/wp-content/uploads/2014/03/Model-Proton-Beam-Therapy-Policy-3-31-2014.pdf accessed December 7, 2014.

94 Ben Hall, "Emails Reveal Strategy To Pass Proton Therapy Bill," News Channel 5 Network, March 26, 2014. http://www.newschannel5.com/story/25084015/emails-reveal-strategy-to-pass-proton-therapy-bill accessed November 19, 2014.

95 Jake Anderson, "Mayo Clinic Seeks Private, Public Funds for $6B Initiative," *Twin Cities Business Magazine* January 30, 2013. http://tcbmag.com/News/Recent-News/2013/January/Mayo-Clinic-Seeks-Private,-Public-Funds-for-$6B-In accessed February 9, 2013.

96 IOP (Institute of Physics) Publishing, "Newsfeed: IBA to Install Dedicated Proton Therapy Centre in Sweden," March 17, 2011. http://medicalphysicsweb.org/cws/article/newsfeed/45412 accessed July 22, 2016.

97 Varian Medical Systems, "Cancer Patients Gain Greater Access to Intensity Modulated Proton Therapy Treatments at Leading German Clinic," press release January 19, 2010. http://newsroom.varian.com/pressreleases accessed August 12, 2016.

98 Hans Rinecker and Ursula Friedsam, "Rinecker Proton Therapy Center: A New Chance to Fight Cancer," *Medical Tourism Magazine* May/June (2009): 51.

99 KFW IPEX-Bank, "Syndicate Financing: West German Proton Therapy Centre Acquired in Full by Essen University Hospital," March 26, 2014. https://www.kfw-ipex-bank.de/International-financing/KfW-IPEX-Bank/Presse/News/Newsdetails_194049.html accessed June 13, 2016.

100 IBA, "IBA Signs Contract with UZ Leuven to Install the First Proton Therapy Center in Belgium," press release, March 25, 2016http://www.iba-worldwide.com/uploads/articles/article_en_pdf/282/PR%20UZ_Leuven-EN-25.03.16.pdf accessed August 13, 2016.

101 Mevion Medical Systems, "Mevion Medical Systems to Install a Proton Therapy System in Switzerland," press release, October 8, 2015. http://www.mevion.com/newsroom/news accessed July 9, 2016.

102 Amanda Pedersen, "Sour IPO Transforms into Sweet JV: Mevion Scraps IPO Plans but Raises $200M and Strikes a JV Deal with Chinese Investors," *Medical Device Daily*, August 5, 2015.http://medicaldevicedaily.com/servlet/com.accumedia.web.Dispatcher?next=bioWorldHeadlines_article&forceid=90458 accessed July 22, 2016.

103 *Business Wire*, "ProNova Delivers Cyclotron to First Dual-Accelerator Clinical Proton Center in the World," September 15, 2014. http://www.businesswire.com/news/home/20140915005225/en/ProNova-Delivers-Cyclotron-Dual-Accelerator-Clinical-Proton-Center#.VISW2GeuSSoaccessed February 13, 2015.

104 Larisa Brass, "Provision Grows Proton Therapy in China," press release, June 3, 2016. http://provisionproton.com/blog/2016/06/03/provision-grows-in-china/ accessed June 15, 2016.

105 National Radiotherapy Advisory Group, *Radiotherapy: Developing a World Class Service for England* Report to Ministers, February 26, 2007.

106 Varian Medical Systems, "Varian Medical Systems Selected to Equip Two National Proton Therapy Centers in England," press release, March 11, 2015. http://newsroom.varian.com accessed August 12, 2016.

107 Allison Connolly and Andrea Gerlin, "Proton-Beam Cancer Sites to Get $380 Million From U.K." Bloomberg, July 31, 2013.http://www.bloomberg.com/news/articles/2013-07-31/proton-beam-cancer-sites-to-get-380-million-from-u-k- accessed July 9, 2016.

108 Rebecca Ratcliffe, "UK to Get First Three Proton Beam Therapy Centres in Cancer Care Milestone," *The Guardian* April 4, 2015.

109 G. B. Coutrakon, "Accelerators for Heavy-charged Particle Radiation Therapy," *Technology in Cancer Research & Treatment* 6 (2007): 49–54.

110 Proton Therapy Center, "Operating Clinical Proton Centres," Prague: not dated. http://www.proton-cancer-treatment.com/proton-therapy/proton-therapy-around-the-world/operating-clinical-proton-centres/ accessed August 13, 2016.

111 Elisabeth Steinert, "Putting Profits Before Health: Siemens Abandons Cancer Therapy Project," World Socialist web site, February 2, 2012. https://www.wsws.org/en/articles/2012/02/siem-f02.html accessed August 10, 2016.

112 Daniela Schulz-Ertner and Hirohiko Tsujii, "Particle Radiation Therapy Using Proton and Heavier Ion Beams," *Journal of Clinical Oncology* 25 (2007): 953–964; Teruhiko Terasawa, Tomas Dvorak, Stanley Ip, Gowri Raman, and Joseph Lau, "Systematic Review: Charged-Particle Radiation Therapy for Cancer," *Annals of Internal Medicine* 151 (2009): 556–565.

113 Yves Lemoigne, ed., *Radiotherapy and Brachytherapy* (Archamps, France: NATO Advanced Study Institute on Physics of Modern Radiotherapy & Brachytherapy, 2009), 173.

114 Paul Litt, *Isotopes and Innovation: MDS Nordion's First Fifty Years, 1946–1996* (Montreal: Published for MDS Nordion by McGill-Queen's University Press, 2000), 226, 210.

115 Young Hoon Ji, Haijo Jung, Kwangmo Yang, Chul Koo Cho, Seong Yul Yoo, Hyung Jun Yoo, Kum Bae Kim, and Mi Sook Kim, "Trends for the Past 10 Years and International Comparisons of the Structure of Korean Radiation Oncology," *Japanese Journal of Clinical Oncology* 40 (2010): 470–475.

116 G. Sahani, M. Kumar, P. K. Dash Sharma, R. Kumar, K Chhokra, B. Mishra, S. P. Agarwal and R. K. Kher, "Compliance of Bhabhatron-II Telecobalt Unit with IEC Standard-radiation Safety," *Journal of Applied Clinical Medical Physics* 10 (2009): 120–130.

117 Jake Van Dyk and Jerry J. Battista, "Cobalt-60: An Old Modality, A Renewed Challenge," (London, Ontario: London Regional Cancer Centre, not dated, citations through mid-1990s). http://www.theratronics.ca/press/VanDyk.pdf accessed November 17, 2012.

10 Rationalizing Radiation Therapy, Reforming Health Care

The history of radiation therapy exemplifies how economic interests have shaped the development of medical specialties, particularly technology-oriented ones, and how they have promulgated policies that reinforce facility growth. As discussed in the second part of this chapter, the policies pertain to payment for services, treatment effectiveness, capital investment, patient safety, and professional conflicts of interest. Another way to control medical care is to define its *quality*. The radiation oncology specialty illustrates the measurement of quality in terms of improved patient outcomes and/or conformance to professional standards and how the two approaches can contradict each other.

Taking the Measure of Cancer and Radiation Therapy

Professional Standards

Specialty associations assumed the mantle of defining and measuring medical care quality in order to improve their services and at the same time maintain control over them. Portraying itself in competition with government and health-maintenance organizations (HMOs) as the arbiter of quality, the American College of Radiology (ACR) asserted in its Patterns of Care Study that standardizing "optimal" characteristics would improve services.[1] As the study defined them, optimal meant availability of full-time radiation oncologists and physicists, computerized treatment planning, formal quality assurance programs, and the highest-powered equipment.[2] Smaller hospitals and freestanding services with less powerful equipment and personnel did not meet professional standards by definition. Departments that did meet the standards had to continually purchase new equipment to maintain their compliance.

The multireport Patterns of Care Study claimed that ACR standards improved patient outcomes. Selecting only cases referred to radiation oncologists and not using controls, the reports held (without claiming higher survival rates) that patients treated in facilities with linear accelerators or betatrons had better local tumor control than patients treated in facilities whose "best" equipment was cobalt-60. Their data revealed, however, that statistically improved local control held only when comparing linear accelerators (linacs) to a subset of less powerful cobalt devices representing a minority of cobalt installations.[3] Moreover, initial reports rationalized their attribution of better local control to linac availability without ascertaining whether the patients with better control were the ones actually treated on the linacs.

Nor did the Patterns of Care studies consider alternative explanations. Patients in highly equipped institutions may have had less advanced cancers to begin with—which is not as paradoxical as it may sound. Professional policy encouraged referring patients with better prognoses to highly equipped centers while permitting local services to perform palliative treatments. Such a practice could mean—as is so often the case in evaluation studies—that outcome measures related more to input characteristics than to applied interventions. In short, the methodologies used in the initial studies could not support their advice that patients with Hodgkin's, cervical, and prostate cancers required the most complex radiation technology to attain optimal outcomes.[4]

Patterns studies that took actual treatments into account reported some survival gains, although they tended to overstate the contribution of radiation. One study claimed a "strong argument for the long-term cure of prostate cancer by external beam radiation," but it did not compare external radiation to surgical treatment, brachytherapy, or active surveillance.[5] A study of stage III cervical cancer treatment found increased survival rates, and in this case it did attribute the gain to a resurgence in brachytherapy.[6] Hodgkin's studies reported that 5-year relapse-free survival rates continued to rise and that for stage III disease, they paralleled improvements in chemotherapy.[7]

The widely-published Patterns project shaped national and international policy, despite its methodological weaknesses, and it took (partial) credit for shifting practice away from cobalt-60 and to the linear accelerator.[8] The American College of Radiology followed up with its Quality Research in Radiation Oncology (QRRO™) project, which reduced measures of outcome and more explicitly applied managerial methods designed to improve physician productivity and compliance with practice standards.[9] The fact that national cancer mortality rates were finally falling appeared to support the specialty's claims of rising treatment effectiveness.

Cancer Data, Screening, and Radiation Treatment

After a relentless rise that progressed throughout the growth of 20th-century medicine, total US cancer *mortality* rates started declining in the 1990s. The reductions were not for the most part due to advances in cancer treatment but to decreased *incidence* of several particularly lethal cancers and early diagnosis of a few others. Stomach-cancer incidence continued its century-long decline, and lung-cancer incidence, which had surged (among men) starting in the 1940s and had multiplied 15-fold, also started dropping.[10] Besides warning about dangers of tobacco, medical care played a small role in these declines.

The medical profession can take a fair amount of credit for earlier diagnosis and treatment of a few other critical cancers. Pap smears and stool blood screening seem to have contributed to declines in mortality from cervical and colo-rectal cancers. Extending screening to other cancers has been problematic, however. As discussed in Chapter 9, there is growing medical consensus that prostate-specific antigen (PSA) screening for prostate cancer has led to more harm than good. It remains a matter of debate whether X-ray screening of the lungs of heavy smokers benefits that population.

Taking advantage of special funding in the Affordable Care Act, radiation oncologists proposed building a nationwide fleet of CT scanning procedure units to screen the 10 million American smokers at highest risk of developing lung cancer.[11] (It was an advertisement of one such unit that popped up on my computer beside the *New York Times* article criticizing overuse of high-cost technology, as described in the introduction to this book.) Researchers had already questioned the wisdom of a process that generated a large number of false positives and inflicted significant patient harm through follow-up biopsies in order to identify a relatively small number of new cancers, but other reports were more positive.[12] In contrast to screening, which assumes the availability of effective treatment, public health initiatives have tried to reduce lung-cancer incidence by reducing use of cancer-causing tobacco products.

Organized public health efforts have also promoted breast-cancer screening. The mammography movement may have decreased mortality from this cancer, although how much and at what cost to women's future health remain in contention.[13] While breast-cancer mortality rates did decline following initiation of widespread screening, the reduction was due in part to a measurement change. Mammography had led to a diagnostic "epidemic" by revealing noninvasive (or at least noninvad*ing*) bumps and diagnosing them as cancer. The "apparent efficacy of treatment" increased as *in situ* lesions rose from 6 percent of all breast cancer diagnoses in 1975 to 36 percent in 2011.[14] The diagnostic change in itself reduced measured breast-cancer mortality rates by inflating the total number of cases with noninvasive growths. Strikingly, however, 5-year mortality rates from invasive breast cancers also started declining in the 1990s, suggesting treatment gain. It is difficult to identify which treatments may have contributed to this gain and under what conditions—the fragmented US health care system does not measure medical treatment very well. No one really knows, for example, how many people receive radiation therapy, and estimated rates vary widely.

ACR's Patterns of Care Study reported in the 1980s that "approximately 48% of newly accessioned cancer patients in radiation therapy practice are treated with curative intent."[15] But counting only patients admitted to radiation oncology practices yields artificially high radiation treatment rates for all cancer patients. The Institute of Medicine estimated in the 1990s that 41 percent of all new cancer patients received radiation.[16] The following decade, the American College of Surgeons–sponsored National Cancer Data Base, covering 70 percent of all newly diagnosed cancer patients and most major cancers, reported that 34 percent of patients received radiation in the first course of treatment, with that figure declining from 36 percent in 2003 to 32 percent in 2013.[17] Added to the newly diagnosed patients counted in each of these studies, uncounted numbers receive radiation after initial treatment failure. Despite the limitations of these measurements, the estimated percentages of cancer patients receiving radiation (especially ACR estimates) have served as the basis of national and international policies regarding the necessary supply of radiation services to treat cancer. Professional views of which cancers respond to radiation also shape policy.

A small number of cancer types make up most of the radiation therapy market. Breast cancer alone represented 41 percent of newly diagnosed National Cancer Data Base patients treated with radiation in the first decade of the 2000s, and breast, prostate, and lung cancer added up to 89 percent. From a patient point of view, roughly 60 percent of those with cervical cancer could expect to receive radiation (with or without other treatments), 50 percent of those with breast cancer, 40 percent with non-small-cell (the more common) lung cancer, 40 percent with prostate cancer, 5 percent with kidney cancer, and 2 percent with colon cancer.[18] This practice spread suggests that expectations of the impact of radiation therapy on survival vary widely according to type of cancer.

Survival rates offer important (if still limited) patient outcome measures, and they seem to show some improvements in cancer treatment over the past few decades. The total 5-year cancer survival rate rose in the United States from 49 percent of patients diagnosed in 1975 to 69 percent of those diagnosed in 2008.[19] Measured 5-year survival rates for prostate cancer rose from 66 to 99 percent in the same span of years, invasive breast cancer from 75 to 91 percent, Hodgkin's from 70 to 90 percent, cervical cancer from 68 to 69 percent, colorectal cancer from 49 to 67 percent, and lung cancer from 11 to 19 percent.

Although the survival gains offer considerable hope, caution must guide their interpretation. The figures do not reveal the extent to which the gains were due to earlier diagnosis within the invasive disease category. Longer measured survival rates do not necessarily mean that patients live longer—it means they live longer after their cancer diagnoses. Earlier diagnosis starts the clock earlier in the disease progression and means that more patients reach the widely-accepted 5-year mark before (in some cases) succumbing to their cancers. Five-year survival rates are not "cure rates," although they are often identified as such. Attaining cure-rate measures requires scientific study.

Scientific Research on Radiation Treatment Effectiveness

Most patients believe there is reasonably good evidence they will benefit from their radiation treatments—as do their doctors. The American Society for Radiation Oncology's 1985 gold medalist claimed that radiotherapy cured 12 percent of all cancer patients and 25 percent of curable cancer patients.[20] The basis for these figures is a mystery, however. The accompanying table did not provide data to support the claim, nor did the paper referenced in the table, nor the two cited in that paper. Such a chain of assertions spinning out of an original undocumented claim is—unfortunately—not uncommon in medicine. It was a leap of faith for one of the cited papers to assert that survival gains in patients with localized cancers over the previous three decades were "primarily due to widespread use of increasingly sophisticated radiotherapy equipment."[21]

It is true that medicine grew technologically and institutionally complex and that it gained much scientific knowledge and even some wisdom—which is one meaning of *sophisticated*. But the word also means to become complex whether or not that complexity is based on knowledge (or wisdom), and a *sophist* argument employs pseudoscientific reasoning. Modern medical care is sophisticated in all of these senses: it is complex, not all of its complexity is knowledge based, and its leaders sometimes obscure the latter fact with specious argument.

Prospective randomized controlled trials (RCTs) arguably offer the best means to date of determining medical effectiveness. The ongoing United Kingdom–based Cochrane Collaboration provides cumulative sets of systematic or metareviews of controlled medical trials. While summarizing the best available evidence at the time of each report, Cochrane reviews are not the last word; they offer only the latest word, and this is subject to change. The reviews are limited by the number and quality of available randomized controlled trials and are themselves of uneven quality. The bottom line is that we do not really know how effective radiation therapy is. Table 10.1 briefly summarizes Cochrane findings as of mid-2016 on the cancers most subject to radiation treatment. It exemplifies the incomplete knowledge of radiotherapy efficacy for all remaining stages, conditions, and treatment combinations.

Although Table 10.1 illustrates giant holes in the fabric of evidence, as of 2016, radiation was found to improve outcomes under certain conditions of patients with Hodgkin's, cervical, breast, and prostate cancers. As radiation was often used in conjunction with other treatments, it is difficult to tease out its contribution relative to those of surgery, chemotherapy, and hormone therapy.

Cochrane reviews have corroborated long-standing observations that radiation can play an important role in pain reduction and other palliative measures. Finding single radiation treatments to be as effective as multiple ones in relieving pain from bone metastases, one Cochrane review held that many radiation oncologists, particularly those in the United States, prescribed excessive palliative radiation.[22] Irradiation of cancer metastases—which potentially offers a huge expansion in the radiation therapy market—has had mixed outcomes. Although whole brain radiation reduced the size of metastases in the brain, a Cochrane study found that it also reduced brain function.[23] Another review found that irradiating metastases in the liver could acutely damage that organ.[24]

It has long been clear that radiation therapy comes with a trade-off; damaging healthy tissues has always been the specialty's major problem. Radiation is not "noninvasive," as frequently claimed in advertisements; its invasive energy is what kills cancer and other nearby cells in the first place. Studies have reported that radiation treatments to the head and neck can lead to jawbone necrosis, carotid artery stenosis, and cognitive decline.[25] Chest irradiation can damage the heart and lead to progressive peripheral neuropathy.[26] Pelvic irradiation can lead to sexual dysfunction.[27] An estimated 8 percent of new solid cancers developing in

Table 10.1 Cochrane Findings on Radiotherapy of Major Cancer Sites—2016

Uterine cervix

- Women with locally advanced cervical cancer seemed to do equally well when treated with radiotherapy or chemoradiotherapy alone compared with women treated with hysterectomy plus radiotherapy, with or without chemotherapy.[28]
- Surgery and radiation led to equivalent survival rates of women with early squamous cell carcinomas (the majority of cervical cancers).[29]
- Surgery led to higher survival rates than radiation for women with early adenocarcinomas.
- Chemotherapy added to radiation improved overall survival for locally advanced cancers compared to radiation alone.[30]
- Combination treatments led to more complications: 29% of women experienced long-term morbidity after surgery plus radiotherapy, 24% did after surgery alone, and 16% after radiation alone.

Breast

- Adding radiation reduced local cancer recurrence after breast-conserving surgery for ductal carcinoma-in-situ (DCIS).[31]
- Radiation combined with surgery reduced recurrence of localized breast cancer and improved breast-cancer-specific survival without improving overall survival.[32]

Prostate

- Low-dose rate brachytherapy and radical prostatectomy led to equivalent recurrence-free survival rates for localized tumors.[33]
- Brachytherapy led to less urinary incontinence.
- External beam radiation following surgery improved local control and overall long-term survival for cancers that had spread locall [34]

Lung

- Adding postoperative radiotherapy to early-stage non-small-cell lung cancer was detrimental to overall patient survival.[35]
- Short radiotherapy courses reduced cough, breathlessness, and pain as effectively as longer courses and carried fewer side effects.[36]

Hodgkin's Lymphoma

- Radiotherapy added to chemotherapy improved tumor control and overall survival of patients with early-stage Hodgkin's disease.[37]

patients surviving cancer a year or more can be related to the radiation treatment of earlier tumors.[38]

Children are particularly sensitive to radiation, as noted in Chapter 9. Radiation treatments can damage their hearts, lungs, kidneys, and brains; stunt their growth; reduce future fertility; and lead to secondary cancers.[39] Partly for these reasons (but also due to the rise of chemotherapeutic agents), use of radiation on children with cancer has declined in the United States. Irradiation of children with acute lymphoblastic leukemia declined from 57 percent in 1973–1976 to 11 percent in 2005–2008, and radiation rates for retinoblastoma (Stanford's poster boy's cancer) declined from 30 to 2 percent.[40] Irradiation of children with non-Hodgkin's lymphoma declined from 57 to 15 percent, while radiation treatment of those with

Hodgkin's disease remained at 72 percent—although doses had fallen from Henry Kaplan's days.

Although the reported damage *can* occur, it doesn't always, by any means. Excepting higher doses, the situations leading to greater radiation damage are not always clear. Even scrupulous research techniques do not find what they do not look for, and measuring benefits more assiduously than harms favors increased medical intervention.[41] The frequency and severity of radiation damage tend to be underreported. The medical literature also tends to downplay patient experience of debilitating fatigue, nausea, vomiting, diarrhea, skin burn, and emotional distress.[42] Anne seemed pretty upbeat about her radiation treatments, but she described to me how her breast had been so burned that she had burst into tears in a department store dressing room when she couldn't find a bra that didn't hurt.[43]

In sum, patient benefits in the century-long experiment of irradiating people with cancer remain mixed and often ambiguous. As has long been appreciated, radiation can significantly reduce tumor size and accompanying pain. It adds incremental survival gains for a few cancers, giving the gift of reasonably comfortable time, even if sometimes not very much. Radiation can add more than incremental gains, usually when combined with other treatments, for a few more cancers. Radiation alone seldom cures cancer, and it continues to inflict harm. Patients (and their doctors) all hope that they will be in the minority that benefits. Hope plays an important role in coping with cancer and seeking early medical attention.[44] Nonetheless, instilling unwarranted hope exploits patients and can lead to submission to futile and damaging treatments.

On (Not) Measuring Relative Effectiveness of Radiotherapy Devices

Leaders expected throughout the development of radiation therapy that gains in device energy levels would lead to clinical gains. As 2002 American College of Radiation Oncology chairman A. Robert Kagan put it, it is "difficult to debunk the myth that the progress of radiation therapy is measured by improvement in technical equipment."[45] Yet an association between machine power and clinical outcome was rarely demonstrated or even studied. Since controlled trials did not measure the benefits of one teletherapy device over another, it was not scientific evidence that drove their development.

Nonetheless, radiotherapists and manufacturers have continued to dream that the very next device just might shoot the magic bullet. They have compared their cancer guns to rifles, lasers, snipers, and crack combat troops (are drones next?) in order to imply reduced collateral damage. At the same time, leaders have had to acknowledge that their devices continued to fire like shotguns. Each voltage increment and particle seemed to offer new hope, but they continued to disappoint. Having exploited the electromagnetic spectrum for photon energy levels and the periodic table for particles, the profession was running out of bullets. Moreover, biotechnology engineering was replacing electrical and nuclear engineering in cancer investment interest. At the turn of the 21st century, radiation oncologists worried that their specialty might not be sustainable, having placed all its bets on a single technology.

The evidence of limited radiation-therapy effectiveness raised political questions about its continued growth. The private insurance sector—itself standing to gain from lower payments—estimated in 2009 that it could save $5 billion a year by reducing inappropriate radiation treatments (and $13 billion by reducing unnecessary diagnostic radiology procedures).[46] The insurance industry joined a range of interests engaged in broader health care policy and reform.

Health Care Reform

Motivated by a mix of sometimes conflicting goals, including those of distributive justice, professional control, economic gain, market dominance, cost containment, and political mileage, health care reform in the United States has stitched together a patchwork system. The following reform approaches pertain to all of medical care, although many of the examples offered discuss their relationships with radiation therapy.

Payment

Payment is the most common regulatory intrusion in the health care market and is the subject of a large number of health care reform studies. Public payment programs in the United States partially cover medical fees for large numbers of (but far from all) people who would otherwise be priced out of the market. The fact that the private insurance industry covers just one-third of total health care expenditures in the United States means that the nation's health care is a quasi-public system that socializes economic risk and privatizes profit. The US government spends more on medical care per person than the UK government does in a National Health Service (NHS) that offers services to the entire population.[47] Furthermore, the NHS does so with lower administrative costs than those incurred in the vast tangle of US providers and payers.

As frequently noted, the fragmented and hierarchical insurance system leads to significant social inequities. Timing of cancer diagnosis is one such example. Between 2003 and 2013, 42 percent of the US population covered by private insurance had their cancers diagnosed in the two earliest disease stages, compared to 36 percent of people covered by Medicare, 30 percent of those covered by Medicaid, and 27 percent of those with no insurance coverage.[48] The spread from 42 to 27 percent meant that wealthier people were significantly more likely to have their cancers diagnosed at a curable stage than poorer people were. While the different population groups may experience different cancers, similar discrimination showed up within certain cancer types.[49] Reducing timing disparities would improve patient outcomes in many cases—but outcomes also depend on other factors. This book looks beyond payment in the policy debate to health care *organization* and *practice*, starting with treatment effectiveness.

Treatment Effectiveness

The inadequacy of scientific evidence concerning medical effectiveness discussed in the first part of this chapter is not limited to cancer treatment. The appalling implication of the evidence-based medicine movement, which implies a degree of restricting the use of medical procedures and technologies to those circumstances demonstrated to benefit from them, is the extent to which many continuing practices are not based on scientific evidence. Not surprisingly, the concept of evidence-based medicine is intensely political.

The Congressional Office of Technology Assessment (OTA) did not last long after noting in 1984 that rapid growth in the medical-device industry had led to excessive use of its products.[50] Technology assessment led organized medicine to fear government intrusion on its authority, manufacturers to fear decreased sales, financiers to fear reduced returns on investments, and disease advocacy groups to fear restricted access to the latest innovations.[51] After OTA fell, the Medicare Payment Advisory Commission later charged, many new medical technologies moved straight into routine clinical use despite inadequate scientific evidence.[52] The US Agency for Healthcare Research and Quality (AHRQ) continues a concern with medical evidence—and it remains a political target.

Although all new medical treatments are necessarily experimental, they can be initiated in ways that limit the number of patients that are subjected to experiment and inform future practices. One such approach would randomize all patients from the beginning of each new treatment, as Morton Kligerman (Chapter 8) and others have suggested. While it has to be recognized that some patients would suffer from not receiving an effective treatment, it is likely that many more patients would benefit from not receiving ineffective and possibly harmful treatments. One study found that most new radiation-therapy treatments had fewer benefits than the ones they were designed to replace.[53]

Yet many doctors have resisted randomized controlled trials (RCTs), as discussed in Chapter 9. They assert that outcomes studies are dated the minute they come out (true) and that the very latest technology or technique renders all earlier studies inoperative. In place of RCTs, Barron Lerner maintained in *Breast Cancer Wars*, doctors have tended to assume that the most radical treatments available were the ones most likely to reduce the risk of bad outcomes.[54] Clinicians who reject RCTs as experimenting on groups of patients seem not to perceive their own use of untested treatments as experimenting on individual patients.

Applying evidence-based medicine can be problematic, however. As Table 10.1 demonstrates, even the best evidence is inconsistent and vastly incomplete. Reducing scientific evidence to mathematical formulae or algorithms can be oversimplistic. Furthermore, practice standards often factor in professional and commercial interests. Manufacturing firms have proposed standards that incorporate use of their products. Specialty associations have built high employment of their members and technologies into their standards. University researchers have proposed standards favoring academic medical centers.

Even when initiated for the purpose of diffusing knowledge, many medical journals have flourished by their contributions to professional prestige and product promotion. Esteemed journals like the *New England Journal of Medicine* and *JAMA*, the Journal of the American Medical Association, accused John Abramson in *Overdo$ed America*, have published articles that hyped selected outcomes and neglected to report inconvenient ones.[55] Radiation oncologists have accused cancer treatment reports of spinning small gains into big claims and intentionally obscuring treatment failures and complications.[56]

Claims of positive outcomes are often more exaggerated when business engages in medical research.[57] Drawing attention to the fact that the manufacturer had funded most of the randomized controlled trials of the drug he was purportedly evaluating, a physician writing a Cochrane review acknowledged that his team was reduced to carefully analyzing market-oriented studies.[58] By the early 2000s, industry was paying for nearly 60 percent of all biomedical research in the United States, and the device industry was rapidly increasing its stakes in the game.[59] One commercial research firm even advertised that it was in the business of developing evidence that supported its clients' product approval and reimbursement goals.[60] Commercial funders of evidence studies sought to expand investment in their products.

Controlling Capital Investment

The 1974–1986 national health planning program primarily sought to control capital investment in high-cost medical care. Its efforts were based on concerns that public reimbursements, research grants, loan guarantees, and tax-exempt bonds raised the costs of medical care and fueled excess capacity.[61] Health planning used the separately legislated Certificate of Need (CoN) process to try to hold back the flood of capital into high-tech specialty services (as described in Chapters 8 and 9). CoN is a potentially formidable tool that could, as its name implies, use population need as a guide to investment in health care services and equipment.

Instead of using illness and effectiveness measures, however, Certificate of Need applied professional trade associations' economic goals. The *National Guidelines for Health Planning* adopted the American College of Radiology and National Electrical Manufacturer's Association joint standard that every megavoltage unit should treat at least 300 patients a year in order to break even financially. The guidelines reiterated the professional assertion that half of all new cancer patients "require megavoltage therapy" and that many returning patients also did.[62] The standards portended a large radiotherapy market.

Ostensibly a corrective to market forces, health planning itself blew with the winds of market ideology. A multiedition planning textbook came to advise health care institutions to invest only in technologies and services with the "potential for growth and profitability."[63] Following market precepts to their logical end, in 1986, the Reagan administration eliminated the national health planning program and the federal Certificate of Need mandate. The hospital industry appreciated CoN protection from instabilities of competition, however, and most states chose to retain (often an attenuated version of) it. At the same time, device companies like Varian Associates prepared to take advantage of postplanning rebound growth in equipment purchase.[64]

Market advocates continued to challenge Certificate of Need. A 2006 voice in the chorus to abolish CoN in Washington State asserted, incredibly, that the market would provide necessary health care, just as food, housing, and transportation were "bountifully provided through vigorous competition in the free market."[65] The US Federal Trade Commission once again applied antitrust law to medical care, this time to challenge Certificate of Need.[66] But CoN looked more appealing after the market failures of 2007–08, and some policy leaders turned back to it. Market ideology remained dominant, however, and it threatened patient safety.

Patient Safety

Many people assume that the medical profession and/or government take responsibility for ensuring that medical care is as safe as possible. Neither does.

Following earlier precedent, Congress established the Food and Drug Administration (FDA) during the New Deal to oversee the safety of food, drugs, and cosmetics marketed in interstate commerce. Medical devices were added only after publicity about patient deaths due to pacemaker malfunctions and intra-uterine device (IUD) complications. In passing the 1976 law, Congress seemed to require that higher-risk devices undergo a (moderately) rigorous premarket *approval* process. The law, however, permitted a less stringent approach. Purportedly a temporary measure, the 510(k) *notification* process permitted the FDA to skip the testing and inspections and pass a device on the basis of "substantial equivalence" to a device that had been marketed prior to the medical device act (and therefore itself never subject to safety evaluation). The FDA has used this process to pass the vast majority of devices.

In 1983, Congress contended that FDA use of the 510(k) process constituted a "bureaucratic neglect for public health and safety that shocks the conscience."[67] Congressional conscience appeared to have little impact on FDA behavior, however. Over the following decades, the FDA "cleared for market" over 90 percent of medical-device applications on the grounds that they had the same intended use and the same technical characteristics as a "predicate" device.[68] While many of the devices fell into the tongue depressor category, some cleared under the 510(k) process were complex radiation machines advertised to the profession and to the public as new technologies.

The FDA employed its 510(k) process to pass the variety of proton teletherapy devices, calling them substantially equivalent to Loma Linda University's instrument. But the FDA web site also reported that the agency cleared the Loma Linda device on the basis of substantial equivalence.[69] Equivalent to what, one might ask? The web site did not divulge that information, nor did a direct enquiry. It took a Freedom of Information request to (partially) reveal that the FDA had determined the Loma Linda device to be "substantially equivalent to devices marketed in interstate commerce prior to May 28, 1976," tersely naming "Synchrocyclotron—Harvard University" as the predicate device.[70] The digital copy sent to me in the name of freedom of information blacked out approximately 150 pages, presumably protecting proprietary information claimed by the company developing the Loma Linda/Fermilab device. Nowhere in the readable pages is the Harvard machine again mentioned to justify determination of substantial equivalence, nor is it acknowledged that Harvard built its machine for nuclear physics research and did not market it for clinical purposes. In effect, the 510(k) process circumvented safety determination of proton-beam therapy.

Although a 1990 amendment of the Safe Devices Act required that evidence of equivalence be made publicly available, it has not been enforced—and it was not evident in the material sent to me.[71] In 2011, the Institute of Medicine recommended the elimination of the 510(k) bypass.[72] But the FDA did not appear to have the staffing capacity or the leadership to review higher-risk medical devices according to the law. Moreover, financial firms appreciated that the 510(k) process served as an imprimatur that reduced their risk of investing in high-tech medical devices.[73] FDA regulation, in this case at least, seemed to protect investors more than consumers.

Abdication of responsibility for public safety is consistent with market theory rejection of public policy and regulation. Encouraging widespread use of the 510(k) process is only one way that industry has used government regulation to protect the medical-business system. Fully half of FDA advisory committee members in the early 2000s had ties in the forms of stock ownership, research grants, and/or consulting arrangements with companies directly involved in the decisions the committees were making.[74] Conjunctions like these constitute serious conflicts of interest. Conflicts of interest also arise in interspecialty relations.

Specialist Supply and Conflicts of Interest

The national supply of medical specialists is not a product of measured (or even assumed) population need for their treatments. It is a product of hospital specialty department needs and aspirations and what the government pays for residency training (around $15 billion a year).[75] Specialist supply has long been a focus of professional policy, since too many as well as too few practitioners relative to demand threaten a specialty's economic viability. The American Society for Radiation Oncology suggested in the mid-1990s that an oversupply of radiation oncologists and their devices had led to excessive costs and excessive use of radiation treatments. The United States had 1.5 times more radiation oncologists per million people compared to Europe and Canada, its study revealed, plus 2.5 times more megavoltage machines.[76] Without explicitly using intervention levels in health-maintenance organizations as benchmarks of appropriate care (a common, if not unchallenged, practice in health-services research), the study drew attention to a 35 percent radiation treatment rate of cancer patients in managed care settings compared to the 50–60 percent reported by the American College of Radiology's Patterns of Care project.

Ironically, a number of European radiotherapy leaders turned the argument around and used the ACR reports to allege that their countries lagged behind global (US) standards. Having worried as recently as 1996 that the country's 30–32 percent radiation therapy rate might indicate overutilization for some cancers, the Swedish Council on Technology Assessment in Health Care shifted gears in 2003. The council at that time announced that Sweden had nearly achieved the "internationally recommended level" of treating half of all cancer cases with radiation.[77] UK radio-oncologists similarly argued a few years later that they had "significantly underestimated" the need for their services and that they needed to irradiate more patients in order to attain "world class service."[78] Despite the fact that some European radiotherapists criticized the "rather crude assumptions" that led to "the almost mythical 50%,"[79] international specialists used specialty-reported intervention rates in the United States as their strategic goal.

Besides augmenting the market for radiation treatments, specialty-based policies sought to maintain professional monopoly over them. While the American College of Radiology's policy that "referring physicians should not have a direct or indirect financial interest in diagnostic or therapeutic facilities to which they refer patients" appeared to take a strong stand against ownership and overtreatment incentives, it was primarily an anticompetitive tactic.[80] In defining the problem as "self-referring" physicians in other specialties, the ACR excluded the situation in which radiologists and radiation oncologists benefited financially from treating patients on equipment that they themselves owned.[81] Concerned that other specialties were infringing on its technology and its market, organized radiology turned to government for protection.

ACR took its complaints to the US Department of Health and Human Services, which issued a broader report accusing physician-owned services of overtreating and overcharging.[82] Profiting from medical-service ownership gave doctors "powerful incentives to bend their professional judgments," *New England Journal of Medicine* editor Arnold Relman told a reporter when the government report was released.[83] California Congressman Pete Stark took up the baton—and ACR's "self-referral" tactic—and the 1989 Ethics in Patient Referrals Act prohibited referral of Medicare and Medicaid patients to clinical laboratories in which the referring physician (or family member) held a financial interest in terms of ownership, investment, or compensation.

Since the (first) Stark law did not cover its specialty, the American College of Radiology continued its campaign. The college blamed excessive utilization and costs in radiation therapy in one state (Florida) on the high proportion of nonradiologists with ownership interests in radiation facilities.[84] Rejoinders to the Florida study criticized its methodology and reported that an examination of actual figures showed that prices, procedure intensity, and net revenues were higher in the services owned by radiologists and radiation oncologists.[85] Nonetheless, the ACR paper was influential in adding its specialty areas to the Stark law and in restricting their competition.[86]

New Stark legislation followed ACR's advice to specifically prohibit nonradiologists' self-referring to radiation equipment in which they held economic interest and also in exempting "in-office ancillary services" from the prohibition.[87] The exemption permitted physicians to profit from treating patients on their own equipment and on that of their group. It supported a surge of equipment purchase in private radiology and radio-oncology offices and freestanding centers—not to mention a broadening of the definition of *group*. In what was perhaps an extreme example of such broadening, physician management company 21st Century Oncology would argue that the company did not violate Stark law when its specialists benefitted financially from referring patients to other 21st Century specialists on the grounds that the entire company comprised a medical group.[88]

ACR's and Stark law's definition of conflict of interest in terms of one specialty benefitting financially from using technology staked out by another specialty blurred conflicts of interest inherent in physician ownership *per se*. Banning all physician ownership of medical services, a representative of the Bank of America advised a policy group, would instantly eliminate such ownership conflicts.[89] (He neglected to mention its potential for shifting medical ownership to bank-financed investors.) Radiation oncologists continued to battle incursions on their turf, and they continued to accuse urologists of owning radiation therapy devices and using them excessively on prostate-cancer patients.[90] While Congressman Stark had tried to reduce physician conflicts of interest, the issue was a political football from the beginning.

Many other professional conflicts of interest remain in addition to loopholes in the Stark laws; they include numerous ties between medicine and industry. Specialty associations build their Washington, DC area lobbying headquarters with corporate funding. Pharmaceutical and device companies enrich specialists with highly paid consultancies, research grants, stock options, and direct payments for using company products. Interconnections like these, an Institute of Medicine committee accused in 2009, threatened the "integrity of scientific investigations, the objectivity of medical education, the quality of patient care, and the public's trust in medicine."[91]

Institutional conflicts of interest arise when employee activities affect a university's or a hospital's grant-garnering capacity, the market value of its financial holdings, or returns on its investments.[92] Even as researchers affirm they have "no relevant financial relationship" with the work they are publishing, their university compensation is not irrelevant; their salaries and promotions are often contingent on performing research that brings in funding. Academia's dual role of using research to generate income as well as knowledge is a conflict of interest in itself. So is conducting research on patients for purposes other than potential clinical benefit.

Egregious Experiment or Standard Practice?

Having unleashed nuclear energy with the atomic bomb, the United States sought to develop it after the war. National leaders asked medical researchers to estimate potential radiation dangers to military personnel and industrial employees.

When Martha Stephens, an English professor at the University of Cincinnati, read in the *Village Voice* in 1971 that her institution was subjecting cancer patients to high-dose total body irradiation (TBI) in order to quantify radiation damage to the human body, she thought it could not be true. Not only was it true, but Stephens also found that the experiment escalated doses to points expected to be lethal and that some patients suffered severe radiation sickness before they died. A *Washington Post* article on the report she coauthored attracted the attention of US Senator Mike Gravel, who asked the College of Radiology to investigate.[93]

The College set up a three-man committee—which included Stanford's Henry Kaplan—and the ACR president subsequently wrote Gravel that the committee had found the Cincinnati TBI project to be "validly conceived, stated, executed, controlled and followed up," and that its procedures were "consistent with accepted good clinical and scientific practice."[94] The nature of cancer, the ACR president argued, often called for "drastic or radical treatments not commonly accepted as reliable or efficacious."

The ACR committee's conclusion was consistent with contemporary clinical practice that accepted radical treatment as going beyond scientific evidence. It seemed to imply that the TBI experiments did not look so very different from Henry Kaplan's and Gilbert Fletcher's wide-field and total-body irradiation treatments of the time—which were themselves reporting serious radiation damage.[95] Radiation physicist and historian Gerald Kutcher later suggested that the ACR representatives had not challenged the Cincinnati experiments because the treatments were uncomfortably close to standard practice in the field and that the experts "would have (at least in part) been questioning their own scientific and ethical probity."[96] Even as radiologists defended the total-body irradiation treatments, Cincinnati's own Institutional Review Board severely criticized them, and the university seemed uneasy about their public exposure.[97] After Stephens publicized the Cincinnati experiments, the university agreed to terminate them, Congress agreed not to hold hearings on them, and the issue was (temporarily) buried.

Cincinnati's was the culmination in a series of similar experiments. Robert Stone had sponsored TBI studies at New York's Memorial Hospital, the Chicago Tumor Clinic, and his own department at the University of California as part of his work on the Manhattan project. His California group reported their total-body irradiations as "part of the normal therapy" of the patients involved.[98] After the war, however, Stone's funding agency (the Atomic Energy Commission) criticized ongoing TBI treatments in his department. Government had some scientific and ethical responsibility for the clinical care it was paying for, an AEC committee chairman wrote Stone, stating that the TBI treatments did not meet scientific standards.[99] Stone vigorously defended medical autonomy in response, and this idea of public responsibility for medical treatment fell by the wayside. The military continued to sponsor studies inflicting radiation damage on human bodies, particularly those of low-income and minority people.[100] The Air Force used its connections with M. D. Anderson Hospital to determine, as Fletcher's team candidly reported in a professional journal, the "dose level beyond which serious acute disturbances must be expected to appear."[101]

Twenty years after the Cincinnati turmoil, public outcry erupted once again when a newspaper article identified some of the patients who had been experimentally injected with plutonium (to see how it affected the body's metabolism).[102]

Political response this time around set up a short-term Advisory Committee on Human Radiation Experiments (ACHRE), held Congressional hearings, and declassified voluminous files covering hitherto little-known radiation experiments. President Clinton charged ACHRE with determining whether the experiments met "ethical and scientific standards, including standards of informed consent, that prevailed at the time of the experiments and that exist today."[103] The committee's purview explicitly excluded "common and routine clinical practices"—just what most patients thought they were receiving. The distinction would be problematic.

ACHRE defined government's ethical responsibility in instrumental terms of reinforcing government policies and medicine's ethical responsibility in instrumental terms of reinforcing medical practice standards. The medical definition was consistent with a long-standing use of deviation from standard practice as the yardstick of social, ethical, and legal malpractice.[104] American College of Radiology spokesman James Cox (who had himself used TBI) testified in the Congressional hearings that the Cincinnati and other TBI studies had been consistent with practice standards of the time.[105] Although ACHRE did conclude that the total-body irradiation studies failed to follow the (inadequate) informed consent procedures of the time of the experiments, it could not agree on the ethics of the treatment/experiments themselves. Stephens suggested that the radiologists on the committee were primarily concerned with damage control and professional solidarity.[106] Did the radiation experiments still seem uncomfortably close to contemporary practices?

The radiation studies and ACHRE's consternation over them challenge the basic premise of a dividing line between medical practice and experiment. Given wide variations in disease virulence and biological response, the history of medicine can be seen as a series of trial-and-error processes that have (necessarily) made patients research subjects. This book has shown how the introduction of each new radiation technology and upgraded device entailed patient experimentation. ACHRE's mandated separation of experiment and practice created an impasse.

Committee members may have been shocked by the 800-pound gorilla at the conference table. It is a simple syllogism:

> IF standard practice is the basis of ethical determination, and
> IF radiation experiments are consistent with standard practice,
> THEN radiation experiments are ethical.

Basing ethical judgment on deviation from common practice, as ACHRE was charged to do, places standard practices (and practice standards) beyond the sphere of public accountability. Although ACHRE offered an "intent to benefit" to mitigate ethical taint,[107] beneficent intentions are insufficient; they can still lead to more harm than good. Experiments to determine how much radiation the human body can tolerate, while crucially different in intent, are not so different—from the patients' point of view—from radical treatments designed to approach maximum tolerance. Similarities between radiation experiments and standard radiation therapy practices meant that organized medicine could not condemn the experiments as unethical—or even as bad medicine—when the issue erupted in the 1970s, again in the 1980s, and again in the 1990s.

What does it mean for a society when its experts cannot come to a consensus on whether doctors' knowingly giving to unwitting patients severely debilitating doses of radiation that cannot possibly cure is unethical? Standard medical practice is the larger issue that is crying out for investigation. Hippocrates' admonition, "First, do no harm," would seem to offer a good starting point. But, as a temporary advisory committee, ACHRE may have hit the limits of government involvement in the economic and professional environment of the 1990s.

All of the health care reform efforts discussed in this chapter are partial responses to serious issues. None fully addressed the problems at stake in radiation therapy or other specialty services, and most served multiple interests. While payment programs reduce inequities, they may also promote excessive medical-facility growth. While restricting growth in one area may use public monies more efficiently, it may redirect capital flows to more speculative ventures. Selectively permitting medical-service ownership confers competitive advantage on the people selected. Regulating product safety can protect consumer health, but its weak enforcement protects the health of medical industries.

Reforms to alleviate conflicts of interest and strengthen equitable access, product safety, capital controls, effective intervention, and ethical treatment would go a very long way toward building a better health care system. But the job is tricky, and it may be impossible in the current market-driven system. A market-oriented politics has strangled reform efforts to safeguard health and continues to build a medical business system that chooses wealth over health.

Notes

1 Simon Kramer and David F. Herring, "The Patterns of Care Study: A Nationwide Evaluation of the Practice of Radiation Therapy in Cancer Management," *International Journal of Radiation Oncology Biology Physics* 1 (1976): 1231–1236; Lawrence R. Coia and Gerald E. Hanks, "Quality Assessment in the USA: How the Patterns of Care Study Has Made a Difference," *Seminars in Radiation Oncology* 7 (1997): 146–156.

2 G. Stephen Brown, David F. Herring, William E. Powers, Simon Kramer, Lawrence W. Davis, Charles J. MacLean, "Patterns of Care in American Radiation Therapy 1973–1975," *International Journal of Radiation Oncology Biology Physics* 7 supplement 1 (1981): 105–106; Jean B. Owen and Lawrence R. Coia, "The Changing Structure of Radiation Oncology: Implications for the Era of Managed Care," *Seminars in Radiation Oncology* 7 (1997): 108–113.

3 Gerald E. Hanks, James J. Diamond, and Simon Kramer, "The Need for Complex Technology in Radiation Oncology: Correlations of Facility Characteristics and Structure with Outcome," *Cancer* 55 (1985): 2198–2201. The subset comprised instruments that operated at a source-to-skin distance of less than 80 cm.

4 Gerald E. Hanks, James J. Diamond, Simon Kramer, "The Need for Complex Technology in Radiation Oncology: Correlations of Facility Characteristics and Structure with Outcome," *Cancer* 55 (1985): 2198–2201.

5 Gerald E. Hanks, John M. Krall, Alexandra L. Hanlon, Sucha O. Asbell, Miljenko V. Pilepich, and Jean Owen, "Patterns of Care and RTOG Studies in Prostate Cancer: Long

Term Survival, Hazard Rate Observations, and Possibilities of Cure," *International Journal of Radiation Oncology Biology Physics* 28 (1994): 39–46.

6 Rachelle Lanciano, Gillian Thomas, and Patricia J. Eifel, "Over 20 Years of Progress in Radiation Oncology: Cervical Cancer," *Seminars in Radiation Oncology* 7 (1997): 121–126. Use of brachytherapy on cervical cancer doubled from 6 percent in 2000 to 12 percent in 2009 (that figure can not be updated, as the data set dropped cervical cancer). Brachytherapy use rose in breast cancer from 0.1 percent in 2000 to 3.8 percent in 2009, and it declined to 2.8 percent in 2012. Brachytherapy use declined in prostate cancer from 14.2 percent in 2000 to 8.6 percent in 2009 and to 5.9 percent in 2012. Brachytherapy accounted for 2.9 percent of all measured radiation treatments in 2000 and 2.1 percent in 2012. American College of Surgeons, National Cancer Data Base (NCDB) Public Benchmark Reports. https://www.facs.org accessed March 20, 2013 and March 18, 2015.

7 Melanie C. Smitt, Jan Buzydlowski, and Richard T. Hoppe, "Over 20 Years of Progress in Radiation Therapy: Hodgkin's Disease," *Seminars in Radiation Oncology* 7 (1997): 127–134.

8 Gustavo S. Montana, A. L. Hanlon, T. J. Brickner, J. E. Owen, G. E. Hanks, C. C. Ling, R. Komaki, V. A. Marcial, G. M. Thomas, and R. Lanciano, "Carcinoma of the Cervix: Patterns of Care Studies: Review of 1978, 1983, and 1988–1989 Surveys," *International Journal of Radiation Oncology Biology Physics* 32 (1995): 1481–1486.

9 J. Frank Wilson and Jean Owen, "Evolutionary Phases in Quality Research in Radiation Oncology over the Last 35 Years," *International Journal of Radiation Oncology Biology Physics* 72, supplement S (2008): S426; Jean B. Owen, Julia R. White, Michael J. Zelefsky, and J. Frank Wilson, "Using QRRO™ Survey Data to Assess Compliance with Quality Indicators for Breast and Prostate Cancer," *Journal of the American College of Radiology* 6 (2009): 442–447.

10 National Cancer Institute, "Age-Adjusted Rates By Data Type All Sites, All Ages, All Races, Both Sexes 1975–2011," Surveillance, Epidemiology, and End Results Program. http://seer.cancer.gov/faststats accessed April 2, 2015.

11 Andrea McKee and Andrew Salner, "A Cancer Battle We Can Win," *New York Times* September 22, 2014, A25; The National Lung Screening Trial Research Team, "Reduced Lung-Cancer Mortality with Low-Dose Computed Tomographic Screening," *New England Journal of Medicine* 365 (2011): 395–409.

12 H. Gilbert Welch, Steven Woolshin, and Lisa M. Schwartz, "How Two Studies on Cancer Screening Led to Two Results," *New York Times* March 13, 2007, D5, D8; Paula Span, "Assessing the Value of Lung Cancer Screening," *New York Times* May 12, 2005, D6.

13 Peter C. Gøtzsche and Karsten Juhl Jørgensen, "Screening for Breast Cancer with Mammography," *Cochrane Library* June 2013. http://onlinelibrary.wiley.com/doi/10.1002/14651858.CD001877.pub5/full accessed November 8, 2016.

14 Robert A. Aronowitz, *Unnatural History: Breast Cancer and American Society* (Cambridge: Cambridge University Press, 2007), 161, 258–259; National Cancer Institute, "Age-Adjusted SEER Incidence Rates by Cancer Site All Ages, All Races, Female 1975–2011 (SEER 9)," http://seer.cancer.gov/faststats accessed April 2, 2015.

15 Simon Kramer, Gerald E. Hanks, David F. Herring, and Lawrence W. Davis, "Summary Results from the Facilities Master List Surveys Conducted by the Patterns of Care Study," *International Journal of Radiation Oncology Biology Physics* 8 (1982): 883–888. Radiation is also used on some noncancerous lesions such as arteriovenous malformations in the brain.

16 Institute of Medicine Committee for Review and Evaluation of the Medical Use Program of the Nuclear Regulatory Commission, *Radiation in Medicine: A Need for Regulatory Reform* (Washington, DC: National Academy Press, 1996), 65.

17 American College of Surgeons, National Cancer Data Base (NCDB) Public Benchmark Reports. https://www.facs.org accessed May 8, 2013 and May 12, 2016.While ACR Patterns of Care surveys overrepresented cancers treated with radiation, the American

College of Surgeons data base may overrepresent hospital-based treatments and cancers treated with surgery.

18 American College of Surgeons, National Cancer Data Base NCDB Public Benchmark Reports.https://www.facs.org accessed May 6, 2013.

19 National Cancer Institute, Surveillance Epidemiology and End Results Program. http://seer.cancer.gov/faststats/ accessed May 12, 2016.

20 Philip Rubin, "The Emergence of Radiation Oncology as a Distinct Medical Specialty," *International Journal of Radiation Oncology Biology Physics* 11 (1985): 1247–1270.

21 Vincent T. DeVita, Jane E. Henney, and Susan M. Hubbard, "Estimation of the Numerical and Economic Impact of Chemotherapy in the Treatment of Cancer," in Joseph H. Burchenal and Herbert F. Oettgen, eds., *Cancer: Achievements, Challenges, and Prospects for the 1980s, Volume 2* (New York: Grune & Stratton, 1981), 859–880.

22 Marko Popovic, Mariska den Hartogh, Liying Zhang, Michael Poon, Henry Lam, Gillian Bedard, Natalie Pulenzas, Breanne Lechner, and Edward Chow, "Review of International Patterns of Practice for the Treatment of Painful Bone Metastases with Palliative Radiotherapy from 1993 to 2013," *Radiotherapy and Oncology* 111 (2014): 11–17.

23 May N. Tsao, Nancy Lloyd, Rebecca K. S. Wong, Edward Chow, Eileen Rakovitch, Normand Laperriere, Wei Xu, and Arjun Sahgal, "Whole Brain Radiotherapy for the Treatment of Newly Diagnosed Multiple Brain Metastases," *Cochrane Library* April 18, 2012. http://onlinelibrary.wiley.com/doi/10.1002/14651858.CD003869.pub3/abstract accessed January 8, 2015.

24 Morten Hoyer, Anand Swaminath, Sean Bydder, Michael Lock, Alejandra Méndez Romero, Brian Kavanagh, Karyn A. Goodman, Paul Okunieff, and Laura A. Dawson, "Radiotherapy for Liver Metastases: A Review of Evidence," *International Journal of Radiation Oncology Biology Physics* 82 (2012): 1047–1057.

25 Kiki C. A. L. Cheriex, Tim H. J. Nijhuis, and Marc A. M. Mureau, "Osteoradionecrosis of the Jaws: A Review of Conservative and Surgical Treatment Options," *Journal of Reconstructive Microsurgery* 29 (2013): 69–75; Veeru Kasivisvanathan, Ankur Thapar, Kerry J. Davies, et al., "Periprocedural Outcomes after Surgical Revascularization and Stenting for Postradiotherapy Carotid Stenosis," *Journal of Vascular Surgery* 56 (2012): 1143–1152.e2; Martin Klein, "Neurocognitive Functioning in Adult WHO Grade II Gliomas: Impact of Old and New Treatment Modalities," *Neuro-Oncology* 14 (2012): 17–24.

26 Daniel S. Ong, Robert A. Aertker, Alexandra N. Clark, et al., "Radiation-Associated Valvular Heart Disease," *Journal of Heart Valve Disease* 22 (2013): 883–892; Sylvie Delanian, Jean-Louis Lefaix, and Pierre-Francois Pradat, "Radiation-induced Neuropathy in Cancer Survivors," *Radiotherapy and Oncology* 105 (2012): 273–282.

27 Luca Incrocci and Pernille Tine Jensen, "Pelvic Radiotherapy and Sexual Function in Men and Women," *Journal of Sexual Medicine* 10 Special Issue S1 (2013): 53–64.

28 Fani Kokka, Andrew Bryant, Elly Brockbank, Melanie Powell, and David Oram, "Hysterectomy with Radiotherapy or Chemotherapy or Both for Women with Locally Advanced Cervical Cancer," *Cochrane Library* April 2015. http://onlinelibrary.wiley.com/doi/10.1002/14651858.CD010260.pub2/full accessed July 12, 2016.

29 Astrid Baalbergen, Yerney Veenstra, and Lukas Stalpers, "Primary Surgery versus Primary Radiotherapy with or without Chemotherapy for Early Adenocarcinoma of the Uterine Cervix," *Cochrane Library* January, 2013. http://onlinelibrary.wiley.com/doi/10.1002/14651858.CD006248.pub3/full accessed August 1, 2014. This study reviewed only one RCT.

30 John A. Green, John J. Kirwan, Jayne Tierney, Paul Symonds, Lydia Fresco, C. Williams, and M. Collingwood, "Concomitant Chemotherapy and Radiation Therapy for Cancer of the Uterine Cervix," *Cochrane Library* July, 2005. http://onlinelibrary.wiley.com/doi/10.1002/14651858.CD002225.pub2/full accessed August 1, 2014.

31 Annabel Goodwin, Sharon Parker, Davina Ghersi, and Nicholas Wilcken, "Post-operative Radiotherapy for Ductal Carcinoma in Situ of the Breast," *Cochrane Library* November, 2013. http://onlinelibrary.wiley.com/doi/10.1002/14651858.CD000563.pub7/full accessed June 18, 2014.

32 Early Breast Cancer Trialists' Collaborative Group (EBCTCG), "Effect of Radiotherapy after Breast-conserving Surgery on 10-year Recurrence and 15-year Breast Cancer Death: Meta-analysis of Individual Patient Data for 10,801 Women in 17 Randomised Trials," *The Lancet* 378 (2011): 1707–1716; Brigid E. Hickey, Daniel P. Francis, and Margot Lehman, "Sequencing of Chemotherapy and Radiotherapy for Early Breast Cancer," *Cochrane Library* April, 2013. http://onlinelibrary.wiley.com/doi/10.1002/14651858.CD005212.pub3/full accessed August 1, 2014.

33 Frank Peinemann, Ulrich Grouven, Lars G. Hemkens, et al., "Low-dose Rate Brachytherapy for Men with Localized Prostate Cancer," *Cochrane Library* July, 2011. http://onlinelibrary.wiley.com/doi/10.1002/14651858.CD008871.pub2/fullaccessed August 1, 2014.

34 Tiffany Daly, Brigid E. Hickey, Margot Lehman, et al., "Adjuvant Radiotherapy Following Radical Prostatectomy for Prostate Cancer," *Cochrane Library* December, 2011.http://onlinelibrary.wiley.com/doi/10.1002/14651858.CD007234.pub2/abstrac-taccessed August 1, 2014.This review curiously concluded that although radiation could lead to urinary stricture and incontinence, there was "no detriment to quality of life."

35 PORT Meta-analysis Group, "Postoperative Radiotherapy for Non-small Cell Lung Cancer," *Cochrane Library* April 2005.http://onlinelibrary.wiley.com/doi/10.1002/14651858.CD002142.pub2/full accessed August 1, 2014.

36 Jason F. Lester, Fergus Macbeth, Elizabeth Toy, and Bernadette Coles, "Palliative RadiotherapyRegimensforNon-smallCellLungCancer,*CochraneLibrary*October,2006. http://onlinelibrary.wiley.com/doi/10.1002/14651858.CD002143.pub2/full accessed August 1, 2014; Rosemary Stevens, Fergus Macbeth, Elizabeth Toy, et al., "Palliative Radiotherapy Regimens for Patients with Thoracic Symptoms from Non-small Cell Lung Cancer, *Cochrane Library* January 1, 2015. http://onlinelibrary.wiley.com/doi/10.1002/14651858.CD002143.pub3/abstract accessed January 8, 2015

37 Christine Herbst, Fareed Ahmed Rehan, Nicole Skoetz, et al., "Chemotherapy Alone versus Chemotherapy Plus Radiotherapy for Early Stage Hodgkin Lymphoma," *Cochrane Library* February, 2011. http://www.cochranelibrary.com/topic/Cancer/Haematological%20malig-nancies/Hodgkin%E2%80%99s%20lymphoma/ accessed July 12, 2016.

38 Amy Berrington de Gonzalez, Rochelle E. Curtis, Stephen F. Kry, Ethel Gilbert, Stephanie Lamart, Christine D. Berg. Marilyn Stovall, and Elaine Ron, "Proportion of Second Cancers Attributable to Radiotherapy Treatment in Adults: A Cohort Study in the US SEER Cancer Registries," *Lancet Oncology* 12 (2011): 353–60. The new tumor incidence ranged from 4 percent following irradiation of cancers of the eye to 24 percent following irradiation of testicular cancer.

39 Tobias Boelling, Stefan Koenemann, Iris Ernst, and Normann Willich, "Late Effects of Thoracic Irradiation in Children," *Strahlentherapie und Onkologie* 184 (2008): 289–295; Sebastiaan L. Knijnenburg, Renée L. Mulder, Antoinette Y. N. Schouten-Van Meeteren, et al., "Early and Late Renal Adverse Effects after Potentially Nephrotoxic Treatment for Childhood Cancer," *Cochrane Library* October 2013. http://onlinelibrary.wiley.com/doi/10.1002/14651858.CD008944.pub2/abstract accessed August 1, 2014.

40 Vikram Jairam, Kenneth B. Roberts, and James B. Yu, "Historical Trends in the Use of Radiation Therapy for Pediatric Cancers: 1973–2008," *International Journal of Radiation Oncology Biology Physics* 85 (2013): e151–155.

41 David S. Jones, *Broken Hearts: The Tangled History of Cardiac Care* (Baltimore: Johns Hopkins University Press, 2013), 20.

42 Julie B. Schnur, Suzanne C. Ouellette, Dana H. Bovbjerg, and Guy H. Montgomery, "Breast Cancer Patients' Experience of External-Beam Radiotherapy," *Qualitative Health Research* 19 (2009): 668–676.
43 Anne Cassia, personal communication, November 18, 2016.
44 David Cantor. "Cancer, Quackery and the Vernacular Meanings of Hope in 1950s America," *Journal of the History of Medicine and Allied Sciences* 61 (2006): 324–368.
45 A. Robert Kagan, "Chairman's Address: A Description and Critical History of Modern Radiation Oncology," *ACRO Bulletin* (Summer, 2002): 12–13.http://www.acro.org/pdf/publications/bulletins/summer2002.pdf accessed June 10, 2007.
46 United Health Center for Health Reform and Modernization, "Federal Health Care Cost Containment—How in Practice Can it be Done?" *Working Paper 1* May 2009, 2.
47 World Bank, "Health Expenditure per Capita (Current US$)." http://data.worldbank.org/indicator/SH.XPD.PCAP accessed June 30, 2013. The NHS is currently succumbing to cuts driven by market ideology and economic turmoil.
48 American College of Surgeons, "Stage by Insurance Status of All Sites Cancer Diagnosed in 2003 to 2013," National Cancer Data Base (NCDB) Public Benchmark Reports.https://www.facs.org accessed May 13, 2016.Data through 2010 that divided the Medicare population into those who purchased a private supplement and those who did not found higher early cancer diagnoses among the former.
49 Twenty-eight percent of the Medicare population had their non-small-cell lung cancers diagnosed in the earliest stages, for example, compared to 23 percent of those privately insured, 17 percent of those receiving Medicaid, and 12 percent of uninsured people. American College of Surgeons, National Cancer Data Base (NCDB) Benchmark Reports, https://www.facs.org accessed October 6, 2014. Updated May 15, 2016.
50 US Congress Office of Technology Assessment, *Federal Policies and the Medical Device Industry* (Washington, DC: 1984), 37.
51 Bryan Luce and Rebecca Singer Cohen, "Health Technology Assessment in the United States," *International Journal of Technology Assessment in Health Care* 25 Supplement 1 (2009): 33–41.
52 Medicare Payment Advisory Commission, *Report to the Congress: Promoting Greater Efficiency in Medicare* (Washington, DC: The Commission, 2007), xii.
53 Heloisa P. Soares, Ambuj Kumar, Stephanie Daniels, et al., "Evaluation of New Treatments in Radiation Oncology: Are They Better Than Standard Treatments?" *JAMA* 293 (2005): 970–978.
54 Barron H. Lerner, *The Breast Cancer Wars: Hope, Fear, and the Pursuit of a Cure in Twentieth-Century America* (New York, NY: Oxford University Press, 2001), 125–126.
55 John Abramson, *Overdo$ed America: The Broken Promise of American Medicine* (New York, NY: HarperCollins, 2004), 37–38.
56 F. E. Vera-Badillo, R. Shapiro, A. Ocana, et al., "Bias in Reporting of End Points of Efficacy and Toxicity in Randomized: Clinical Trials for Women with Breast Cancer," *Annals of Oncology* 24 (2013):1238–1244.
57 Julie Anderson, Francis Neary, and John V. Pickstone in collaboration with James Raferty, *Surgeons, Manufacturers and Patients* (Basingstoke, Hampshire: Palgrave Macmillan, 2007), 118.
58 Abraham M. Nussbaum, *The Finest Traditions of My Calling: One Physician's Search for the Renewal of Medicine* (New Haven, CT: Yale University Press, 2016), 95–96.
59 Hamilton Moses, E. Ray Dorsey, David H. M. Matheson, and Samuel O. Thier, "Financial Anatomy of Biomedical Research," *JAMA* 294 (2005): 1333–1342.
60 eResearch Technology Inc., self-description, Genstar Capital. http://www.gencap.com/portfolio/ert.php accessed August 23, 2014.
61 US Bureau of Health Facilities, *Health Capital Is$ues* (Washington, DC: US Department of Health and Human Services, 1981), viii–ix.
62 US Department of Health, Education, and Welfare, *National Guidelines for Health Planning* (Hyattsville, MD: 1978), 13–14.

63 Philip N. Reeves and Russell C. Coile, *Introduction to Health Planning* (Arlington, VA: Information Resources Press, 1989), 54.
64 Varian Associates, *1986 Annual Report.* Russell and Sigurd Varian Papers, SC 345, Varian Associates Series, Box 2. Special Collections and University Archives, Stanford University Libraries.
65 John Barnes, *Failure of Government Central Planning: Washington's Medical Certificate of Need Program* (Seattle, WA: Washington Policy Center, 2006), 8.
66 US Federal Trade Commission and US Department of Justice, *Improving Health Care: A Dose of Competition* (Washington, DC: 2004), 22.
67 John D. Dingell, "Letter of Transmittal," for *Medical Device Regulation: The FDA's Neglected Child* (Washington, DC: USGPO, 1983).
68 Jan B. Pietzsch, Marta G. Zanchi, and John H. Linehan, "Medical Device Innovators and the 510(k) Regulatory Pathway: Implications of a Survey-Based Assessment of Industry Experience—Part 2: Medical Device Ecosystem and Policy," *Journal of Medical Devices* 7 (2013): 021003-1–021003-5.
69 US Food and Drug Administration, "Loma Linda University Proton Beam Therapy System," K872369.http://www.accessdata.fda.gov/scripts/cdrh/cfdocs/cfpmn/pmn_template.cfm?id=k872369 accessed June 30, 2013.
70 US Food and Drug Administration, File K872369, "510(k) Notification of Intent to Market Loma Linda Proton Beam Therapy System," Rockville, MD: FDA Division of Freedom of Information, July 1, 2013.
71 Diana Zuckerman, Paul Brown, and Aditi Das, "Lack of Publicly Available Scientific Evidence on the Safety and Effectiveness of Implanted Medical Devices," *JAMA Internal Medicine* 174 (2014):1781–1787.
72 Institute of Medicine, *Medical Devices and the Public's Health: The FDA 510(k) Clearance Process at 35 Years* (Washington, DC: National Academies Press, 2011).
73 Z. Ayca Altintig, Hsin-Hui Chiu, and M. Sinan Goktan, "How Does Uncertainty Resolution Affect VC Syndication?" *Financial Management* 42 (2013): 611–646.
74 Richard A. Deyo, "Gaps, Tensions, and Conflicts in the FDA Approval Process: Implications for Clinical Practice," *Journal of the American Board of Family Practice* 17 (2004): 142–149; Dominique A. Tobbell, *Pills, Power, and Policy: The Struggle for Drug Reform in Cold War America and its Consequences* (Berkeley, CA: University of California Press, 2012), 126–127. The FDA was not the only government agency with such a conflict of interest.
75 Institute of Medicine Committee on the Governance and Financing of Graduate Medical Education, *Graduate Medical Education That Meets the Nation's Health Needs* (Washington, DC: National Academies Press, July, 2014), 64.
76 David H. Hussey, John L. Horton, Nancy P. Mendenhall, John E. Munzenrider, Christopher M. Rose, and Jonathan H. Sunshine, "Manpower Needs for Radiation Oncology: A Preliminary Report of the ASTRO Human Resources Committee," *International Journal of Radiation Oncology Biology Physics* 35 (1996): 809–820.
77 Ulrik Ringborg, David Bergqvist, Bengt Brorsson, et al., "The Swedish Council on Technology Assessment in Health Care (SBU) Systematic Overview of Radiotherapy for Cancer Including a Prospective Survey of Radiotherapy Practice in Sweden 2001—Summary and Conclusions," *Acta Oncologica* 42 (2003): 357–365.
78 National Radiotherapy Advisory Group, *Radiotherapy: Developing a World Class Service for England* London, report to Ministers, February 26, 2007, 3.
79 Søren M. Bentzen, Germaine Heeren, Brian Cottier, Ben Slotman, Bengt Glimelius, Yolande Lievens, and Walter van den Bogaert, "Towards Evidence-Based Guidelines for Radiotherapy Infrastructure and Staffing Needs in Europe: The ESTRO QUARTS Project," *Radiotherapy and Oncology* 75 (2005): 355–365.
80 Otha W. Linton, *The American College of Radiology: The First 75 Years* (Reston, VA.: American College of Radiology, 1997), 157, 160, 165.

81 Jean M. Mitchell and Jonathan H. Sunshine, "Consequences of Physicians' Ownership of Health Care Facilities—Joint Ventures in Radiation Therapy," *New England Journal of Medicine* 327 (1992): 1497–1501.

82 US Department of Health and Human Services, *Financial Arrangements Between Physicians and Health Care Businesses: Report to Congress* (Washington, DC: USDHHS, 1989), iii.

83 Michael Waldholz and Walt Bogdanich, "Warm Bodies: Doctor-Owned Labs Earn Lavish Profits in a Captive Market," *Wall Street Journal* March 1, 1989, A1.

84 Jean M. Mitchell and Jonathan H. Sunshine, "Consequences of Physicians' Ownership of Health Care Facilities—Joint Ventures in Radiation Therapy," *New England Journal of Medicine* 327 (1992): 1497–1501.

85 Stan N. Finkelstein and Kevin Neels, "Self-Referral by Physicians," Kevin F. O'Grady, "Self-Referral by Physicians," *New England Journal of Medicine* 328 (1993): 1274, 1275.

86 Jennifer O'Sullivan, *Report for Congress: Medicare: Physician Self-Referral ("Stark I and II")* (Washington, DC: Congressional Research Service, September 27, 2007), 3.

87 Medicare Payment Advisory Commission, *Report to the Congress: Improving Incentives in the Medicare Program* (Washington, DC: The Commission, 2009), 86.

88 John Carreyrou and Janet Adamy, "Medicare Unmasked: Doctor 'Self-Referral' Thrives on Legal Loophole," *Wall Street Journal* October 23, 2014, A1.

89 Kelly J. Devers, Linda R. Brewster, and Paul B. Ginsburg, "Specialty Hospitals: Focused Factories or Cream Skimmers?" (Washington, DC: Center for Studying Health System Change, April 15, 2003), Gary Taylor in discussion. www.hschange.com, accessed June 20, 2003.

90 Jean Mitchell, "Urologists' Use of Intensity Modulated Radiation Therapy for Prostate Cancer," *New England Journal of Medicine* 369 (2013): 1629–1637.

91 Bernard Lo and Marilyn J. Field, eds., *Conflict of Interest in Medical Research, Education, and Practice* (Washington, DC: National Academies Press, 2009), 1.

92 Ezekiel J. Emanuel and Daniel Steiner, "Institutional Conflict of Interest," *New England Journal of Medicine* 332 (1995): 262–268.

93 Martha Stephens, *The Treatment: The Story of Those Who Died in the Cincinnati Radiation Tests* (Durham, NC: Duke University Press, 2002), 3–6.

94 Robert W. McConnell to Senator Mike Gravel, January 3, 1972. ACHRE No. DOD-042994-A-7. http://www.gwu.edu/~nsarchiv/radiation/dir/mstreet/commeet/meet8/brief8/tab_g/br8gle.txt accessed February 12, 2007

95 Gilbert H. Fletcher, Tongpoon Watanavit, and Felix N. Rutledge, "Whole-Pelvis Irradiation with 4,000 Rads in Stage I and Stage II Cancers of the Uterine Cervix," *Radiology* 86 (1966): 436–443; Henry S. Kaplan and Saul A Rosenberg, "Extended-Field Radical Radiotherapy in Advanced Hodgkin's Disease: Short-Term Results of 2 Randomized Clinical Trials," *Cancer Research* 26 Part I (1966): 1268–1276.

96 Gerald Kutcher, *Contested Medicine: Cancer Research and the Military* (Chicago, IL: University of Chicago Press, 2009), 184.

97 David Egilman, Wes Wallace, Cassandra Stubbs, and Fernando Mora-Corrasco, "A Little Too Much of the Buchenwald Touch? Military Radiation Research at the University of Cincinnati, 1960–1972," *Accountability in Research* 6 (1998): 63–102.

98 Robert S. Stone, *Industrial Medicine on the Plutonium Project: Survey and Collected Papers* (New York, NY: McGraw-Hill, 1951), 338.

99 Alan Gregg to Robert Stone, October 20, 1948. Robert S. Stone papers, 1940–1956, BANC MSS 80/80 c. The Bancroft Library, University of California, Berkeley, CA.

100 The medical profession had felt it "had a right to get some return" from low-income patients, one physician later explained, "since our taxes were paying their hospital bills." Advisory Committee on Human Radiation Experiments, *Final Report of the Advisory Committee on Human Radiation Experiments* (New York, NY: Oxford University Press, 1996), 83.

101 Lowell S. Miller, Gilbert H. Fletcher, and Herbert B. Gerstner, "Radiobiologic Observations on Cancer Patients Treated with Whole-body X-irradiation," *Radiation Research* 4 (1958): 150–165.

102 Eileen Welsome, *The Plutonium Files: America's Secret Medical Experiments in the Cold War* (New York: NY: Dial Press, 1999), 2–7.

103 Advisory Committee on Human Radiation Experiments, *Final Report of the Advisory Committee on Human Radiation Experiments* (New York, NY: Oxford University Press, 1996), 554–555.

104 Sydney A. Halpern, *Lesser Harms: The Morality of Risk in Medical Research* (Chicago, IL: University of Chicago Press, 2004), 107–114.

105 Roger W. Byhardt, James D. Cox, J. Frank Wilson, Joseph Libnoch, and Richard S. Stein, "Total Body Irradiation vs. Chemotherapy as a Systemic Adjuvant for Small Cell Carcinoma of the Lung," *International Journal of Radiation Oncology Biology Physics* 5 (1979): 2043–2048; James D. Cox, testimony, "Radiation Experiments Conducted by the University of Cincinnati Medical School with Department of Defense Funding," Hearing, Committee of the Judiciary, US House of Representatives, Washington, DC, April 11, 1994.

106 Martha Stephens, *The Treatment: The Story of Those Who Died in the Cincinnati Radiation Tests* (Durham, NC: Duke University Press, 2002), 116.

107 Advisory Committee on Human Radiation Experiments, *Final Report of the Advisory Committee on Human Radiation Experiments* (New York, NY: Oxford University Press, 1996), 228.

11 Choosing Health Over Wealth

Market forces, assumptions, and policies have shaped medical delivery. Medical specialties together with their institutions, suppliers, and financiers have consequently become big businesses in themselves. Using radiation therapy as a case study of this development, *Cancer, Radiation Therapy, and the Market* shows how it competed with surgery, gynecology, urology, and other specialties in treating cancer patients with X-rays, radioactive materials, and particle beams. Its leaders coordinated the work of enterprising university and medical-school departments, hospitals, manufacturing companies, and financial firms to competitively build more and more powerful radiation devices. In the process, they wove elements of the market economy into the fabric of medical care.

Although it may be more reassuring for doctors and policy makers to believe that the present medical delivery business arose from economic shifts starting around 1965 or 1970, market-driven medicine has a much older history. It has shaped all of medical care as we know it. Medical care emulated entrepreneurial, competitive, and financial organization throughout the 20th century. Re-forming health care to correspond with health needs and scientific evidence of effectiveness requires challenging the market strategies that drove this development.

Market Strategies

Market strategies embedded in medical delivery have expanded professional and institutional returns on investment as well as economic returns. They have helped build powerful research universities, specialty-based hospital complexes, and prestigious academic medical centers. Specialties initially established themselves by carving out selected populations, diseases, and/or technologies and establishing monopoly control over them, as Table 11.1 notes. Together with hospital administrators, specialists designed clinical interventions for the market and built special procedure units for them. The administrators selectively invested in high-cost technologies, converted services into revenue-generating entities, and employed methods of business management to enhance procedure unit productivity. The financial industry and wealthy foundations, joined by government programs, expanded hospital supply and consolidated medical services in institutions serving large market areas. Financiers used insurance and debt to integrate medical care into the financial industry. Providers used media stories and advertising to

Table 11.1 Market Strategies in Medical Care

- Monopolize populations, diseases, and technologies
- Design high-cost technologies and revenue-generating procedures for the market
- Build high-tech institution-based and freestanding procedure units
- Apply business-management methods to enhance productivity in medical delivery
- Consolidate services in hospital complexes serving large market areas
- Convert medical services into or merge with profit-making corporations
- Invest in services with high monetary and professional returns
- Compete for patients and doctors using technology and advertising
- Integrate medical care into finance via insurance and debt
- Assign financial risk to government, delegate regulation to trade associations

solicit patients and to expand their demand for new technologies. Government assumed considerable financial risk but delegated major regulatory powers to professional trade associations.

Describing in large part how modern medical systems operate, market strategies have drawn the medical care map. They have built hospitals and high-tech specialty units at the expense of primary care. They have carved out surgical and technological procedures and developed them as independent businesses.[1] They have neglected social and environmental factors impacting health, finding more reward in disease *treatment* than in its *prevention.*[2] They have incurred excessive costs and excessive intervention rates relative to available scientific evidence. By and large, market strategies have favored large providers, insurers, and investors over small providers, patients and other people.

While policy makers need to scrutinize market strategies for negative consequences, the strategies may sometimes have positive effects. Some may assist in raising efficiency and value for money in public systems. Medicine's government-granted monopoly status may help protect patients from unqualified practitioners, although it raises questions about who decides what professions do with their monopoly privileges. Consolidating services in institutions can take steps toward integrating clinical care, although it tends to remain departmentalized. Freestanding procedure units specializing in a few technologies may individually provide more efficient individual services at lower cost, although they tend to lower systemic efficiency and raise total costs. Integrating finance with delivery, as in health maintenance organizations (HMOs) and national health services, may rationalize total investment, but it may also impose rules of finance.

Market strategies have gained political ascendancy far beyond their potential benefits, however, and they have had many negative consequences. Theories of *competition* have become the rationale for business management, debt financing, and corporate ownership of medical care. Although there can be little *price* competition in an economy subsidized by insurance plans and government programs, investors and other economic interests have inflated technological capacity and luxury accommodation in the name of competition. The technology inflation has increased the risk of providers using the technologies excessively in order to keep their devices and themselves fully employed.

Defining all social problems in terms of market solutions, neoliberal theory since the 1960s has intensified market strategies and required that all human services conform to market principles. Its free-trade precept, which prohibits public policies that might threaten potential corporate profits, even to benefit peoples' health, subjugates social institutions (and peoples' health) to the interests of commerce. The Federal Trade Commission (FTC), for example, warned the American College of Radiology (ACR) that manufacturers of a radiation device had complained that ACR critique of the effectiveness of the device constituted restraint of trade.[3] The Ninth US Circuit Court extended the trade approach by upholding an argument that Certificate of Need imposed an unreasonable burden on commerce by impeding hospital participation in the medical market.[4]

The market revolution in medical care is a capital coup. The financial industry has expanded its insurance products, investments, bank loans, bond issues, and public offerings. It has required providers to make managerial decisions on the basis of financial analysis. It has privatized services, promoted conversion to for-profit status, and—where feasible—encouraged going "public" by selling stock on Wall Street. It was not surprising, a management professor wrote in 2003, that creditors, stockholders, and commercial sources of capital were actively reconfiguring medical care by forcing mergers, bankruptcies, and reorganizations.[5] Commercial financing meant that even nonprofit services put themselves "'in play' in the market for corporate control," the professor held, whether they realized it or not.

There is less of a boundary between for-profit and not-for-profit medical care than conventionally thought. Not-for-profit providers act like for-profit ones when they develop services and hire staff on the basis of revenue-generating potential, neglect nonremunerative services (and patients), debt finance growth, spin off for-profit entities, and invest surplus revenues in the financial markets. Financial rules requiring that each service unit support itself with its own revenues prioritize the bottom line: "No Margin, No Mission," as the aphorism goes. Yet margin building can sabotage missions and warp medical ethics itself.[6] Defining *value* in terms of technological and capital intensity has blocked dialogue and even thought about human *need*. The market valuation of everything sanctifies property rights over human rights.[7] Market strategies have undermined public policy and stifled alternative visions. Reforms that re-evaluate and offer alternatives to the market strategies are pivotal in creating better health care systems.

Re-Forming Health Care

Many books analyzing social problems end with an "obligatory prescription that is utopian, banal, unhelpful or out of tune with the rest of the book," an essayist once criticized.[8] Authors may neglect implications of their analyses because they have not (or have) recognized how deep the problems lay. Or they have discovered the extent to which change threatens powerful interests. Perhaps they are further advised that a less-than-upbeat conclusion might not market well. My conclusion (in tune with the rest of the book) is that democratic health reform needs to challenge the market strategies and reconstruct health care systems based on people's health needs and measured treatment effectiveness.

In contrast, contemporary US health policy is an assortment of professional aspirations, business interests, and market ideologies. Financial industry tactics have in large part substituted for public policy. With the "power to invest in or withdraw capital funds from the hospital industry," business school professor Patricia Arnold noted in 1991 (5 years after the demise of the national health planning program), "'Wall Street' became the new health planning agency."[9]

Financial interest in maintaining the private insurance industry and in sustaining the role that its bond purchases and service reimbursements play in directing the flow of capital in medical care have long dominated health-reform agendas. The Committee on the Costs of Medical Care in 1932 called for expanded private health insurance to pay for specialty services for middle-class populations.[10] Congress rejected a profusion of national health insurance bills up through the 1970s, after which reform proposals—including the Clinton administration's managed competition, the two Bush administrations' proposals, and Obamacare (the only one to pass after Medicare and Medicaid in 1965)—added complex epicycles to a fragmented insurance system that did not work well in the first place.

Although the Affordable Care Act (ACA, or Obamacare) reportedly added 20 million people to government and insurance rosters, many insured as well as uninsured Americans continued to experience frustration, anger, and stress when navigating the maze of health care plans, going into debt to pay medical bills and doing without needed care. Yet, in the economic climate of the early 21st century, national health insurance, not to mention a national health service, is almost unthinkable. Instead of national coordination, the United States has a set of weak regulatory tools (partially described in Chapter 10) at which opponents continually chip away—or worse. Public health reformers have generally favored incremental reforms implementing market-based strategies over "regime change,"[11] while ideologues have called for dismantling safety regulation and excluding large segments of the population.

Even when inspired by ideals of equity in terms of justice, many health care reforms have augmented investor equity. Obamacare was "going to make some people *very* rich," a former director of the Centers for Medicare and Medicaid Services enthused at a meeting of large investors.[12] Provisions that benefited companies designed to profit from the law, he advised, would transfer billions of dollars from Washington to Wall Street. This is just one of many examples of how the medical business converts our taxes into private wealth instead of public health. Revolving doors between business and governmental agencies such as the Centers for Medicare and Medicaid Services and the Food and Drug Administration inject business spokespeople and values directly into policy making and strongly impact health care regulation and reform. Wall Street is not only a major planning agent but is also a major beneficiary of the health care system. Debt financing is an important tactic for bringing services into the domain of capital. Large capital expenditures required by new hospitals and proton centers confer power on Wall Street to shape the organization, practice, and even the purpose of medical care. Reforms to expand public health would have to control capital investment.

"But that's not democratic!" an economist ejaculated when I informed him that state Certificate of Need (CoN) programs could deny costly hospital capital investments. He was committing a not uncommon fallacy of conflating *democracy* with protection of *free trade* and *private property*. (CoN does in fact aspire to democratic process when it names consumer majorities on its committees—although that is not enough.) The economist's concern was that CoN challenges the premise that privately owned hospitals (accepting public monies, which is virtually all of them) can invest in anything they find profitable.

Nonetheless, Certificate of Need programs can only react to hospital proposals to buy high-cost technologies or build high-cost services. In place of CoN's case-by-case review process, health reform could develop budget-based national, state-wide, and/or HMO-type delivery systems. Despite the present-day market ideology backlash against it, government is the route most open to reforming medical delivery along these lines. Private insurance, in contrast, has served to maintain the medical *status quo* and the interests of the financial industry. Government already is a major force in health care, paying for large portions of it and bestowing on it licensing, patenting, and bankruptcy protections.

The simplest system-wide reform would include everyone in a publicly administered and funded Medicare-type single-payer system. Single payer could advance equality of access while eliminating the confusion and high administrative costs of existing insurance products.[13] But—although it would be a major accomplishment—it would not be sufficient. It would still need to ensure effectiveness and safety. Effectiveness-based health reform would ask what kinds and what combination of services best contribute to people's health. Addressing these issues would be a major accomplishment.

Initiating such an undertaking means asking fundamental questions about the structure of the existing medical care system: How might health care personnel and services be better organized? How many and which categories of specialists should be trained? Are the most highly specialized and highly equipped services best? What would be an appropriate ratio of medical specialists to primary care personnel, including nurses and other health care professionals? What accountability should be required in exchange for the grant of professional monopoly? How many and which specialty procedure units should be provided in hospitals, outside of hospitals, or as hospitals in themselves? What does the evidence show about consolidating services in large complexes? Should health care institutions design their services for the purpose of generating income? If not, how do they survive? What would be required to control excessive medical care growth? How can conflicts of interest be mitigated (or eliminated)? Should the diffusion of medical devices be regulated? How many of which devices do nations really need? What would it take to align medical intervention with scientific evidence? How can services become more effective *and* more equitably distributed? What is the evidence regarding the effect of competition on health care? How do we educate ourselves about health and health care in the face of misleading advertisements? Should law require truth in hospital and medical advertising? Can private insurance companies and private medical facilities meet health needs? Should investors, corporations, universities, and/or physicians own medical facilities? And, finally, who should control capital investment in health care and how? While these questions may invoke the specter of *rationing* in the sense of reducing oversupply, overtreatment, and luxury accoutrements, they challenge the current use of *price* as a ruthless rationing tool.

In addition to engaging in public policy debate as health care citizens, we can participate in our personal care choices as consumers in the marketplace and as medical patients. We might ask doctors questions such as: How do you know the treatment you use is a good idea? What is the evidence of benefit? What are the risks? What outcomes do your patients experience? Would they choose the treatment again? What are your specialty's practice standards and what evidence supports them? Doctors need to develop a willingness to discuss such questions with patients (without writing "troublemaker" into their medical records). At the same time, doctors as well as patients recognize that they often have to make critical choices on the basis of inadequate evidence.

Open to some of these questions, at least, Meaghan's radiation oncologist told her that it was not clear whether she'd benefit from radiation after her mastectomy because the pathologist had reported breast-cancer cells in adjacent lymph nodes. Since different doctors recommend different protocols under these circumstances, the oncologist said, the decision was Meaghan's call. Having rapidly become a well-informed patient, Meaghan knew she was weighing potential long-term radiation damage to her lungs, heart, and bones against the anxiety that she might not have done all she could to treat her cancer. She chose to have the treatment, after which her chest tissues were so damaged from radiation that they broke down and became seriously infected following an implant, leading to hospitalization and several more reconstructive surgeries.[14]

With little other recourse available, some patients (and their lawyers) resort to suing doctors and/or hospitals when they suffer harm from medical treatment. But malpractice claims must be based on negligence, which is defined as deviation from standard practice. This provision (partly) protects doctors from lawsuits regarding adverse patient outcomes beyond their control. While errors make the news and can generate huge monetary settlements, many adverse outcomes in medical care result not from deviance but from standard practices themselves.

There is a tension, even a discord, between decision making at the individual level and at the population level. It's one thing to hold that most patients under particular circumstances should or should not receive radiation. It's quite another to identify which patients. Even in situations of inadequate evidence—which describes large segments of medical care—individual doctors and individual patients must decide whether or not to choose particular treatments. The default position in these situations should not necessarily be in favor of treatment. Doctors (and their consensus development conferences) have generally not perceived the extent to which medical specialties have historically been built on (or despite) insufficient evidence, as this history describes for one specialty.

Perhaps many of us would prefer to trust that our doctors have a solid knowledge of all the relevant evidence and the ability to apply it judiciously. But this is asking a lot; it may be asking too much of a technology-based profession where hidden assumptions lie beneath evidence interpretations and practice standards. Rather than putting the entire burden on individual doctors and patients, we need to build ways to bring physician, patient, and public health representatives together to develop (flexible) ways to handle complex clinical situations.

Tackling the individual and institutional questions also requires confronting market strategies. Patients might further ask their doctors: Who is benefitting financially from my getting the recommended treatment? Do you get paid more if you perform a particular procedure on me? Have you or any of your partners invested financially in the equipment you use or refer patients to? Do you or the institutions you affiliate with receive any compensation from companies that sell medical supplies, devices, or drugs that you use? Do your specialty group, hospital department, academic practice plan, and/or corporate organization pressure you to increase your productivity? Do they encourage you to use more surgical or technological procedures? Has your medical group or institution borrowed heavily to purchase equipment? Since most of the market strategies are structural, however, they are beyond the scope of questions of individuals. (Emphasis on individual patient questions in fact reinforces a market/consumer approach.) Furthermore, market systems offer no accountable agents to direct questions to.

Although market advocates employ the phrase "consumer-driven," they do not mean people actively demanding answers to questions like the ones listed here or participating in decision making about health care. Instead, they mean people passively shaping health care via purchasing decisions. Market theories camouflage the role of *power*. What leaders really mean by market reform is control by the most powerful and wealthy interests in the market. In the case of medical care, this means control by major medical centers, research universities, specialty associations, manufacturers, insurance companies, corporate employers, and financial firms—along with their think tanks and lobby groups.

In concentrating the power and wealth of providers, payers, and investors, market strategies have diminished the capacity of a nation's people to build a system dedicated to their health. Noting that the strategies listed in Table 11.1 remain incompletely implemented, market advocates have continued to prescribe them. They have continued to promote managerial and financial methods and to champion the assimilation of medical care into the corporate domain.

Health care reform finally needs to ask wider questions: Who benefits from the contemporary medical business system, and how can we build more effective, equitable, and efficient health care systems? Collectively, we can put efficacy and population need on the reform agenda. Although medical care was never as different from the commercial economy as it likes to think, it has nonetheless expressed visions and values of *service*. Patients, physicians, and the public working together democratically just might be able to redirect national investment toward effective health care as well as toward educational and employment opportunities that so strongly impact people's health. Yet it is all too easy to fall into the current of dominant thought. As warned in the book *Healthy, Wealthy, and Fair*, "market thinking filters into the calculations of the very interests who normally lead the charge for social justice."[15] I can only hope that we will empower ourselves to overthrow the market strategies and choose health over wealth.

Notes

1 Stuart Friedman, "Market Memo: Opportunities for Growth Exist amid Niche Facilities, (Carve Outs)," *Health Care Strategic Management* 20 (2002): 1, 17–19.

2 An estimated 29 percent of all US cancer deaths have been attributed to smoking. *New York Times* November 1, 2016, D3. A suggestion at a meeting of the National Cancer Advisory Board of the National Cancer Institute that it take a stand against NIH funding of universities accepting money from the tobacco industry resulted only in nervous laughter. 141st Meeting, Bethesda, MD, February 6, 2007.

3 Otha W. Linton, *The American College of Radiology: The First 75 Years* (Reston, VA: ACR, 1997), 151.

4 Anna Oh, "Ninth Circuit Rules that State Certificate of Need Laws May Unconstitutionally Burden Interstate Commerce," *American Journal of Law & Medicine* 37 (2011): 684–686.

5 J. B. Silvers, "The Role of the Capital Markets in Restructuring Health Care," In Peter J. Hammer, Deborah Haas-Wilson, Mark A. Peterson, and William M. Sage, eds., *Uncertain Times: Kenneth Arrow and the Changing Economics of Health Care* (Durham, NC: Duke University Press, 2003), 156–166.

6 Barbara Bridgman Perkins, "Accumulating Resources in Perinatal Intensive Care Centers," *Business and Professional Ethics Journal* 12 (1993): 51–66; Robert Martinsen, "The History of Bioethics: An Essay Review," *Journal of the History of Medicine and Allied Sciences* 56 (2001): 168–175.

7 Kean Birch and Vlad Mykhnenko, eds., *The Rise and Fall of Neoliberalism: The Collapse of an Economic Order?* (London: Zed Books, 2010), 8; Colin Crouch, *The Strange Non-Death of Neoliberalism* (Cambridge: Polity, 2011), 16, 167, 176.

8 David Greenberg, "No Exit," *New York Times Book Review* March 20, 2011, 31.

9 Patricia J. Arnold, "The Invisible Hand in Health Care: The Rise of Financial Markets in the U.S. Hospital Industry," In John L. Campbell, J. Rogers Hollingsworth, and Leon N. Lindberg, eds., *Governance in the American Economy* (Cambridge: Cambridge University Press, 1991), 293–316.

10 Barbara Bridgman Perkins, "Economic Organization of Medicine and the Committee on the Costs of Medical Care," *American Journal of Public Health* 88 (1998): 1721–1726.

11 Carl E. Ameringer, *The Health Care Revolution: From Medical Monopoly to Market Competition* (Berkeley, CA: University of California Press, 2008), 205–208.

12 Adam Davidson, "Who is Betting on Obamacare?" *New York Times Magazine* November 3, 2013, 36–39, 57, 60, 63, emphasis original.

13 Steffie Woolhandler, Terry Campbell, and David U. Himmelstein, "Costs of Health Care Administration in the United States and Canada," *New England Journal of Medicine* 349 (2003): 768–775.

14 Meaghan Campbell, personal communication, November 29, 2016.

15 James A. Morone and Lawrence R. Jacobs, *Healthy, Wealthy, and Fair: Health Care and the Good Society* (Oxford: Oxford University Press, 2005), 11.

Acknowledgments

I would especially like to thank Guy Alchon, Howard Berliner, Theodore Brown, Meaghan Campbell, Anne Cassia, Juliana Froggatt, Jennifer Gunn, Debora Holmes, George Irwin, Bruce Jennings, Gretchen Kruger, Gerald Kutcher, Martha Livingston, Cheri Lucas-Jennings, Penny MacElveen-Hoehn, Joan Marx, Ivan Perkins, John Perkins, Karen Reeds, Barbara Katz Rothman, Rosemary Stevens, and the late John Pickstone and Renate Wilson for their encouragement and engagement one way or another with this work. Thanks also to the helping librarians and archivists at Harvard University; Massachusetts Institute of Technology; National Library of Medicine; New York Academy of Medicine; Schenectady Museum Archives; Stanford University; University of California, Berkeley; University of California, Los Angeles; University of California, San Francisco; University of Washington; and Wellcome Library. Finally, I am grateful for the public availability of the Internet.

Selected Bibliography

I list here archival collections (first section) and printed scholarly publications (second section). Online sources, specific archival items, and magazine, newspaper, and newsletter articles may be found in the notes.

Archival Collections

American Research and Development Corporation. MC 495. Institute Archives and Special Collections. Massachusetts Institute of Technology, Cambridge, MA.

Buechner, William W., Papers, 1928–1978. MC 229. Institute Archives and Special Collections. Massachusetts Institute of Technology, Cambridge, MA.

General Electric Archives. Schenectady Museum Archives, Schenectady, NY.

Ginzton, Edward, Papers. SC 330. Special Collections and University Archives. Stanford University Libraries, Palo Alto, CA.

Harvard University Cancer Commission. Publications for the Collis P.Huntington Memorial Hospital, 1913–1952. HUF 260.875. Harvard University Archives, Cambridge, MA.

Health and Hospital Planning Council of Southern New York Collection. Rare Book Room, New York Academy of Medicine, New York, NY.

High Voltage Engineering Corporation Records. MC153. Institute Archives and Special Collections. Massachusetts Institute of Technology, Cambridge, MA.

Kaplan, Henry S., Papers. SC 317. Special Collections and University Archives. Stanford University Libraries, Palo Alto, CA.

Lawrence, Ernest O., Papers. BANC FILM 2248. The Bancroft Library. University of California, Berkeley, CA.

Puget Sound Health Systems Agency Archives. Special Collections Division. University of Washington Libraries, Seattle, WA.

Stone, Robert S., Papers, 1940–1956. BANC MSS 80/80 c. The Bancroft Library. University of California, Berkeley, CA.

Terman, Frederick Emmons, Papers. SC160. Special Collections and University Archives. Stanford University Libraries, Palo Alto, CA.

Trump, John, Papers, 1937–1981. MC 223. Institute Archives and Special Collections. Massachusetts Institute of Technology, Cambridge, MA

Twight, Janet Dana, Papers. Special Collections Division. University of Washington Libraries, Seattle, WA.

Varian, Russell and Sigurd, Papers. SC 345. Special Collections and University Archives. Stanford University Libraries, Palo Alto, CA.

Varian, Inc., Records. SC 889. Special Collections and University Archives. Stanford University Libraries, Palo Alto, CA.

Young, Owen D., Papers. Schenectady Museum Archives, Schenectady, NY.

Books, Chapters, Dissertations, Journal Articles, and Reports

Ablin, Richard J. *The Great Prostate Hoax: How Big Medicine Hijacked the PSA Test and Caused a Public Health Disaster*. With Ronald Piana. New York: Palgrave Macmillan, 2014.

Abramson, John. *Overdo$ed America: The Broken Promise of American Medicine*. New York: HarperCollins, 2004.

Ackerly, D. Clay, Ana M. Valverde, Lawrence W. Diener, K. L. Dossary, and K. A. Schulman. "Fueling Innovation in Medical Devices (and Beyond): Venture Capital in Health Care." *Health Affairs* 28 (2009): w68–w75.

Adair, F. E. "The Results of Treatment of Mammary Carcinoma by Surgical and Irradiation Methods at the Memorial Hospital, New York City, during the Decade 1916 to 1926." *Annals of Surgery* 95 (1932): 410–424.

Advisory Committee on Human Radiation Experiments. *Final Report of the Advisory Committee on Human Radiation Experiments*. New York: Oxford University Press, 1996.

Allen, Aaron M., Todd Pawlicki, Lei Dong, et al. "An Evidence Based Review of Proton Beam Therapy: The Report of ASTRO's Emerging Technology Committee." *Radiotherapy and Oncology* 103 (2012): 8–11.

Allt, W. E. C. "Supervoltage Radiation Treatment in Advanced Cancer of the Uterine Cervix." *Canadian Medical Association Journal* 100 (1969): 792–797.

Almond, Peter R. *Cobalt Blues: The Story of Leonard Grimmett, the Man behind the First Cobalt-60 Unit in the United States*. New York: Springer, 2013.

Altintig, Z. Ayca, Hsin-Hui Chiu, and M. Sinan Goktan. "How Does Uncertainty Resolution Affect VC Syndication?" *Financial Management* 42 (2013): 611–646.

American College of Radiology, "Guidelines for Determining Standards of Radiotherapy in Approved Cancer Centers," Chicago: American College of Radiology, 1964.

Ameringer, Carl E. *The Health Care Revolution: From Medical Monopoly to Market Competition*. Berkeley: University of California Press, 2008.

Andersen, Ronald, and John F. Newman. "Societal and Individual Determinants of Medical Care Utilization in the United States." *Milbank Quarterly* 83 (2005): 1–28.

Anderson, Julie, Francis Neary, and John V. Pickstone. *Surgeons, Manufacturers and Patients*. In collaboration with James Raferty. Basingstoke, Hampshire: Palgrave Macmillan, 2007.

Ante, Spencer E. Creative Capital: Georges Doriot and the Birth of Venture Capital. Boston: Harvard Business Press, 2008.

Arnold, Patricia J. "The Invisible Hand in Health Care: The Rise of Financial Markets in the U.S. Hospital Industry." In *Governance in the American Economy*, ed. John L. Campbell, J. Rogers Hollingsworth, and Leon N. Lindberg, 293–316. Cambridge: Cambridge University Press, 1991.

Arns, Robert G. "The High-Vacuum X-Ray Tube: Technological Change in Social Context." *Technology and Culture* 38 (1997): 852–890.

Aronowitz, Jesse N., and Roger F. Robison. "Howard Kelly Establishes Gynecologic Brachytherapy in the United States." *Brachytherapy* 9 (2010): 178–184.

Aronowitz, Robert. "'Screening' for Prostate Cancer in New York's Skid Row: History and Implications." *American Journal of Public Health* 104 (2014): 70–76.

Aronowitz, Robert. *Unnatural History: Breast Cancer and American Society*. Cambridge: Cambridge University Press, 2007.

Arrow, Kenneth J. "Uncertainty and the Welfare Economics of Medical Care." *American Economic Review* 53 (1963): 941–973.

Bagshaw, Malcolm A., and Henry S. Kaplan. "Supervoltage Linear Accelerator Radiation Therapy VIII: Retinoblastoma." *Radiology* 86 (1966): 242–246.

Barnes, John. *Failure of Government Central Planning: Washington's Medical Certificate of Need Program*. Seattle: Washington Policy Center, 2006.

Barnhard, Howard J. "Supervoltage Therapy Comes of Age: A Report for the Practicing Physician." *New England Journal of Medicine* 258 (1958): 275–277.

Barr, Donald A. *Introduction to U.S. Health Policy: The Organization, Financing, and Delivery of Health Care in America*. Baltimore: Johns Hopkins University Press, 2011.

Bentzen, Søren M., Germaine Heeren, Brian Cottier, Ben Slotman, Bengt Glimelius, Yolande Lievens, and Walter van den Bogaert. "Towards Evidence-Based Guidelines for Radiotherapy Infrastructure and Staffing Needs in Europe: The ESTRO QUARTS Project." *Radiotherapy and Oncology* 75 (2005): 355–365.

Berenson, Robert A., Thomas Bodenheimer, and Hoangmai H. Pham. "Specialty-Service Lines: Salvos in the New Medical Arms Race." *Health Affairs* 25 (2006): w337–w343.

Berman, L. Todd, and G. Pierce Taylor. *Radiation Therapy in Connecticut*. North Haven: Connecticut Hospital Planning Commission, 1972.

Berwick, Donald M., and Andrew D. Hackbarth. "Eliminating Waste in U.S. Health Care." *JAMA* 307 (2012): 1512–1516.

Berlant, Jeffrey Lionel. *Profession and Monopoly: A Study of Medicine in the United States and Great Britain*. Berkeley: University of California Press, 1975.

Berrington de Gonzalez, Amy, Rochelle E. Curtis, Stephen F. Kry, Ethel Gilbert, Stephanie Lamart, Christine D. Berg. Marilyn Stovall, and Elaine Ron. "Proportion of Second Cancers Attributable to Radiotherapy Treatment in Adults: A Cohort Study in the US SEER Cancer Registries." *Lancet Oncology* 12 (2011): 353–360.

Birch, Kean, and Vlad Mykhnenko, eds. The Rise and Fall of Neoliberalism: The Collapse of an Economic Order? London: Zed Books, 2010.

Birr, Kendall. Pioneering in Industrial Research: The Story of the General Electric Research Laboratory. Washington DC: Public Affairs, 1957.

Blume, Stuart S. Insight and Industry: On the Dynamics of Technological Change in Medicine. Cambridge, MA: MIT Press, 1992.

Boelling, Tobias, Stefan Koenemann, Iris Ernst, and Normann Willich. "Late Effects of Thoracic Irradiation in Children." *Strahlentherapie und Onkologie* 184 (2008): 289–295.

Boice, John D., and Lois B. Travis. "Body Wars: Effect of Friendly Fire (Cancer Therapy)." *Journal of the National Cancer Institute* 87 (1995): 705–706.

Boone, Max L. M., John H. Lawrence, William G. Connor, Richard Morgado, John A. Hicks, and Richard C. Brown. "Introduction to the Use of Protons and Heavy Ions in Radiation Therapy: Historical Perspective." *International Journal of Radiation Oncology Biology Physics* 3 (1977): 65–69.

Borchmann, Peter, Dennis A. Eichenauer, and Andreas Engert. "State of the Art in the Treatment of Hodgkin Lymphoma." *Nature Reviews Clinical Oncology* 9 (2012): 450–459.

Bosk, Charles. *Forgive and Remember: Managing Clinical Failure*. Chicago: University of Chicago Press, 1979.

Brada, Michael, Madelon Pijls-Johannesma, and Dirk De Ruysscher. "Proton Therapy in Clinical Practice: Current Clinical Evidence." *Journal of Clinical Oncology* 25 (2007): 965–970.

Brady, Luther W., Simon Kramer, Seymour H. Levitt, R. G. Parker, and W. E. Powers. "Radiation Oncology: Contributions of the United States in the Last Years of the 20th Century." *Radiology* 219 (2001):1–5.

Brawley, Otis Webb. *How We Do Harm: A Doctor Breaks Ranks about Being Sick in America*. With Paul Goldberg. New York: St. Martin's Griffin, 2011.

Brecher, Ruth, and Edward Brecher. *The Rays: A History of Radiology in the United States and Canada*. Baltimore: Williams and Wilkins, 1969.

Brown, A. P., M. M. Urie, R. Chisin, , and H. D. Suit . "Proton Therapy for Carcinoma of the Nasopharynx: A Study in Comparative Treatment Planning." *International Journal of Radiation Oncology Biology Physics* 16 (1989): 1607–1614.

Brown, Frank A., and Henry S. Kaplan. "Hodgkin's Disease: A Revised Clinical Classification and an Approach to the Treatment of Its Localized Form." *Stanford Medical Bulletin* 15 (1957): 183–192.

Brown, G. Stephen, David F. Herring, William E. Powers, Simon Kramer, Lawrence W. Davis, Charles J. MacLean. "Patterns of Care in American Radiation Therapy, 1973–1975." *International Journal of Radiation Oncology Biology Physics* 7, supplement 1 (1981): 105–106.

Brownlee, Shannon. *Overtreated: Why Too Much Medicine Is Making Us Sicker and Poorer*. New York: Bloomsbury, 2007.

Bruce, W. R., and C. L. Ash. "Survival of Patients Treated for Cancer of the Breast, Cervix, Lung, and Upper Respiratory Tract at the Ontario-Cancer-Institute (Toronto) from 1930 to 1957." *Radiology* 81 (1963): 861–870.

Bruère, Robert W. "The Swope Plan and After." *Survey* 67 (1932): 583–585, 647–648, 653.

Burchenal, Joseph H. and Herbert F. Oettgen, eds. *Cancer: Achievements, Challenges, and Prospects for the 1980s, volume 2*. New York: Grune and Stratton, 1981.

Burr, R. C., E. N. MacKay, and A. H. Sellers. "Radiation Therapy in Treatment of Carcinoma of Lung." *Canadian Medical Association Journal* 88 (1963): 1181–1184.

Burrill, E. Alfred. "Van de Graaff Accelerators for Radiation Research and Applications." In *Radiation Sources*, ed. A. Charlesby, 85–127. New York: Macmillan/ Pergamon, 1964.

Busby, S. M. "The Cobalt Bomb in the Treatment of Bladder Tumours." *Canadian Medical Association Journal* 73 (1955): 872–875.

Buschke, Franz, ed. *Progress in Radiation Therapy*. New York: Grune and Stratton, 1958.

Buschke, Franz, Simeon T. Cantril, and Herbert M. Parker. *Supervoltage Roentgentherapy*. Springfield, IL: Charles C. Thomas, 1950.

Buschke, Franz, and George Jack. "Twenty-Five Years' Experience with Super-voltage Therapy in the Treatment of Transitional Cell Carcinoma of the Bladder." *American Journal of Roentgenology, Radium Therapy, and Nuclear Medicine* 99 (1967): 387–392.

Byhardt, Roger W., James D. Cox, J. Frank Wilson, Joseph Libnoch, and Richard S. Stein. "Total Body Irradiation vs. Chemotherapy as a Systemic Adjuvant for Small Cell Carcinoma of the Lung." *International Journal of Radiation Oncology Biology Physics* 5 (1979): 2043–2048.

California Tumor Registry. *Cancer Registration and Survival in California*. Berkeley: State of California Department of Public Health, 1963.

Campbell, John L., J. Rogers Hollingsworth, and Leon N. Lindberg, eds. *Governance in the American Economy*. Cambridge: Cambridge University Press, 1991.

Cantor, David. "Cancer, Quackery and the Vernacular Meanings of Hope in 1950s America." *Journal of the History of Medicine and Allied Sciences* 61 (2006): 324–368.

Cantor, David. "Radium and the Origins of the National Cancer Institute." In *Biomedicine in the Twentieth Century:* Practices, *Policies, and Politics*, ed. Caroline Hannaway, 95–146. Amsterdam: IOS, 2008.

Carpender, J. W. J. "Supervoltage: Should We Junk 250 kv? A Symposium." *Radiology* 67 (1956): 481–515.

Case, James T. "The Early History of Radium Therapy and the American Radium Society." *American Journal of Roentgenology, Radiation Therapy and Nuclear Medicine* 82 (1959): 574–585.

Case, James T. "History of Radiation Therapy." In *Progress in Radiation Therapy*, ed. Franz Buschke, 13-41. New York: Grune and Stratton, 1958.

Case, James T. "Some Early Experiences in Therapeutic Radiology: Formation of the American Radium Society." *American Journal of Roentgenology and Radium Therapy* 70 (1953): 487–491.

Caulfield, Catherine. *Multiple Exposures: Chronicles of the Radiation Age.* Chicago: University of Chicago Press, 1989.

Chandler, Alfred D. *The Visible Hand: The Managerial Revolution in American Business.* Cambridge, MA: Harvard University Press, 1977.

Charlesby, A., ed. *Radiation Sources*. New York: Macmillan/Pergamon, 1964.

Charlton, E. E., W. F. Westendorp, L. E. Dempster, and George Hotaling. "A Million-Volt X-Ray Unit." *Radiology* 35 (1940): 585–597.

Cheriex, Kiki C. A. L., Tim H. J. Nijhuis, and Marc A. M. Mureau. "Osteoradionecrosis of the Jaws: A Review of Conservative and Surgical Treatment Options." *Journal of Reconstructive Microsurgery* 29 (2013): 69–75.

Childs, Herbert. *An American Genius: The Life of Ernest Orlando Lawrence*. New York: E. P. Dutton, 1968.

Chou, Roger, Jennifer M. Croswell, Tracy Dana, et al. "Screening for Prostate Cancer: A Review of the Evidence for the U.S. Preventive Services Task Force." *Annals of Internal Medicine* 155 (2011): 762–771.

Clark, R. Lee. and Clifton D. Howe. *Cancer Patient Care at M. D. Anderson Hospital and Tumor Institute*. Chicago: Year Book Medical Publishers, 1976.

Cleveland Hospital Council. *Cleveland Hospital and Health Survey, Part Ten: Hospitals and Dispensaries*. Cleveland: Cleveland Hospital Council, 1920.

Cochran, Thomas C. *The American Business System: A Historical Perspective, 1900–1955.* New York: Harper and Row, 1957.

Coia, Lawrence R., and Gerald E. Hanks. "Quality Assessment in the USA: How the Patterns of Care Study Has Made a Difference." *Seminars in Radiation Oncology* 7 (1997): 146–156.

Committee for Radiation Therapy Studies. *A Proposal for Integrated Cancer Management in the United States: The Role of Radiation Oncology*. Bethesda, MD: National Cancer Institute, 1972.

Committee for Radiation Therapy Studies. *A Prospect for Radiation Therapy in the United States, Final Report*. Bethesda, MD: National Institutes of Health, 1968.

Connors, Joseph M. Review of *Henry Kaplan and the Story of Hodgkin's Disease*, by Charlotte DeCroes Jacobs. *Journal of the History of Medicine and Allied Sciences* 67 (2012): 501–504.

Coolidge, W. D. "The Development of Modern Roentgen-Ray Generating Apparatus." *American Journal of Roentgenology and Radium Therapy* 24 (1930): 605–620.

Cooter, Roger. "The Politics of a Spatial Innovation: Fracture Clinics in Inter-war Britain." In *Medical Innovations in Historical Perspective*, ed. John V. Pickstone, 146–164. New York: St. Martin's, 1992.

Costolow, William E. "Radiation Therapy in Extensive Bladder Carcinoma." *California and Western Medicine* 56 (1942): 247–248.

Coutrakon, G. B. "Accelerators for Heavy-Charged Particle Radiation Therapy." *Technology in Cancer Research and Treatment* 6 (2007): 49–54.

Cox, James D., and Simon Kramer. "Strategic Plan for Radiologic Sciences: Outcome Analysis." *Cancer Treatment Symposia* 1 (1984): 169–175.

Creager, Angela N. H. *Life Atomic: A History of Radioisotopes in Science and Medicine*. Chicago: University of Chicago Press, 2013.

Crouch, Colin. *The Strange Non-death of Neoliberalism*. Cambridge: Polity, 2011.

Daly, Jeanne. *Evidence-Based Medicine and the Search for a Science of Clinical Care*. Berkeley: University of California Press, 2005.

Davis, Devra. *The Secret History of the War on Cancer*. New York: Basic Books, 2007.

Davis, Karen, Kristof Stremikis, David Squires, and Cathy Schoen. *Mirror, Mirror, on the Wall: How the U.S. Health Care System Compares Internationally*. New York: Commonwealth Fund, 2014.

Davis, Michael M., and Mary C. Jarrett. *A Health Inventory of New York City*. New York: Welfare Council of New York City, 1929.

Delaney, Thomas F., and Hanne M. Kooy, eds. *Proton and Charged Particle Radiotherapy*. Philadelphia: Wolters Kluwer, 2008.

Delanian, Sylvie, Jean-Louis Lefaix, and Pierre-Francois Pradat. "Radiation-Induced Neuropathy in Cancer Survivors." *Radiotherapy and Oncology* 105 (2012): 273–282.

Delclos, Luis, and Edward J. Quinlan. "Malignant Tumors of the Ovary Managed with Postoperative Megavoltage Irradiation." *Radiology* 93 (1969): 659–663.

Del Regato, Juan A. "Albert Soiland and the Early Development of Therapeutic Radiology in the United States." *International Journal of Radiation Oncology Biology Physics* 9 (1983): 243–254.

Del Regato, Juan A. *Radiological Oncologists: The Unfolding of a Medical Specialty*. Reston, VA: Radiology Centennial, 1993.

DeVita, Vincent T., and Elizabeth DeVita-Raeburn. *The Death of Cancer*. New York: Farrar, Straus and Giroux, 2015.

DeVita, Vincent T., Jane E. Henney, and Susan M. Hubbard. "Estimation of the Numerical and Economic Impact of Chemotherapy in the Treatment of Cancer." In *Cancer: Achievements, Challenges, and Prospects for the 1980s*, ed. Joseph H. Burchenal and Herbert F. Oettgen, vol. 2, 859–880. New York: Grune and Stratton, 1981.

Deyo, Richard A. "Gaps, Tensions, and Conflicts in the FDA Approval Process: Implications for Clinical Practice." *Journal of the American Board of Family Practice* 17 (2004): 142–149.

Diller, Wendy. "How Varian Medical Stays on Top." *Windhover's In Vivo: The Business and Medicine Report* 21 (2003): 1–8.

Dingell, John D. "Letter of Transmittal." For *Medical Device Regulation: The FDA's Neglected Child*. Washington DC: USGPO, 1983.

Domhoff, G. William. *The Bohemian Grove and Other Retreats: A Study in Ruling-class Cohesiveness*. New York: Harper and Row, 1974.

Dommann, Monika. "From Danger to Risk: The Perception and Regulation of X-Rays in Switzerland, 1896–1970." In *The Risks of Medical Innovation: Risk Perception and*

Assessment in Historical Context, ed. Thomas Schlich and Ulrich Tröhler, 93–115. London: Routledge, 2006.

Donzé, Pierre-Yves. "Making Medicine a Business in Japan: Shimadzu Co. and the Diffusion of Radiology (1900–1960)." *Gesnerus* 67 (2010): 241–262.

Dresser, Richard, and Jack Spencer. "Physical and Clinical Observations on the Use of Million-Volt X-Rays." *New England Journal of Medicine* 218 (1938): 415–417.

Drucker, Peter F. *Innovation and Entrepreneurship: Practices and Principles*. New York: Harper and Row, 1985.

Early Breast Cancer Trialists' Collaborative Group [EBCTCG]. "Effect of Radiotherapy after Breast-Conserving Surgery on 10-Year Recurrence and 15-Year Breast Cancer Death: Meta-analysis of Individual Patient Data for 10,801 Women in 17 Randomised Trials." *Lancet* 378 (2011): 1707–1716.

Ebert, Robert H. "The Role of the Medical School in Planning the Health-Care System." *Journal of Medical Education* 42 (1967): 481–488.

Edwards, Rebecca. *New Spirits: Americans in the Gilded Age, 1865–1905*. New York: Oxford University Press, 2006.

Egilman, David, Wes Wallace, Cassandra Stubbs, and Fernando Mora-Corrasco. "A Little Too Much of the Buchenwald Touch? Military Radiation Research at the University of Cincinnati, 1960-1972." *Accountability in Research* 6 (1998): 63–102.

Ellwood, Paul M., Walter J. McClure, and John C. Rosala. *How Business Interacts with the Health Care System*. Washington DC: National Chamber Foundation, 1978.

Emanuel, Ezekiel J., and Victor R. Fuchs. "The Perfect Storm of Overutilization." *JAMA* 299 (2008): 2789–2791.

Emanuel, Ezekiel J., and Daniel Steiner. "Institutional Conflict of Interest." *New England Journal of Medicine* 332 (1995): 262–268.

Etzkowitz, Henry. *MIT and the Rise of Entrepreneurial Science*. New York: Routledge, 2002.

Evans, Thomas W. *The Education of Ronald Reagan: The General Electric Years and the Untold Story of His Conversion to Conservatism*. New York: Columbia University Press, 2006.

Ewing, James. "Early Experiences in Radiation Therapy." *American Journal of Roentgenology and Radium Therapy* 31 (1934): 153–163.

Ewing, James. "Radium Therapy in Cancer." *Journal of the American Medical Association* 68 (1917): 1238–1247.

Falit, Benjamin P., Cary P. Gross, and Kenneth B. Roberts. "Integrated Prostate Cancer Centers and Over-utilization of IMRT: A Close Look at Fee-for-Service Medicine in Radiation Oncology." *International Journal of Radiation Oncology Biology Physics* 76 (2010): 1285–1288.

Farmer, F. T. "Supervoltage Therapy—a Review of Present Day Facilities and Techniques." *Physics in Medicine and Biology* 6 (1962): 505–531.

Farrell, Diana, Eric Jensen, and Bob Kocher. *Accounting for the Cost of Health Care in the United States: A New Look at Why Americans Spend More*. New York, McKinsey Global Institute, 2008.

Findley, Palmer. "Complications and Disappointments in Radium Therapy for Cancer of the Uterus." *Canadian Medical Association Journal* 32 (1935): 154–161.

Finkelstein, Stan N., and Kevin Neels. "Self-Referral by Physicians." *New England Journal of Medicine* 328 (1993): 1274.

Fishman, Elliot A. "MIT Patent Policy, 1932–1946: Historical Precedents in University-Industry Technology Transfer." PhD diss., University of Pennsylvania, 1996.

Fletcher, Gilbert H. "Cobalt-60 in Management of Cancer." *Journal of the American Medical Association* 183 (1963): 103–108.

Fletcher, Gilbert H. "Present Status of Cobalt-60 Teletherapy in the Management of the Cancer Patient." *Journal of the American Medical Association* 164 (1957): 244–248.

Fletcher, Gilbert. "Supervoltage Roentgentherapy: Clinical Evaluation Based on 2,000 Cases." *Texas State Journal of Medicine* 55 (1959): 676–683.

Fletcher, Gilbert H. *Textbook of Radiotherapy*. Philadelphia: Lea and Febiger, 1966.

Fletcher, Gilbert H., and Felix N. Rutledge. "Over-all Results in Radiotherapy for Carcinoma of the Cervix." *Clinical Obstetrics and Gynecology* 10 (1967) 958–964.

Fletcher, Gilbert H., and Edgar C. White. "Possibilities of Supervoltage Roentgenotherapy in the Management of Cancer of the Breast." *Southern Medical Journal* 52 (1959): 805–812.

Fletcher, Gilbert H., Tongpoon Watanavit, and Felix N. Rutledge. "Whole-Pelvis Irradiation with 4,000 Rads in Stage I and Stage II Cancers of the Uterine Cervix." *Radiology* 86 (1966): 436–443.

Freedman, Benjamin. "Equipoise and the Ethics of Clinical Research." *New England Journal of Medicine* 317 (1987): 141–145.

Freidson, Eliot. *Profession of Medicine: A Study of the Sociology of Applied Knowledge*. New York: Harper and Row, 1970.

Friedman, Milton. "Concepts of Radical Irradiation Therapy." *CA: A Cancer Journal for Clinicians* 5 (1955): 20–28.

Friedman, M. "The Light Is Better Here." *American Journal of Roentgenology, Radium Therapy and Nuclear Medicine* 102 (1968): 3–7.

Friedman, Milton. "Supervoltage (One Million Volt) Roentgen Therapy at Walter Reed General Hospital." *Surgical Clinics of North America* 24 (1944): 1424–1432.

Friedman, Milton, Marshall Brucer, and Elizabeth Anderson, eds. *Roentgens, Rads, and Riddles, a Symposium on Supervoltage Radiation Therapy*. Oak Ridge, TN: Medical Division, Oak Ridge Institute of Nuclear Studies, 1956.

Friedman, Stuart. "Market Memo: Opportunities for Growth Exist amid Niche Facilities, (Carve Outs)." *Health Care Strategic Management* 20 (2002): 1, 17–19.

Fuller, Lillian M. "Results of Large Volume Irradiation in the Management of Hodgkin's Disease and Malignant Lymphomas Originating in the Abdomen." *Radiology* 87 (1966) 1058–1064.

Fuller, Lillian M., and Gilbert H. Fletcher. "The Radiotherapeutic Management of the Lymphomatous Diseases." *American Journal of Roentgenology, Radium Therapy and Nuclear Medicine* 88 (1962): 909–923.

Gabriel, Joseph M. *Medical Monopoly: Intellectual Property Rights and the Origins of the Modern Pharmaceutical Industry*. Chicago: University of Chicago Press, 2014.

Galison, Peter, and Bruce William Hevly. *Big Science: The Growth of Large-Scale Research*. Stanford, CA: Stanford University Press, 1992.

Gaudillière, Jean-Paul. "Hormones at Risk: Cancer and the Medical Uses of Industrially-Produced Sex Steroids in Germany, 1930–1960." In *The Risks of Medical Innovation: Risk Perception and Assessment in Historical Context*, ed. Thomas Schlich and Ulrich Tröhler, 148–169. London: Routledge, 2006.

Gawande, Atul. *Complications: A Surgeon's Notes on an Imperfect Science*. New York: Picador, 2002.

Geiger, Roger L. *To Advance Knowledge: The Growth of American Research Universities, 1900–1940*. New York: Oxford University Press, 1986.

Gilbert, James. *Designing the Industrial State: The Intellectual Pursuit of Collectivism in America, 1880–1940*. Chicago: Quadrangle Books, 1972.

Gillmor, C. Stewart. *Fred Terman at Stanford: Building a Discipline, a University, and Silicon Valley*. Stanford, CA: Stanford University Press, 2004.

Ginzburg [sic for Ginzberg], Eli, ed. *Regionalization and Health Policy*. Washington DC: U.S. Department of Health, Education, and Welfare, 1977.

Ginzton, E. L. "The $100 Idea." *IEEE Spectrum* 12 (1975): 30–39.

Ginzton, Edward L., and Craig S. Nunan. "History of Microwave Electron Linear Accelerators for Radiotherapy." *International Journal of Radiation Oncology Biology Physics* 11 (1985): 205–216.

Glatstein, Eli. "Intensity-Modulated Radiation Therapy: The Inverse, the Converse, and the Perverse." *Seminars in Radiation Oncology* 12 (2002): 272–281.

Goffman, Thomas E., and Eli Glatstein. "The Vulnerability of Radiation Oncology within the Medical Industrial Complex." *International Journal of Radiation Oncology Biology Physics* 59 (2004): 1–3.

Goitein, Michael, and James D. Cox. "Should Randomized Clinical Trials Be Required for Proton Radiotherapy?" *Journal of Clinical Oncology* 26 (2008): 175–176.

Goitein, Michael, and John Munzenrider. "Proton Therapy: Good News and Big Challenges." *International Journal of Radiation Oncology Biology Physics* 10 (1984): 319–320.

Goldberg, Daniel S. "Suffering and Death among Early American Roentgenologists: The Power of Remotely Anatomizing the Living Body in Fin de Siècle America." *Bulletin of the History of Medicine* 85 (2011): 1–28.

Goldsmith, Jeff. "Death of a Paradigm: The Challenge of Competition." *Health Affairs* 3 (1984): 5–19.

Gompers, Paul A. "The Rise and Fall of Venture Capital." *Business and Economic History* 23 (1994): 1–16.

Goodman, Jordan, Anthony McElligott, and Lara Marks, eds. *Useful Bodies: Humans in the Service of Medical Science in the Twentieth Century*. Baltimore: Johns Hopkins University Press, 2003.

Gottlieb, Symond R. "A Brief History of Health Planning in the United States." In *Regulating Health Facilities Construction*, ed. Clark C. Havighurst, 7–25. Washington DC: American Enterprise Institute for Public Policy Research, 1974.

Governor's Committee on Hospital Costs. *Report of the Governor's Committee on Hospital Costs*. New York: The Committee, 1965.

Gray, Bradford H. *The Profit Motive and Patient Care*. Cambridge, MA: Harvard University Press, 1991.

Green, D. T., and R. F. Errington. "1000 Curie Cobalt Units for Radiation Therapy. III. Design of a Cobalt 60 Beam Therapy Unit." *British Journal of Radiology* 25 (1952): 309–313.

Greene, Jeremy. *Prescribing by Numbers: Drugs and the Definition of Disease*. Baltimore: Johns Hopkins University Press, 2007.

Greene, Jeremy A., and David Herzberg. "Hidden in Plain Sight: Marketing Prescription Drugs to Consumers in the Twentieth Century." *American Journal of Public Health* 100 (2010): 793–806.

Grubbé, Emil. *X-Ray Treatment: Its Origin, Birth, and Early History*. Saint Paul: Bruce, 1949.

Gustavson, Anita, Birgitta Osterman, and Eva Cavallin-Ståhl. "A Systematic Overview of Radiation Therapy Effects in Hodgkin's Lymphoma." *Acta Oncologica* 42 (2003): 589–604.

Haas, Lewis L., and Roger A. Harvey. "Clinical Aspects of Betatron Irradiation." *American Journal of Roentgenology, Radium Therapy and Nuclear Medicine* 76 (1956): 905–918.

Hall, Stephen S. *A Commotion in the Blood: Life, Death, and the Immune System.* New York: Henry Holt, 1997.

Halpern, Sydney A. *Lesser Harms: The Morality of Risk in Medical Research.* Chicago: University of Chicago Press, 2004.

Hammer, Peter J., Deborah Haas-Wilson, Mark A. Peterson, and William M. Sage, eds. *Uncertain Times: Kenneth Arrow and the Changing Economics of Health Care.* Durham, NC: Duke University Press, 2003.

Hanks, Gerald E., James J. Diamond, and Simon Kramer. "The Need for Complex Technology in Radiation Oncology: Correlations of Facility Characteristics and Structure with Outcome." *Cancer* 55 (1985): 2198–2201.

Hanks, Gerald E., John M. Krall, Alexandra L. Hanlon, Sucha O. Asbell, Miljenko V. Pilepich, and Jean Owen. "Patterns of Care and RTOG Studies in Prostate Cancer: Long Term Survival, Hazard Rate Observations, and Possibilities of Cure." *International Journal of Radiation Oncology Biology Physics* 28 (1994): 39–46.

Hannaway, Caroline, ed. *Biomedicine in the Twentieth Century: Practices, Policies, and Politics.* Amsterdam: IOS, 2008.

Hanson, Gerald Peter. "Organization of Radiation Therapy Services Related to Outcome." PhD diss., University of California, Los Angeles, 1971.

Hanson, William. *The Edge of Medicine: The Technology That Will Change Our Lives.* New York: Palgrave Macmillan, 2008.

Harvey, Roger A. "X-Ray Requirements for the Smaller Hospital." In *Transcript of the Institute on Hospital Planning.* Chicago: American Hospital Association, 1948.

Hasan, Malik M. "Sounding Board: Let's End the Nonprofit Charade." *New England Journal of Medicine* 334 (1996): 1055–1057.

Havighurst, Clark C. *Deregulating the Health Care Industry: Planning for Competition.* Cambridge, MA: Ballinger, 1982.

Havighurst, Clark C., ed. *Regulating Health Facilities Construction.* Washington DC: American Enterprise Institute for Public Policy Research, 1974.

Hayman, James, Jane Weeks, and Peter Mauch. "Economic Analyses in Health Care: An Introduction to the Methodology with an Emphasis on Radiation Therapy." *International Journal of Radiation Oncology Biology Physics* 35 (1996): 827–841.

Hayter, Charles. *An Element of Hope: Radium and the Response to Cancer in Canada, 1900–1940.* Montreal: McGill-Queen's University Press, 2005.

Hayter, Charles. "Tarnished Adornment: The Troubled History of Quėbec's Institute du Radium." *Canadian Bulletin of Medical History* 20 (2003): 343–365.

Healy, William P. "Evaluation of Radiation Therapy in Malignant Disease of the Female Generative Tract." *American Journal of Obstetrics and Gynecology* 26 (1933): 789–803.

Healy, William P. "Radiation Therapy in Cancer of the Cervix." *Canadian Medical Association Journal* 32 (1935): 647–651.

Heilbron, J. L., and Robert W. Seidel. *Lawrence and His Laboratory: A History of the Lawrence Berkeley Laboratory.* Vol. 1. Berkeley: University of California Press, 1989.

Heilbroner, Robert, and Aaron Singer. *The Economic Transformation of America: 1600 to the Present. Fort Worth*: Harcourt Brace, 1994.

Herken, Gregg, *Brotherhood of the Bomb.* New York: Henry Holt, 2002.

Herzlinger, Regina E. *Market-Driven Health Care: Who Wins, Who Loses in the Transformation of America's Largest Service Industry.* Reading, MA: Addison-Wesley, 1997.

Hevly, Bruce. “Stanford’s Supervoltage X-Ray Tube.” *Osiris* 9 (1994): 85–100.

Heyman, J., ed. *Annual Report on the Results of Radiotherapy in Carcinoma of the Uterine Cervix*. Geneva: League of Nations, 1937.

Hocker, Alfred F., and Ruth J. Guttman. “Three and One Half Years’ Experience with the 1,000 Kilovolt Roentgen Therapy Unit at Memorial Hospital.” *American Journal of Roentgenology and Radium Therapy* 51 (1944): 83–94.

Hodges, Fred J., “The Section on Radiology.” *Journal of the American Medical Association* 95 (1930): 833–834.

Hodges, Fred J., “X-ray Facilities for the General Hospital,” *Architectural Record* 101 (1947): 141–142.

Hoffman, Beatrix. *The Wages of Sickness: The Politics of Health Insurance in Progressive America*. Chapel Hill: University of North Carolina Press, 2001.

Holmes, George W., and Milford D. Schulz. “Supervoltage Radiation: A Review of the Cases Treated during an Eight Year Period (1937–1944 Inclusive).” *American Journal of Roentgenology and Radium Therapy* 60 (1946): 533–554.

Hoppszallern, Suzanna, and Christine M. Hughes. *Outpatient Radiology Service: Successful Business Strategies*. Chicago: American Hospital Association, 1988.

Houston, C. Stuart. *Steps on the Road to Medicare: Why Saskatchewan Led the Way*. Montreal: McGill-Queens University Press, 2002.

Howell, Joel D. *Technology in the Hospital: Transforming Patient Care in the Early Twentieth Century*. Baltimore: Johns Hopkins University Press, 1995.

Hoyer, Morten, Anand Swaminath, Sean Bydder, Michael Lock, Alejandra Méndez Romero, Brian Kavanagh, Karyn A. Goodman, Paul Okunieff, and Laura A. Dawson. “Radiotherapy for Liver Metastases: A Review of Evidence.” *International Journal of Radiation Oncology Biology Physics* 82 (2012): 1047–1057.

Hussey, David H., John L. Horton, Nancy P. Mendenhall, John E. Munzenrider, Christopher M. Rose, and Jonathan H. Sunshine. “Manpower Needs for Radiation Oncology: A Preliminary Report of the ASTRO Human Resources Committee.” *International Journal of Radiation Oncology Biology Physics* 35 (1996): 809–820.

Hutton, Eric. “The Atom Bomb That Saves Lives.” *Maclean’s* February 15, 1952.

Iglehart, John K. “Health Insurers and Medical-Imaging Policy—A Work in Progress.” *New England Journal of Medicine* 360 (2009): 1030–1037.

Incrocci, Luca, and Pernille Tine Jensen. “Pelvic Radiotherapy and Sexual Function in Men and Women.” *Journal of Sexual Medicine* 10, supplement S1 (2013): 53–64.

Innes, G. S. “The One Million Volt X-Ray Therapy Equipment at St. Bartholomew’s Hospital, 1936–1960.” In “Megavoltage Radiotherapy, 1937–1987,” ed. P. N. Plowman and A. N. Harnett, supplement no. 22, *British Journal of Radiology* (1988): 11–16.

Institute of Medicine (US). *Graduate Medical Education That Meets the Nation’s Health Needs*. Washington DC: National Academies, 2014.

Institute of Medicine (US). *Medical Devices and the Public’s Health: The FDA 510(k) Clearance Process at 35 Years*. Washington DC: National Academies, 2011.

Institute of Medicine (US). *Radiation in Medicine: A Need for Regulatory Reform*. Washington DC: National Academy, 1996.

Institute of Medicine (US). *Value in Health Care: Accounting for Cost, Quality, Safety, Outcomes, and Innovation*. Washington DC: National Academies, 2009.

International Atomic Energy Agency. *Directory of High-Energy Radiotherapy Centres*. Vienna: IAEA, 1968.

International Atomic Energy Agency. *Radioisotope Teletherapy Equipment: International Directory*. Vienna: IAEA, 1959.

International Atomic Energy Agency. *Use of Radioisotopes and Supervoltage Radiation in Radioteletherapy*. Vienna: IAEA, 1960.

International Symposium on Hodgkin's Disease. National Cancer Institute Monograph 36. Bethesda, MD: National Cancer Institute, 1973.

Jacobs, Charlotte DeCroes. *Henry Kaplan and the Story of Hodgkin's Disease*. Stanford, CA: Stanford University Press, 2010.

Jairam, Vikram, Kenneth B. Roberts, and James B. Yu. "Historical Trends in the Use of Radiation Therapy for Pediatric Cancers: 1973–2008." *International Journal of Radiation Oncology Biology Physics* 85 (2013): e151–e155.

Janeway, Henry H. *Radium Therapy in Cancer at the Memorial Hospital in New York*. New York: Paul B. Hoeber, 1917.

Jarosek, Stephanie, Sean Elliott, and Beth A. Virnig. *Proton Beam Therapy in the U.S. Medicare Population: Growth in Use between 2006 and 2009*. Rockville, MD: Agency for Healthcare Research and Quality, 2012.

Jessop, Bob. "From Hegemony to Crisis? The Continuing Ecological Dominance of Neoliberalism." In *The Rise and Fall of Neoliberalism: The Collapse of an Economic Order?* ed. Kean Birch and Vlad Mykhnenko, 171–187. London: Zed Books, 2010.

Ji, Young Hoon, Haijo Jung, Kwangmo Yang, Chul Koo Cho, Seong Yul Yoo, Hyung Jun Yoo, Kum Bae Kim, and Mi Sook Kim. "Trends for the Past 10 Years and International Comparisons of the Structure of Korean Radiation Oncology." *Japanese Journal of Clinical Oncology* 40 (2010): 470–475.

Johns, H. E., and T. A. Watson. "The Cobalt-60 Story." *Cancer in Ontario* (Toronto: Ontario Cancer Treatment and Research Foundation 1982): 20–24.

Johnstone, P., J. Kerstiens, M. Williams, and R. Helsper. "Proton Facility Economics: The Essential Role of Prostate Cancer (CaP)." *International Journal of Radiation Oncology Biology Physics* 78 (2010): S564.

Jones, Arthur. "The Development of Megavoltage X-Ray Therapy at St. Bartholomew's Hospital." In "Megavoltage Radiotherapy, 1937–1987," ed. P. N. Plowman and A. N. Harnett, supplement no. 22, *British Journal of Radiology* (1988): 3–10.

Jones, David S. *Broken Hearts: The Tangled History of Cardiac Care*. Baltimore: Johns Hopkins University Press, 2013.

Jones, David S. and Robert L. Martensen, "Human Radiation Experiments and the Formation of Medical Physics at the University of California, San Francisco and Berkeley, 1937–1962," In *Useful Bodies: Humans in the Service of Medical Science in the Twentieth Century*, ed. Jordan Goodman, Anthony McElligott, and Lara Marks, 81–108. Baltimore: Johns Hopkins University Press, 2003.

Jongen, Yves. "Review on Cyclotrons for Cancer Therapy." In *Proceedings of Cyclotrons 2010*, [Conference Proceedings] 398–403. Lanzhou, China.

Kaiser, David, ed. *Becoming MIT*. Cambridge, MA: MIT Press, 2010.

Kalanithi, Paul. *When Breath Becomes Air*. New York: Random House, 2016.

Kaplan, Henry S. "Clinical Evaluation and Radiotherapeutic Management of Hodgkin's Disease and the Malignant Lymphomas." *New England Journal of Medicine* 278 (1968): 892–899.

Kaplan, Henry S. "Current Status of Radiotherapy for Neoplastic Disease." *DM Disease-a-Month* 11 (1965): 1–56.

Kaplan, Henry S. "Early Microscopic Diagnosis of Lymphosarcoma In Situ in Thymus of Irradiated Mice." *Federation Proceedings* 19 (1960): 399.

Kaplan, Henry S. "Historic Milestones in Radiobiology and Radiation Therapy." *Seminars in Oncology* 6 (1979): 479–489.

Kaplan, Henry S. "Hodgkin's Disease." *Current Problems in Radiology* 1 (1971): 1–39.

Kaplan, Henry S. *Hodgkin's Disease*. 2nd ed. Cambridge, MA: Harvard University Press, 1980.

Kaplan, Henry S. "New Horizons in Radiotherapy of Malignant Disease." *Journal of the American Medical Association* 171 (1959): 133–138.

Kaplan, Henry S. "The Radical Radiotherapy of Regionally Localized Hodgkin's Disease." *Radiology* 78 (1962): 553–569.

Kaplan, Henry S. "Radiotherapeutic Advances in the Treatment of Neoplastic Disease." *Israel Journal of Medical Sciences* 13 (1977): 808–814.

Kaplan, Henry S. "Recent Experimental Contributions to Radiotherapy." *American Journal of Roentgenology, Radium Therapy and Nuclear Medicine* 80 (1958): 822–832.

Kaplan, Henry S., ed. *Research in Radiology: Proceedings of an Informal Conference*. Washington DC: National Research Council (US), 1958.

Kaplan, Henry S., and Saul A Rosenberg. "Extended-Field Radical Radiotherapy in Advanced Hodgkin's Disease: Short-Term Results of 2 Randomized Clinical Trials." *Cancer Research* 26, pt. 1 (1966): 1268–1276.

Kaplan, Henry S., H. Alan Schwettman, William M. Fairbank, Douglas Boyd, and Malcolm A. Bagshaw. "A Hospital-Based Superconducting Accelerator Facility for Negative Pi-Meson Beam Radiotherapy." *Radiology* 108 (1973): 159–172.

Kaplan, Henry S., and Hugh M. Wilson. "The Present Status of Radiation Therapy of Cancer." *Connecticut State Medical Journal* 10 (1946): 183–186.

Kaplan, Ira I. "Radiotherapeutics: A Foreword and an Editorial," In *The 1932 Year Book of Radiology*, ed. Charles A. Waters and Ira I. Kaplan, 345–349. Chicago: Year Book Medical Publishers, 1932.

Kargon, Robert, and Elizabeth Hodes. "Karl Compton, Isaiah Bowman, and the Politics of Science in the Great Depression." *Isis* 76 (1985): 300–318.

Kasivisvanathan, Veeru, Ankur Thapar, Kerry J. Davies, et al. "Periprocedural Outcomes after Surgical Revascularization and Stenting for Postradiotherapy Carotid Stenosis." *Journal of Vascular Surgery* 56 (2012): 1143–1152.e2.

Keene, Floyd E., and Robert A. Kimbrough. "End-Results of Radium Therapy in Carcinoma of the Cervix." *American Journal of Obstetrics and Gynecology* 23 (1932): 838–841.

Keith, D. Y. "The Present Status of Radiation Therapy." *Kentucky Medical Journal* 20 (June 1922): 411–418.

Kelly, Howard A. "Radium in the Treatment of Menstrual Disorders." *Journal of the American Medical Association* 97 (1931): 760–763.

Kelsey, Chris R., Anne W. Beaven, Louis F. Diehl, and Leonard R. Prosnitz. "Combined-Modality Therapy for Early-Stage Hodgkin Lymphoma: Maintaining High Cure Rates While Minimizing Risks." *Oncology—New York* 26 (2012): 1182–1193.

Kenney, Martin, and W. Richard Goe. "The Role of Social Embeddedness in Professorial Entrepreneurship: A Comparison of Electrical Engineering and Computer Science at UC Berkeley and Stanford." *Research Policy* (2004) 33: 691–707.

Kevles, Bettyann Holtzmann. *Naked to the Bone: Medical Imaging in the Twentieth Century*. Reading, MA: Addison-Wesley, 1997.

Kirk, Jeffrey. *Machines in Our Hearts: The Cardiac Pacemaker, the Implantable Defibrillator, and American Health Care*. Baltimore: Johns Hopkins University Press, 2001.

Klein, Martin. "Neurocognitive Functioning in Adult WHO Grade II Gliomas: Impact of Old and New Treatment Modalities." *Neuro-oncology* 14 (2012): 17–24.

Kligerman, Morton M. "High Voltage Radiation Therapy." *Annual Review of Medicine* 11 (1960): 303–314.

Kotliar, Alan. "A Marketing Study of the Medical Electronics Industry." MBA thesis, University of Pennsylvania, 1959.

Kotz, David M. *The Rise and Fall of Neoliberal Capitalism*. Cambridge, MA: Harvard University Press, 2015.

Kramer, Simon, Gerald E. Hanks, David F. Herring, and Lawrence W. Davis. "Summary Results from the Facilities Master List Surveys Conducted by the Patterns of Care Study." *International Journal of Radiation Oncology Biology Physics* 8 (1982): 883–888.

Kramer, Simon, and David F. Herring. "The Patterns of Care Study: A Nationwide Evaluation of the Practice of Radiation Therapy in Cancer Management." *International Journal of Radiation Oncology Biology Physics* 1 (1976): 1231–1236.

Krippner, Greta R. *Capitalizing on Crisis: The Political Origins of the Rise of Finance*. Cambridge, MA: Harvard University Press, 2011.

Kumar, Sameer, and Jeffrey L. Ricker. "General Electric, a Model of Corporate Citizenship and Business Evolution." *International Journal of Energy Technology and Policy* 2 (2004): 354–368.

Kutcher, Gerald. *Contested Medicine: Cancer Research and the Military*. Chicago: University of Chicago Press, 2009.

Lanciano, Rachelle, Gillian Thomas, and Patricia J. Eifel. "Over 20 Years of Progress in Radiation Oncology: Cervical Cancer." *Seminars in Radiation Oncology* 7 (1997): 121–126.

Landa, Edward R. "A Brief History of the American Radium Industry and Its Ties to the Scientific Community of Its Early Twentieth Century." *Environment International* 19 (1993): 503–508.

Landa, Edward R. "Buried Treasure to Buried Waste: The Rise and Fall of the Radium Industry." *Colorado School of Mines Quarterly* 82 (1987): i–viii, 1–76.

Landa, Edward R. "The First Nuclear Industry." *Scientific American* 247 (November 1982): 180–193.

Lane-Claypon, Janet E. *Cancer of the Uterus: A Statistical Inquiry into the Results of Treatment, Being an Analysis of the Existing Literature*. Reports on Public Health and Medical Subjects, no. 40. London: Ministry of Health, 1927.

Laramore, George E. "The Use of Neutrons in Cancer Therapy: A Historical Perspective through the Modern Era." *Seminars in Oncology* 24 (1997): 672–685.

Laramore, George E., Robert Emery, David Reid, Stefani Banerian, Ira Kalet, Jonathan Jacky, and Ruedi Risler. "University of Washington Clinical Neutron Facility: Report on 26 Years of Operation." *AIP Conference Proceedings* 1412 (2011): 311–318.

Laughlin, John S., Radhe Mohan, and Gerald J. Kutcher. "Choice of Optimum Megavoltage for Accelerators for Photon Beam Treatment." *International Journal of Radiation Oncology Biology Physics* 12 (1986): 1551–1557.

Lave, Judith R., and Lester B. Lave. *The Hospital Construction Act: An Evaluation of the Hill–Burton Program, 1948–1973*. Washington DC: American Enterprise Institute for Public Policy Research, 1974.

Lavine, Matthew. "The Early Clinical X-Ray in the United States: Patient Experiences and Public Perceptions." *Journal of the History of Medicine and Allied Sciences* 67 (2012): 587–625.

Lawrence, Ernest O. "Nuclear Physics and Biology." In *Molecular Films, the Cyclotron, and the New Biology*, by Hugh Stott Taylor, Ernest O. Lawrence, and Irving Langmuir, 63-91. New Brunswick, NJ: Rutgers University Press, 1942.

Lécuyer, Christophe. "The Making of a Science Based Technological University: Karl Compton, James Killian, and the Reform of MIT, 1930–1957." *Historical Studies in the Physical and Biological Sciences* 23 (1992): 153–180.

Lécuyer, Christophe. *Making Silicon Valley: Innovation and the Growth of High Tech, 1930–1970.* Cambridge, MA: MIT Press, 2006.

Lécuyer, Christophe. "Patrons and a Plan." In *Becoming MIT*, ed. David Kaiser, 59–80. Cambridge, MA: MIT Press, 2010.

Lederman, Manuel. "The Early History of Radiotherapy: 1895–1939." *International Journal of Radiation Oncology Biology Physics* 7 (1981): 639–648.

Lee, Burton J. "The Therapeutic Value of Irradiation in the Treatment of Mammary Cancer: A Survey of Five-Year Results in 355 Cases Treated at the Memorial Hospital of New York." *Annals of Surgery* 88 (1928): 26–47.

Lemoigne, Yves, ed. *Radiotherapy and Brachytherapy.* Archamps, France: NATO Advanced Study Institute on Physics of Modern Radiotherapy and Brachytherapy, 2009.

Leopold, Ellen. *Under the Radar: Cancer and the Cold War.* New Brunswick, NJ: Rutgers University Press, 2009.

Leopold, George R. "The ABCs of Radiology." *Radiology* 198 (1996): 45A–47A.

Lerner, Barron H. *The Breast Cancer Wars: Hope, Fear, and the Pursuit of a Cure in Twentieth-Century* America. New York: Oxford University Press, 2001.

Leszczynski, Konrad, and Susan Boyko. "On the Controversies Surrounding the Origins of Radiation Therapy." *Radiotherapy and Oncology* 42 (1997): 213–217.

Leucutia, T. "The American Radium Society and the Journal: Fifty Years of Scientific Advancement." *American Journal of Roentgenology, Radium Therapy and Nuclear Medicine* 96 (1966): 804–806.

Levitt, Theodore. *The Marketing Imagination.* New York: Free Press, 1986.

Linton, Otha W. *The American College of Radiology: The First 75 Years.* Reston, VA: American College of Radiology, 1997.

Linton, Otha W. *Radiology at Massachusetts General Hospital, 1896–2000.* Boston: The General Hospital, 2001.

Linton, Otha W. Radiology at Memorial Sloan-Kettering Cancer Center. New York: Department of Radiology, Memorial Sloan-Kettering Cancer Center, 2006.

Linton, Otha W. *The World of Stanford Radiology: 1901–2006.* Palo Alto: Departments of Radiology and Radiation Oncology, Stanford University, 2006.

Litt, Paul. *Isotopes and Innovation: MDS Nordion's First Fifty Years, 1946–1996.* Montreal: Published for MDS Nordion by McGill-Queen's University Press, 2000.

Lo, Bernard, and Marilyn J. Field, eds. *Conflict of Interest in Medical Research, Education, and Practice.* Washington DC: National Academies, 2009.

Lodge, Mark, Madelon Pijls-Joannesma, Lisa Stirk, Alastair J. Munro, Dirk De Ruysscher, and Tom Jefferson. "A Systematic Literature Review of the Clinical and Cost-Effectiveness of Hadron Therapy in Cancer." *Radiotherapy and Oncology* 83 (2007): 110–122.

Long, M. F., and P. J. Feldstein. "Economics of Hospital Systems: Peak Loads and Regional Coordination." *American Economic Review* 57 (1967): 119–129.

Lowen, Rebecca S. *Creating the Cold War University: The Transformation of Stanford.* Berkeley: University of California Press, 1997.

Löwy, Ilana. "Knife, Rays and Women: Controversies about the Uses of Surgery versus Radiotherapy in the Treatment of Female Cancers in France and in the US, 1920–1960." In *Cancer Patients, Cancer Pathways*, ed. Carsten Timmermann and Elizabeth Toon, 103–129. Basingstoke, Hampshire: Palgrave Macmillan, 2012.

Löwy, Ilana. *A Woman's Disease: The History of Cervical Cancer.* Oxford: Oxford University Press, 2011.

Lubenau, Joel O., and Richard F. Mould. "The Roller Coaster Price of Radium." *Journal of Oncology* 59 (2009): 148e–154e.

Lucas, Charles DeForest. "The Therapeutic and Economic Indications for Teleradium and the Supervoltage X-ray Machine." *Radiology* 34 (1940): 193–199.

Luce, Bryan, and Rebecca Singer Cohen. "Health Technology Assessment in the United States." *International Journal of Technology Assessment in Health Care* 25, supplement 1 (2009): 33–41.

Macbeth, Fergus R., and Michael V. Williams. "Proton Therapy Should Be Tested in Randomized Trials," *Journal of Clinical Oncology* 26 (2008): 2590–2591.

Mackenzie, Sholto. *Cancer: An Inquiry into the Extent to Which Patients Receive Treatment*. Reports on Public Health and Medical Subjects No. 89. London: Ministry of Health, HMSO, 1939.

MacLeod, Gordon, and Mark Perlman. *Health Care Capital: Competition and Control.* Cambridge, MA: Ballinger, 1978.

Maeda, Yasuko, Morten Høyer, Lilli Lundby, and Christine Norton. "Faecal Incontinence Following Radiotherapy for Prostate Cancer: A Systematic Review." *Radiotherapy and Oncology* 98 (2011): 145–153.

Marks, Richard D. "Fourteen Years' Experience with Cobalt-60 Radiation Therapy in the Treatment of Early Cancer of the True Vocal Cords." *Cancer* 28 (1971): 571–576.

Marsh, Henry. *Do No Harm: Stories of Life, Death, and Brain Surgery.* New York: St. Martin's, 2014.

Martinsen, Robert. "The History of Bioethics: An Essay Review." *Journal of the History of Medicine and Allied Sciences* 56 (2001): 168–175.

McCraw, Thomas K., ed. *Creating Modern Capitalism: How Entrepreneurs, Companies, and Countries Triumphed in Three Industrial Revolutions*. Cambridge, MA: Harvard University Press, 1997.

McGrath, Patrick J. *Scientists, Business, and the State, 1890–1960*. Chapel Hill: University of North Carolina Press, 2002.

McQuaid, Kim. "Competition, Cartelization and the Corporate Ethic: General Electric's Leadership during the New Deal Era, 1933–1940." *American Journal of Economics and Sociology* 36 (1977): 417–428.

McQuaid, Kim. "Corporate Liberalism in the American Business Community, 1920–1940." *Business History Review* 52 (1978): 342–368.

M. D. Anderson Foundation, University of Texas, Houston. *Proceedings at the Dedication of the M. D. Anderson Hospital for Cancer Research, Houston*, February 17, 1944 Houston, 1944.

M. D. Anderson Hospital and Tumor Institute. *Annual Report 1953–1954*. Houston: University of Texas, 1954.

M. D. Anderson Hospital and Tumor Institute. The First Twenty Years of the University of Texas M. D. Anderson Hospital and Tumor Institute. Houston: University of Texas, 1964.

M. D. Anderson Hospital and Tumor Institute. *General Report, 1961–1964* Houston: University of Texas, 1964.

M. D. Anderson Hospital and Tumor Institute, *General Report 1968–1970*, Houston: University of Texas, 1970.

"Medical News: New York—Radium Institute of America." *Journal of the American Medical Association* 53 (1909): 1923.

Medical Research Council. *Medical Uses of Radium: Summary of Reports from Research Centres for 1930*. Special Report Series No. 160. London: HMSO, 1931.

Medical Research Council. *Medical Uses of Radium: Summary of Reports from Research Centres for 1938*. Special Report Series No. 236. London: Medical Research Council, HMSO, 1939.

Medicare Payment Advisory Commission. *Report to the Congress: Improving Incentives in the Medicare Program*. Washington DC: The Commission, 2009.

Medicare Payment Advisory Commission. *Report to the Congress: Promoting Greater Efficiency in Medicare*. Washington DC: The Commission, 2007.

Medina Domenech, Rosa M., and Claudia Castañeda. "Redefining Cancer during the Interwar Period: British Medical Officers of Health, State Policy, Managerialism, and Public Health." *American Journal of Public Health* 97 (2007): 1563–1571.

Mercado, Paul, and Jose M. Sala. "Comparison of Conventional and Supervoltage Radiation in the Management of Cancer of the Cervix." *Radiology* 90 (1968): 967–970.

Miller, Lowell S., Gilbert H. Fletcher, and Herbert B. Gerstner. "Radiobiologic Observations on Cancer Patients Treated with Whole-Body X-Irradiation." *Radiation Research* 4 (1958): 150–165.

Mintz, Beth, and Michael Schwartz. "Capital Formation and the United States Health Care System: The Relationship between the Private and the Public Sector." *Research in the Sociology of Health Care* 18 (2000): 229–248.

Mitchell, Jean. "Urologists' Use of Intensity Modulated Radiation Therapy for Prostate Cancer." *New England Journal of Medicine* 369 (2013): 1629–1637.

Mitchell, Jean M., and Jonathan H. Sunshine. "Consequences of Physicians' Ownership of Health Care Facilities—Joint Ventures in Radiation Therapy." *New England Journal of Medicine* 327 (1992): 1497–1501.

Montague, E. D., and G. H. Fletcher. "Curative Value of Irradiation in the Treatment of Nondisseminated Breast Cancer." *Cancer* 46, supplement S4 (1980): 995–998.

Montana, Gustavo S., A. L. Hanlon, T. J. Brickner, J. E. Owen, G. E. Hanks, C. C. Ling, R. Komaki, V. A. Marcial, G. M. Thomas, and R. Lanciano. "Carcinoma of the Cervix: Patterns of Care Studies: Review of 1978, 1983, and 1988–1989 Surveys." *International Journal of Radiation Oncology Biology Physics* 32 (1995): 1481–1486.

Moran, Michael. *Governing the Health Care State*. Manchester: Manchester University Press, 1999.

Morone, James A., and Lawrence R. Jacobs. *Healthy, Wealthy, and Fair: Health Care and the Good Society*. Oxford: Oxford University Press, 2005.

Moscucci, Ornella. "The 'Ineffable Freemasonry of Sex': Feminist Surgeons and the Establishment of Radiotherapy in Early Twentieth-Century Britain." *Bulletin of the History of Medicine* 81 (2007): 139–163.

Moses, Hamilton, E. Ray Dorsey, David H. M. Matheson, and Samuel O. Their. "Financial Anatomy of Biomedical Research." *JAMA* 294 (2005): 1333–1342.

Mould, Richard F. *A Century of X-Rays and Radioactivity in Medicine*. Philadelphia: Institute of Physics Publishing, 1993.

Mowery, David C., et al. *Ivory Tower and Industrial Innovation: University–Industry Technology Transfer before and after the Bayh-Dole Act*. Stanford, CA: Stanford University Press, 2004.

Moyer, Virginia A. "Screening for Prostate Cancer: U.S. Preventive Services Task Force Recommendation Statement." *Annals of Internal Medicine* 157 (2012): 120–134.

Mukherjee, Siddhartha. *The Emperor of All Maladies: A Biography of Cancer*. New York: Scribner, 2010.

Mudd, Seeley G., Clyde K. Emery, Orville M. Meland, and William E. Costolow. "Data Concerning Three Years' Experience with 600 kv (Peak) Roentgen Therapy." *American Journal of Roentgenology, Radium Therapy and Nuclear Medicine* 31 (1934): 520–531.

Murphy, Caroline Claire Scanlon. "A History of Radiotherapy to 1950: Cancer and Radiotherapy in Britain, 1830–1950." PhD thesis, University of Manchester, 1986.

Narang, Amol K., Edwin Lam, Martin A. Makary, et al. "Accuracy of Marketing Claims by Providers of Stereotactic Radiation Therapy." *Journal of Oncology Practice* 9 (2013): 57–62.

National Lung Screening Trial Research Team. "Reduced Lung-Cancer Mortality with Low-Dose Computed Tomographic Screening." *New England Journal of Medicine* 365 (2011): 395–409.

National Radiotherapy Advisory Group. *Radiotherapy: Developing a World Class Service for England*. Report to Ministers. February 26, 2007.

Neil, Russell H., William E. Costolow, and Orville N. Meland. "Design and Construction of a Simple Applicator for 1,000 Curies of Cobalt 60." *Radiology* 61 (1953): 408–410.

Nice, Charles M., and K. Wilhelm Stenstrom. "Irradiation Therapy on Hodgkin's Disease." *Radiology* 62 (1954): 641–653.

Noble, David F. *America by Design: Science, Technology, and the Rise of Corporate Capitalism*. Oxford: Oxford University Press, 1977.

Nussbaum, Abraham M. *The Finest Traditions of My Calling: One Physician's Search for the Renewal of Medicine*. New Haven, CT: Yale University Press, 2016

O'Grady, Kevin F. "Self-Referral by Physicians." *New England Journal of Medicine* 328 (1993): 1275.

Oh, Anna. "Ninth Circuit Rules That State Certificate of Need Laws May Unconstitutionally Burden Interstate Commerce." *American Journal of Law and Medicine* 37 (2011): 684–686.

Ong, Daniel S., Robert A. Aertker, Alexandra N. Clark, et al. "Radiation-Associated Valvular Heart Disease." *Journal of Heart Valve Disease* 22 (2013): 883–892.

Olsen, Dag Rune, Øyvind S. Bruland, Gunilla Frykholm, and Inger Natvig Norderhaug. "Proton Therapy—a Systematic Review of Clinical Effectiveness." *Radiotherapy and Oncology* 83 (2007): 123–132.

Olson, James S. *Bathsheba's Breast: Women, Cancer and History* (Baltimore: Johns Hopkins University Press, 2002.

Olson, James S. *Making Cancer History: Disease and Discovery at the University of Texas M. D. Anderson Cancer Center*. Baltimore: Johns Hopkins University Press, 2009.

O'Sullivan, Jennifer. *Report for Congress: Medicare: Physician Self-Referral ("Stark I and II")*. Washington DC: Congressional Research Service, 2007.

Owen, Jean B., and Lawrence R. Coia. "The Changing Structure of Radiation Oncology: Implications for the Era of Managed Care." *Seminars in Radiation Oncology* 7 (1997): 108–113.

Owen, Jean B., Lawrence R. Coia, and Gerald E. Hanks. "The Structure of Radiation Oncology in the United States in 1994." *International Journal of Radiation Oncology Biology Physics* 39 (1997): 179–185.

Owen, Jean B., Julia R. White, Michael J. Zelefsky, and J. Frank Wilson. "Using QRRO™ Survey Data to Assess Compliance with Quality Indicators for Breast and Prostate Cancer." *Journal of the American College of Radiology* 6 (2009): 442–447.

Panitch, Leo, and Sam Gindlin. *The Making of Global Capitalism: The Political Economy of American Empire*. London: Verso, 2012.

Parker, Robert G., ed. *A Planning Guide for Community Radiation Oncology Facilities*. [np] American College of Radiology, 1974.

Parsons, Charles L., et al. *Extraction and Recovery of Uranium, Radium, and Vanadium from Carnotite*. Washington DC: US Bureau of Mines, 1915.

Perkins, Barbara Bridgman. "Accumulating Resources in Perinatal Intensive Care Centers." *Business and Professional Ethics Journal* 12 (1993): 51–66.

Perkins, Barbara Bridgman. "Designing High-Cost Medicine: Hospital Surveys, Health Planning, and the Paradox of Progressive Reform." *American Journal of Public Health* 100 (2010): 223–233.

Perkins, Barbara Bridgman. "Economic Organization of Medicine and the Committee on the Costs of Medical Care." *American Journal of Public Health* 88 (1998): 1721–1726.

Perkins, Barbara Bridgman. *The Medical Delivery Business: Health Reform, Childbirth, and the Economic Order*. New Brunswick, NJ: Rutgers University Press, 2004.

Perkins, Barbara Bridgman. "Shaping Institution-Based Specialism: Early Twentieth-Century Economic Organization of Medicine." *Social History of Medicine* 10 (1997): 419–435.

Peters, M. Vera. "Prophylactic Treatment of Adjacent Areas in Hodgkin's Disease." *Cancer Research* 26, pt. 1 (1966): 1232–1243.

Peters, M. Vera. "A Study of Survivals in Hodgkin's Disease Treated Radiologically." *American Journal of Roentgenology and Radium Therapy* 63 (1950): 299–311.

Pickles, Tom, George B. Goodman, Chris J. Fryer, Julie Bowen, Andrew J. Coldman, Graeme G. Duncan, Peter H. Graham, Michael Mckenzie, William James Morris, Dorianne E. Rheaume, and Isabel Syndikus. "Pion Conformal Radiation of Prostate Cancer: Results of a Randomized Study." *International Journal of Radiation Oncology Biology Physics* 43 (1999): 47–55.

Pickstone, John V. "Contested Cumulations: Configurations of Cancer Treatments through the Twentieth Century." *Bulletin of the History of Medicine* 81 (2007): 164–196.

Pickstone, John V., ed. *Medical Innovations in Historical Perspective*. New York: St. Martin's, 1992.

Pickstone, John V. *Ways of Knowing: A New History of Science, Technology, and Medicine*. Chicago: University of Chicago Press, 2000.

Pietzsch, Jan B., Marta G. Zanchi, and John H. Linehan. "Medical Device Innovators and the 510(k) Regulatory Pathway: Implications of a Survey-Based Assessment of Industry Experience—Part 2: Medical Device Ecosystem and Policy." *Journal of Medical Devices* 7 (2013): 021003-1–021003-5.

Piketty, Thomas. *Capital in the Twenty-First Century*. Trans. Arthur Goldhammer. Cambridge, MA: Harvard University Press, 2014.

Pinell, Patrice. *The Fight against Cancer: France, 1890–1940*. London: Routledge, 2002.

Plowman, P. N., and A. N. Harnett, eds. "Megavoltage Radiotherapy, 1937–1987, Proceedings of a Conference." Supplement no. 22, *British Journal of Radiology* (1988).

Polanyi, Karl. *The Great Transformation*. Boston: Beacon, 1944.

Popovic, Marko, Mariska den Hartogh, Liying Zhang, Michael Poon, Henry Lam, Gillian Bedard, Natalie Pulenzas, Breanne Lechner, and Edward Chow. "Review of International Patterns of Practice for the Treatment of Painful Bone Metastases with Palliative Radiotherapy from 1993 to 2013." *Radiotherapy and Oncology* 111 (2014): 11–17.

Porter, Glenn. *The Rise of Big Business, 1860–1920*. Arlington Heights, IL: Harlan Davidson, 1992.

President's Commission on Heart Disease, Cancer and Stroke. *Report to the President: A National Program to Conquer Heart Disease, Cancer and Stroke.* Vol. 1. Washington DC: President's Commission on Heart Disease, Cancer and Stroke, 1964.

Proctor, Robert A. *Cancer Wars: How Politics Shapes What We Know and Don't Know About Cancer.* New York, NY: Basic, 1995.

Prosnitz, Leonard R., Rafael L. Montalvo, Diana. B. Fischer, Allen B. Silberstein, and David S. Berger, "Treatment of Stage IIIA Hodgkin's Disease: Is Radiotherapy Alone Adequate?" *International Journal of Radiation Oncology Biology Physics* 4 (1978): 781–787.

Pyle, Gerald F. *Heart Disease, Cancer and Stroke in Chicago: A Geographical Analysis with Facilities, Plans for 1980.* University of Chicago Department of Geography Research Paper No. 134. Chicago: University of Chicago, 1971.

Raju, M. R. "Particle Radiotherapy: Historical Development and Current Status." *Radiation Research* 145 (1996): 391–407.

Rao, Vijay M., and David C. Levin. "The Overuse of Diagnostic Imaging and the Choosing Wisely Initiative." *Annals of Internal Medicine* 157 (2012): 574–576.

Reagan, Patrick D. *Designing a New America: The Origins of New Deal Planning, 1890–1943.* Amherst: University of Massachusetts Press, 1999.

Reeves, Philip N., and Russell C. Coile. *Introduction to Health Planning.* Arlington VA: Information Resources, 1989.

Reich, Leonard S. *The Making of American Industrial Research.* Cambridge: Cambridge University Press, 1985.

Relman, Arnold S. "The New Medical-Industrial Complex." *New England Journal of Medicine* 303 (1980): 963–970.

Rentetzi, Maria. "The U.S. Radium Industry: Industrial In-House Research and the Commercialization of Science." *Minerva* 46 (2008): 437–462.

Richman, Chaim, Henry Aceto, Munduni R. Raju, and Bernard Schwartz. "The Radiotherapeutic Possibilities of Negative Pions." *AJR, American Journal of Roentgenology* 96 (1966): 777–790.

Richtmyer, F. K., H. A. Barton, and M. T. Jones. "A 600 kv X-Ray Plant." *British Journal of Radiology* 5 (1932): 214.

Ringborg, Ulrik, David Bergqvist, Bengt Brorsson, et al. "The Swedish Council on Technology Assessment in Health Care (SBU) Systematic Overview of Radiotherapy for Cancer Including a Prospective Survey of Radiotherapy Practice in Sweden 2001—Summary and Conclusions." *Acta Oncologica* 42 (2003): 357–365.

Roberts, Edward B. *Entrepreneurs in High Technology: Lessons from MIT and Beyond.* New York: Oxford University Press, 1991.

Robinson, James C. *The Corporate Practice of Medicine: Competition and Innovation in Health Care.* Berkeley: University of California Press, 1999.

Robison, Roger. "Historical Vignette: American Radium Engenders Telecurie Therapy during World War I." *Medical Physics* 27 (2000): 1212–1216.

Robison, Roger F. "Howard Atwood Kelly (1858–1943): Founding Professor of Gynecology at Johns Hopkins Hospital and Pioneer American Radium Therapist." *Journal of Oncology* 60 (2010): 21e–35e.

Robison, Roger F. *Mining and Selling Radium and Uranium.* Cham, Switzerland: Springer, 2015.

Robison, Roger F. "The Race for Megavoltage: X-Rays versus Telegamma." *Acta Oncologica* 34 (1995): 1055–1074.

Rollin, Betty. *First, You Cry.* Philadelphia, PA: Lippincott, 1976.

Roqué, Xavier. "Marie Curie and the Radium Industry: A Preliminary Sketch." *History and Technology* 13 (1997): 267–291.

Rosen, George. *The Specialization of Medicine with Particular Reference to Ophthalmology*. New York: Froben, 1944.

Rosenberg, Saul A., and Henry S. Kaplan. "The Evolution and Summary Results of the Stanford Randomized Clinical Trials of the Management of Hodgkin's Disease: 1962–1984." *International Journal of Radiation Oncology Biology Physics* 11 (1985): 5–22.

Rosenthal, Eric T. "How and Why Are Patients Referred for Proton Beam Therapy in the US and What Proven Benefits Does It Really Have?" *Oncology Times UK* 9 (2010): 19, 21.

Rosner, David. *A Once Charitable Enterprise: Hospitals and Health Care in Brooklyn and* New York, *1885–1915*. Cambridge: Cambridge University Press, 1982.

Ross, James W. "A Clinical Study of Cancer of the Uterine Cervix: Summary of the Results Obtained by Various Methods of Treatment." *Canadian Medical Association Journal* 7 (1922): 772–780.

Rubin, Philip. "The Emergence of Radiation Oncology as a Distinct Medical Specialty." *International Journal of Radiation Oncology Biology Physics* 11 (1985): 1247–1270.

Ruggles, Howard E. "A Year's Experience with 800 kv Roentgen Rays." *American Journal of Roentgenology and Radium Therapy* 36 (1936): 366–367.

Sade, Robert M. "Medical Care as a Right: A Refutation." *New England Journal of Medicine* 285 (1971): 1288–1292.

Sagerman, Robert H., Gerald E. Hanks, and Malcolm S. Bagshaw. "Supervoltage Radiation Therapy Use of the Linear Accelerator for Treating Ovarian Adenocarcinoma." *California Medicine* 102 (1965): 118–122.

Sahani, G., M. Kumar, P. K. Dash Sharma, R. Kumar, K. Chhokra, B. Mishra, S. P. Agarwal and R. K. Kher. "Compliance of Bhabhatron-II Telecobalt Unit with IEC Standard-Radiation Safety." *Journal of Applied Clinical Medical Physics* 10 (2009): 120–130.

Sakurai, Hideyuki, W. Robert Lee, and Colin G. Orton. "Point/Counterpoint: We Do Not Need Randomized Clinical Trials to Demonstrate the Superiority of Proton Therapy." *Medical Physics* 39 (2012): 1685–1687.

Sandy, Lewis G., Thomas Bodenheimer, L. Gregory Pawlson, and Barbara Starfield. "The Political Economy of U.S. Primary Care." *Health Affairs* 28 (2009): 1136–1145.

Schafer, James A. *The Business of Private Medical Practice: Doctors, Specialization, and Urban Change in Philadelphia, 1900-1940*. New Brunswick, NJ: Rutgers University Press, 2014.

Schlich, Thomas. *Surgery, Science and Industry: A Revolution in Fracture Care, 1950s–1970s*. Basingstoke, Hampshire: Palgrave Macmillan, 2002.

Schlich, Thomas, and Ulrich Tröhler, eds. *The Risks of Medical Innovation: Risk Perception and Assessment in Historical Context*. London: Routledge, 2006.

Schnur, Julie B., Suzanne C. Ouellette, Dana H. Bovbjerg, and Guy H. Montgomery. "Breast Cancer Patients' Experience of External-Beam Radiotherapy." *Qualitative Health Research* 19 (2009): 668–676.

Schultz, George P. "The Logic of Health Care Facility Planning." *Socio-economic Planning Sciences* 4 (1970): 383–393.

Schulz, Milford D. "The Supervoltage Story." *American Journal of Roentgenology, Radium Therapy and Nuclear Medicine* 124 (1975): 541–559.

Schulz-Ertner, Daniela, and Hirohiko Tsujii. "Particle Radiation Therapy Using Proton and Heavier Ion Beams." *Journal of Clinical Oncology* 25 (2007): 953–964.

Scott, K. G. "Robert Spencer Stone (1895–1966)." *Radiation Research* 33 (1968): 675–676.

Scott, Wendell G. *Planning Guide for Radiologic Installations*. Chicago: Year Book Publishers, 1953 and 1966.

Seidel, Robert W. "Technology Choice in Early High-Energy Physics." *History and Technology* 9 (1992): 175–187.

Sharpe, Virginia A., and Alan I. Faden. *Medical Harm: Historical, Conceptual, and Ethical Dimensions of Iatrogenic Illness*. Cambridge: Cambridge University Press, 1998.

Sheehan, Mark, Claire Timlin, Ken Peach, et al. "Position Statement on Ethics, Equipoise and Research on Charged Particle Radiation Therapy." *Journal of Medical Ethics* 40 (2014): 572–575.

Silvers, J. B. "The Role of the Capital Markets in Restructuring Health Care." In *Uncertain Times: Kenneth Arrow and the Changing Economics of Health Care*, ed. Peter J. Hammer, Deborah Haas-Wilson, Mark A. Peterson, and William M. Sage, 156–166. Durham, NC: Duke University Press, 2003.

Simpson, Burton T., and Melvin C. Reinhard. "Advantages and Disadvantages of Radium Packs." *American Journal of Roentgenology and Radium Therapy* 35 (1936): 513–521.

Sisterson, J. M., and B. Gottschalk. "Hospital-Based Acceleration for Proton Radiotherapy." *International Journal of Radiation Oncology Biology Physics* 10, supplement 2 (1984): 165.

Sixth International Congress of Radiology. *Abstracts of Papers*. London: The Congress, 1950.

Sixth International Congress of Radiology. *Handbook and Guide to the Technical Exhibition*. London: The Congress, 1950.

Sixth International Congress of Radiology. *Preliminary Programme*. London: The Congress, 1950.

Smith, Ivan H. "Cobalt-60 Beam Therapy: Some Impressions after Five Years." *Canadian Medical Association Journal* 77 (1957): 289–297.

Smith, Ivan H., J. C. H. Fetterly, J. S. Lott, J. C. F. MacDonald, Lois M. Myers, P. M. Pfalzner, and D. H. Thomson. *Cobalt-60 Teletherapy: A Handbook for the Radiation Therapist and Physicist.* New York: Harper and Row, Hoeber Medical Division, 1964.

Smith, Thomas J., and Bruce E. Hillner. "Bending the Cost Curve in Cancer Care." *New England Journal of Medicine* 364 (2011): 2060–2065.

Smitt, Melanie C., Jan Buzydlowski, and Richard T. Hoppe. "Over 20 Years of Progress in Radiation Therapy: Hodgkin's Disease." *Seminars in Radiation Oncology* 7 (1997): 127–134.

Soares, Heloisa P., Ambuj Kumar, Stephanie Daniels, et al. "Evaluation of New Treatments in Radiation Oncology: Are They Better Than Standard Treatments?" *JAMA* 293 (2005): 970–978.

Soiland, Albert. "The Therapeutic Aspect of Short Wave X-Rays." *California State Journal of Medicine* 21 (1923): 415–417.

Soiland, Albert. "The Evolution of Roentgen Therapy in Higher Voltages." *California and Western Medicine* 22 (1924): 148–150.

Soiland, Albert. "Radiology." *California and Western Medicine* 26 (1927): 372–373.

Soiland, Albert. "Experimental Clinical Research Work with X-Ray Voltages above 500,000: A Preliminary Statement." *Radiology* 20 (1933): 99–102.

Soiland, Albert, William E. Costolow, Orville N. Meland, and Ludwig Lindberg. "Our Concept of the Management of Cancer Patients by Modern Therapeutic Methods." In *International Congress of Scientific and Social Campaign against Cancer*, 326–338. Brussels, Belgium: Ligue Nationale Belge Contre Le Cancer, 1936.

Stanford Research Institute. A Study of Small Business in the Electronics Industry. Washington DC: Small Business Administration, 1962.

Stanford University Committee on Future Plans, *Stanford Medical School Council Report*. Stanford CA: Stanford University, 1952.

Stark, R. B. "Robert Abbé and His Contributions to Plastic Surgery." *Plastic and Reconstructive Surgery* 12 (1953): 41–58.

Starr, Paul. *The Social Transformation of American Medicine: The Rise of a Sovereign Profession and the Making of a Vast Industry*. New York: Basic Books, 1982.

Steinbach, Herbert L. "History of the Department of Radiology at Baylor University Medical Center." *Baylor University Medical Center Proceedings* 17 (2004): 425–431.

Steinberg, Michael L., and Andre Konski. "Proton Beam Therapy and the Convoluted Pathway to Incorporating Engineering Technology into Routine Medical Care in the United States." *Cancer Journal* 15 (2009): 333–338.

Stephens, Martha. *The Treatment: The Story of Those Who Died in the Cincinnati Radiation Tests*. Durham, NC: Duke University Press, 2002.

Stevens, Robert B., and Rosemary Stevens. *Welfare Medicine in America: A Case Study of Medicaid*. New Brunswick, NJ: Transaction, 2003.

Stevens, Rosemary. *American Medicine and the Public Interest*. Updated ed. Berkeley: University of California Press, 1998.

Stevens, Rosemary. *In Sickness and In Wealth: American Hospitals in the Twentieth Century*. New York: Basic Books, 1989.

Stevens, Rosemary. *The Public–Private Health Care State: Essays on the History of American Health Care Policy*. New Brunswick, NJ: Transaction, 2007.

Stockburger, Wayne T. *Radiology Administration: A Business Guide*. Philadelphia: J. B. Lippincott, 1989.

Stone, Robert S. *Industrial Medicine on the Plutonium Project: Survey and Collected Papers*. New York: McGraw-Hill, 1951.

Stone, Robert. "Neutron Therapy and Specific Ionization." *American Journal of Roentgenology and Radiation Therapy* 59 (1948): 771–785.

Stone, Robert S. "Skin Reactions Caused by 1,000 Kilovolt and 200 Kilovolt Radiations." *Radiology* 30 (1938): 88–93.

Stone, Robert S., and Rose V. Louie. "The Use of a 70-Mev Synchrotron in Cancer Therapy. II. Clinical Aspects." *Radiology* 83 (1964): 797–806.

Stone, Robert S., and J. Maurice Robinson. "Skin Reactions Produced by 200 kv and 1000 kv Radiations: A Comparison." *California and Western Medicine* 55 (1941): 11–14.

Strockbine, M. F., J. E. Hancock, and G. H. Fletcher. "Complications in 831 Patients with Squamous Cell Carcinoma of the Intact Uterine Cervix Treated with 3,000 Rads or More Whole Pelvis Irradiation." *American Journal of Roentgenology, Radium Therapy and Nuclear Medicine* 108 (1970): 293–304.

Strong, M. Stuart, Charles W. Vaughan, Herbert L. Kayne, I. M. Aral, A. Ucmakli, M. Feldman, and G. B. Healy. "A Randomized Trial of Preoperative Radiotherapy in Cancer of the Oropharynx and Hypopharynx." *American Journal of Surgery* 136 (1978): 494–500.

Suit, Herman D., James Becht, Joseph Leong, Michael Stracher, William C. Wood, Lynn Verhey, and Michael Goitein. "Potential for Improvement in Radiation Therapy." *International Journal of Radiation Oncology Biology Physics* 14 (1988): 777–786.

Suit, Herman D., and Jay S. Loeffler. *Evolution of Radiation Oncology at Massachusetts General Hospital*. New York: Springer, 2011.

Sutro, C. J. "The University of Texas MD Anderson Hospital and Tumor Institute: The Southwest's World-Renowned Cancer Center." *CA: A Cancer Journal for Clinicians* 14 (1964): 236–243.

Taylor, Hugh Stott, Ernest O. Lawrence, and Irving Langmuir. *Molecular Films, the Cyclotron, and the New Biology*. New Brunswick, NJ: Rutgers University Press, 1942.

Teitelman, Robert. *Profits of Science: The American Marriage of Business and Technology*. New York: Basic Books, 1994.

Terasawa, Teruhiko, Tomas Dvorak, Stanley Ip, Gowri Raman, and Joseph Lau. "Systematic Review: Charged-Particle Radiation Therapy for Cancer." *Annals of Internal Medicine* 151 (2009): 556–565.

Thwaites, David I., and John B. Tuohy. "Back to the Future: The History and Development of the Clinical Linear Accelerator." *Physics in Medicine and Biology* 51 (2006): R343–R362.

Tiber Group. *Can Local Products Compete in a National Marketplace? The Carve-Out Guide II*. Chicago: Tiber Group, 2000.

Tiber Group. *The "Carve-Out" Guide*. Chicago: Tiber Group, 1997.

Tierney, Thomas M., and Leonard F. Krystynak. *Capital Analysis and Priority Setting: Capital Formation Concerns in the Health Sector*. San Francisco: Western Center for Health Planning, 1981.

Timmermann, Carsten, and Elizabeth Toon, eds. *Cancer Patients, Cancer Pathways*. Basingstoke, Hampshire: Palgrave Macmillan, 2012.

Timmermann, Carsten, and Julie Anderson, eds. *Devices and Designs: Medical Technologies in Historical Perspective*. Basingstoke, Hampshire: Palgrave Macmillan, 2006.

Tobbell, Dominique A. *Pills, Power, and Policy: The Struggle for Drug Reform in Cold War America and Its Consequences*. Berkeley: University of California Press, 2012.

Tod, Margaret. *An Inquiry into the Extent to Which Cancer Patients in Great Britain Receive Radiotherapy*. Altrincham: John Sherratt and Son, 1950.

Tomes, Nancy. *Remaking the American Patient: How Madison Avenue and Modern Medicine Turned Patients into Consumers*. Chapel Hill: University of North Carolina Press, 2016.

Toon, Elizabeth. "Does Bigger Mean Better? British Perspectives on American Cancer Treatment and Research, 1948." *Journal of Clinical Oncology* 25 (2007): 5831–5834.

Transcript of the Institute on Hospital Planning. Chicago: American Hospital Association, 1948.

Trikalinos, Thomas A., Teruhiko Terasawa, Stanley Ip, Gowri Raman, and Joseph Lau, *Particle Beam Radiation Therapies for Cancer: Technical Brief No. 1* (Rockville, MD: Agency for Healthcare Research and Quality, 2009.

Trout, E. Dale. "History of Radiation Sources for Cancer Therapy." In *Progress in Radiation Therapy*, ed. Franz Buschke, 42–61. New York: Grune and Stratton, 1958.

Trout, Hugh H., and C. H. Peterson. "Cancer of the Breast: Use of Radium and Roentgen Therapy in Conjunction with the Radical Operation." *Journal of the American Medical Association* 95 (1930): 1307–1310.

Ueyama, Takahiro, and Christophe Lécuyer. "Building Science-Based Medicine at Stanford: Henry Kaplan and the Medical Linear Accelerator, 1948–1975." In *Devices and Designs: Medical Technologies in Historical Perspective*, ed. Carsten Timmermann and Julie Anderson, 137–155. Basingstoke, Hampshire: Palgrave Macmillan, 2006.

University of California, Berkeley. *Free Enterprise and University Research*. Berkeley: University of California, 1954.

US Bureau of Health Facilities. *Health Capital Is$ues*. Washington DC: US Department of Health and Human Services, 1981.

US Congress Office of Technology Assessment. *Federal Policies and the Medical Device Industry*. Washington DC: US Congress, 1984.

US Department of Health and Human Services. *Financial Arrangements between Physicians and Health Care Businesses: Report to Congress*. Washington DC: US Department of Health and Human Services, 1989.

US Federal Trade Commission and US Department of Justice. *Improving Health Care: A Dose of Competition*. Washington, DC: US Federal Trade Commission and US Department of Justice, 2004.

US Health Resources Administration. *National Guidelines for Health Planning*. Hyattsville, MD: Department of Health, Education, and Welfare, 1978.

US Senate. *Report of the National Panel of Consultants on the Conquest of Cancer*. Washington DC: Committee on Labor and Public Welfare, 1971.

Valier, Helen. "Uncertain Enthusiasm: PSA Screening, Proton Therapy and Prostate Cancer." In *Cancer Patients, Cancer Pathways*, ed. Carsten Timmermann and Elizabeth Toon, 186–203. Basingstoke, Hampshire: Palgrave Macmillan, 2012.

Varian, Dorothy. *The Inventor and the Pilot*. Palo Alto: Pacific Books, 1983.

Vera-Badillo, F. E., R. Shapiro, A. Ocana, et al. "Bias in Reporting of End Points of Efficacy and Toxicity in Randomized: Clinical Trials for Women with Breast Cancer." *Annals of Oncology* 24 (2013): 1238–1244.

Vogel, Morris J. *The Invention of the Modern Hospital, Boston, 1870–1930*. Chicago: University of Chicago Press, 1980.

von Essen, C. F., M. A. Bagshaw, S. E. Bush, A. R. Smith, and M. M. Kligerman. "Long-Term Results of Pion Therapy at Los Alamos." *International Journal of Radiation Oncology Biology Physics* 13 (1987): 1389–1398.

Wailoo, Keith. *How Cancer Crossed the Color Line*. New York: Oxford University Press, 2011.

Wainerdi, Richard E. *Texas Medical Center*. New York: Newcomen Society of the United States, 1993.

Ward, George Gray. "The Complications of Radium Therapy in Gynecology." *American Journal of Obstetrics and Gynecology* 25 (1933): 1–10.

Ward, Charles B., John E. Wirth, and John E. Rose. "One and One Half-Years' Experience with Supervoltage Roentgen Rays." *American Journal of Roentgenology and Radium Therapy* 36 (1936): 368–380.

Warner, John Harley. *The Therapeutic Perspective: Medical Practice, Knowledge, and Identity in America, 1820–1885*. Cambridge, MA: Harvard University Press, 1986.

Warren, S. Reid, and Roderick L. Tondreau. "The Retrospectoscope: The Good Old Days with William J. Hogan." RadioGraphics 6 (1985): 515-20.

Watson, T. A. *Results of Treatment of Cancer in Saskatchewan, 1932–44*. Saskatchewan: Saskatchewan Cancer Commission, 1951.

Watson, T. A. *Results of Treatment of Cancer in Saskatchewan, 1945–52*. Saskatchewan: Saskatchewan Cancer Commission, 1958.

Watson, William L., and Jerome Urban. "Million Volt Roentgen Therapy for Intrathoracic Cancer: Palliative Effects in a Series of Sixty-Three Cases." *American Journal of Roentgenology and Radium Therapy* 49 (1943): 299–306.

Weber Basin Health Planning Council. *Radiation Therapy in Northern Utah*. Ogden, UT: Intermountain Regional Medical Program, 1973.

Weisz, George. *Divide and Conquer: A Comparative History of Medical Specialization*. New York: Oxford University Press, 2006.

Welch, H. Gilbert, Lisa M. Schwartz, and Steven Woloshin. *Overdiagnosed: Making People Sick in the Pursuit of Health*. Boston: Beacon, 2011.

Welsome, Eileen. *The Plutonium Files: America's Secret Medical Experiments in the Cold War*. New York: Dial, 1999.

Wheatley, Steven C. *The Politics of Philanthropy: Abraham Flexner and Medical Education*. Madison, WI: University of Wisconsin Press, 1988.

Wilson, J. Frank "An Historical Perspective: American Radium Society, 1916–1995: Years of Distinction." *American Journal of Clinical Oncology* 20 (1997): 530–535.

Wilson, J. Frank, and Jean Owen. "Evolutionary Phases in Quality Research in Radiation Oncology over the Last 35 Years." *International Journal of Radiation Oncology Biology Physics* 72, supplement S (2008): S426.

Wilson, Richard. *A Brief History of the Harvard University Cyclotrons*. Cambridge, MA: Harvard University Department of Physics, 2004.

Wise, George. *Willis R. Whitney, General Electric, and the Origins of U.S. Industrial Research*. New York: Columbia University Press, 1985.

Wood, Francis Carter. "Recent Cancer Therapy." *Canadian Medical Association Journal* 13 (1923): 152–159.

Woolhandler, Steffie, Terry Campbell, and David U. Himmelstein. "Costs of Health Care Administration in the United States and Canada." *New England Journal of Medicine* 349 (2003): 768–775.

Year Book of Radiology. Chicago: Year Book Medical Publishers, 1932.

Yu, James B., Pamela R. Soulos, Jeph Herrin, Laura D. Cramer, Arnold L. Potosky, Kenneth B. Roberts, and Cary P. Gross. "Proton versus Intensity-Modulated Radiotherapy for Prostate Cancer: Patterns of Care and Early Toxicity." *Journal of the National Cancer Institute* 105 (2013): 25–32.

Zantinga, Arty R., and Max J. Coppes. "James Ewing (1866–1943): 'The Chief.'" *Medical and Pediatric Oncology* 21 (1993): 505–510.

Zuckerman, Diana, Paul Brown, and Aditi Das. "Lack of Publicly Available Scientific Evidence on the Safety and Effectiveness of Implanted Medical Devices." *JAMA Internal Medicine* 174 (2014): 1781–1787.

Index

Milton Keynes UK
Ingram Content Group UK Ltd.
UKHW040105071024
449327UK00019B/817